MOLECULAR
BIOLOGY
INTELLIGENCE
UNIT

INTRATHYMIC T-CELL DEVELOPMENT

Janko Nikolić-Žugić, M.D., Ph.D.
Memorial Sloan-Kettering Cancer Center
and Cornell University Graduate School of Medical Sciences
New York

R.G. LANDES COMPANY
AUSTIN

MOLECULAR BIOLOGY INTELLIGENCE UNIT

INTRATHYMIC T-CELL DEVELOPMENT

R.G. LANDES COMPANY/Austin

CRC Press is the exclusive worldwide distributor of publications
of the Molecular Biology Intelligence Unit.
CRC Press, 2000 Corporate Blvd., NW, Boca Raton, FL 33431. Phone: 407/994-0555.

Submitted: October 1993
Published: January 1994

Production Manager: Carol Harwell
Copy Editor: Constance Kerkaporta

Please address all inquiries to the Publisher:
R.G. Landes Company, 909 Pine Street, Georgetown, TX 78626
or P.O. Box 4858, Austin, TX 78765
Phone: 512/ 863 7762; FAX: 512/ 863 0081

ISBN 1-57059-014-1
CATALOG # LN9014

Library of Congress Cataloging -in-Publication Data

Nikolić-Žugić, Janko, 1960-
    Intrathymic T-cell development / Janko Nikolić-Žugić
       p. cm. -- (Molecular biology intelligence unit)
    Includes bibliographical references and index.
    ISBN 1-57059-014-1 (Hard cover) : $89.95
    1. T cells. 2. T cells--Differentiation. 3. Thymus--Physiology.
I. Title. II. Series.
    [DNLM: 1. T-Lymphocytes. 2. Thymus Gland--anatomy & histology.
3. Thymus Gland--immunology. 4. Cell Differentiation. WH 200
N693i 1993]
QR185.8.T2N55 1993
616.07'9--dc20
DNLM/DLC
for Library of Congress
          93-41387
          CIP

ABBREVIATIONS

CD cluster of differentiation molecules

DN $CD8^-CD4^-$ (double-negative) thymocytes

DP $CD8^+CD4^+$ (double-positive) thymocytes

MHC major histocompatibility complex encoded molecules

SP $CD8^-CD4^+$ or $CD8^+CD4^-$ (single positive) thymocytes

TcR T cell receptor for antigen

TL $CD8^{lo}CD4^{lo}TcR^{lo}$ (triple-low) thymocytes

TN same as DN but TcR^-

CMJ corticomedullary junction

APC antigen-presenting cell

IL interleukin

DC dentritic cells

Tg transgenic

TEC thymic epithelial cell

To Dragana and Tijana, with all my love.

FOREWORD

Why does one write a book? Since I began thinking of editing and writing this monograph, this question was on my mind. Finally, the answer crystallized: I used this monograph as an opportunity to step back and look at the progress of the past thirty-some years, and to admire it; it also allowed me to think of the problems of contemporary thymocyte development, including issues that I do not deal with in everyday laboratory life. This process, although at times overwhelming, was a lot of fun. I hope that the readers will share it.

I have tried to provide a complete set of references for each of the chapters that I wrote. I am aware that, due to time and space constraints, I must have done an imperfect job. Some of my colleagues, therefore, may not be adequately mentioned. I apologize to all of them, and assure them that no malice or arrogance has played a role. I also wish to stress that the interpretations in the chapters I wrote, including the possible misunderstandings of the work of the others, are solely mine. They do not necessarily reflect the original authors' or commonly accepted views. In fact, wherever possible, I tried to provide alternative interpretations and hypotheses.

This book could not have been finished were it not for a number of special people: my co-authors for preparing excellent contributions in a timely fashion; my understanding family that let me take a larger than usual chunk of time away from them in order to complete this work; Dr. Sofija Andjelić, Alberto Molano and Dr. Carolyn Tućek for helpful suggestions and stimulating discussion; Drs. Ulli Hammerling, Howard Petrie, Neal Rosen and Carolyn Tućek for critical reading of the manuscript and language polishing; and my mother, Mirjana Nikolić and my secretary, Anne Kennard, for patient assistance with the references. I thank them all wholeheartedly. I also thank the PEW Charitable Fund and the NIH for support.

Janko Nikolić-Žugić, M.D., Ph.D.
New York, October, 1993

CONTENTS

CONTRIBUTORS

Sofija Andjelic, M.D.
Immunology Program
Memorial Sloan-Kettering Cancer Center
New York

Simon R. Carding, Ph.D.
Department of Microbiology
University of Pennsylvania
Philadelphia

Gregory S. Kelner, Ph.D.
Department of Immunology
DNAX Research Institute
Palo Alto

Elizabeth A. Lacy, Ph.D.
Molecular Biology Program
Memorial Sloan-Kettering Cancer Center
and Cornell University
Graduate School of Medical Sciences
New York

Louis A. Matis, Ph.D.
Alexion Pharmaceuticals
New Haven, Connecticut

Janko Nikolić-Žugić, M.D., Ph.D.
Immunology Program
Memorial Sloan-Kettering Cancer Center
and Cornell University
Graduate School of Medical Sciences
New York

Fred Ramsdell, Ph.D.
Department of Immunobiology
Immunex Research and Development Corp.
Seattle

Sharon R. Seiler, Ph.D.
Molecular Biology Program
Memorial Sloan-Kettering Cancer Center
New York

Jonathan Sprent, M.D., Ph.D.
Department of Immunology
The Scripps Research Institute
La Jolla

Charles D. Surh, Ph.D.
Department of Immunology
The Scripps Research Institute
La Jolla

Tannishtha, B.S.
Department of Microbiology
University of Pennsylvania
Philadelphia

Faith B. Wells, Ph.D.
Biological Carcinogenesis
and Development Program
Program Resources, Inc./Dyncorp
Frederick, Maryland

Albert Zlotnik, Ph.D.
Department of Immunology
DNAX Research Institute
Palo Alto

CHAPTER 1

INTRODUCTION

Janko Nikolić-Žugić

T cells are the major regulatory and a significant effector component of the immune system. Their principal role is to eliminate intracellular foreign invaders (viruses, intracellular bacteria) and tumor cells and to help B cells produce antibodies directed against extracellular pathogens. Over 95% of T cells depend on the thymus as the site of their differentiation. Since the recognition of the thymus as an essential organ for the function of the immune system and the discovery that it represents the site of T-cell maturation,[1] the interest of the immunological community in the thymus has flourished. In over 30 years, thymology has advanced considerably beyond the initial period of phenomenology. Without the pretense of providing a complete history of thymology, I shall briefly mention several landmark discoveries that had major impact on the field.

The discovery of positive intrathymic selection[2,3] and the studies on the kinetics of thymocyte migration and export[4,5] were the major developments in the late seventies. These years also brought the advent of the monoclonal antibody technique.[6] Subsequently, an increased number of antibodies against defined cell surface markers led to extensive mapping of precursor-product relationships between various thymocyte subsets in the mid- and late eighties (reviewed in 7 and 8). At the same time, the technique of fetal thymic organ culture (reviewed in 9) permitted the studies of T-cell development in vitro. The identification of the T-cell receptor (TcR) molecules and genes[10] and the production of monoclonal antibodies to various segments of this receptor, set the stage for the de facto demonstration of intrathymic clonal deletion in normal animals,[11] and for the production of TcR transgenic animals.[12,13,14,15] This, in turn, provided an elegant and simple model to study various aspects of T-cell development. The latest technical tool, the gene "knockout" via homologous recombination,[16] has been widely used in thymus research as of the beginning of this decade.

Despite these advances, several questions have been very difficult to crack. The precise molecular mechanism of commitment to the T-cell lineage, as well as the mechanism of commitment to the αβ or γδ pathway, are not known. The molecular master switches of T-cell development are also obscure, and signals governing early (TcR⁻) thymocytes through proliferative stages, phenotypic changes and TcR gene rearrangement are not known. Thymic epithelial cells are difficult to isolate in appreciable numbers, and our knowledge of their interaction with developing thymocytes is scarce (reviewed in 17, 18). Most importantly, a major mystery remains centered around positive and negative selection: How does a thymocyte know when to die and when to live (be rescued)? A related issue is that of signal transduction in maturing thymocytes. Last but not least, the control of accessory molecule exclusion is complex and far from being resolved.

REFERENCES

1. Davies AJ. The tale of T cells. Immunol Today 1993;14:137-140.

2. Bevan MJ. In a radiation chimera host H-2 antigens determine the immune responsiveness of donor cytotoxic cells. Nature 1977; 269:417-418.

3. Zinkernagel RM, Calahan GN, Klein J et al. Cytotoxic T cells learn specificity for self H-2 during differentiation in the thymus. Nature 1978; 271:251-254.

4. McPhee D, Pye J, Shortman K. The differentiation of T-lymphocytes. V. Evidence for intrathymic death of most thymocytes. Thymus 1979; 1:151.

5. Scollay R, Butcher E, Weissman I. Thymus migration: Quantitative studies on the rate of migration of cells from the thymus to the periphery in mice. Eur J Immunol 1980; 10:210.

6. Kohler G, Milstein C. Continuous cultures of fused cells secreting antibody of predefined specificity. Nature 1975;256: 495-497.

7. Nikolic-Zugic J. Phenotypic and functional stages in thymocyte development. Immunol Today 1991; 12:65-71.

8. Shortman K. Cellular aspects of early T-cell development. Curr Opinion Immunol 1192; 4:140.

9. Jenkinson EJ, Owen JJT. T-cell differentiation in thymus organ cultures. Sem Immunol 1990; 2:51-58.

10. Davis MM, Bjorkman PJ. T-cell antigen receptor genes and T-cell recognition. Nature 1988; 334:395.

11. Kappler JW, Roehm N, Marrack P. T-cell tolerance by clonal elimination in the thymus. Cell 1987; 49:273-281.

12. Teh H-S, Kisielow P, Scott B et al. Thymic major histocompatibility complex antigens and the αβ/T-cell receptor determine the CD4/CD8 phenotype of T cells. Nature 1988; 335:229.

13. Sha WC, Nelson CA, Newberry RD et al. Positive and negative selection of an antigen receptor on T cells in transgenic mice. Nature 1988; 336:73-76.

14. Kaye J, Hsu M-L, Sauron M-E et al. Selective development of CD4⁺ T cells in transgenic mice expressing a class II MHC-restricted antigen receptor. Nature 1989; 341:746.

15. Berg LJ, Pullen AM, Fazekas de StGroth B et al. Antigen/MHC-specific T cells are preferentially exported from the thymus in the presence of their MHC ligand. Cell 1989; 58:1035.

16. Mansour SL, Thomas KR, Capecchi MR. Disruption of the proto-oncogene int-2 in mouse embryo-derived stem cells: a general strategy for targeting mutations to non-selectable genes. Nature 1988; 336:348-352.

17. Boyd RL, Tucek CL, Godfrey DI et al. The thymic microenvironment. Immunol Today 1993; 14:445-459.

18. Ritter M, Boyd RL. Development in the thymus: it takes two to tango. Immunol Today 1993; 14:462-469.

CHAPTER 2

ANATOMY AND HISTOLOGY OF THE THYMUS*

Charles D. Surh

Jonathan Sprent

The thymus is the major site for generation of immunocompetent lymphocytes.[1] T-cell formation in the thymus is controlled by two distinct classes of cells, endogenous epithelial cells (EC) and exogenous bone-marrow (BM) cells. In consort, these parenchymal cells orchestrate the development of thymocytes by providing the appropriate microenvironments and signals necessary for differentiation and maturation of young T cells. In particular, thymic parenchymal cells play a crucial role in shaping the T-cell repertoire and selectively exporting mature T-cell receptor (TcR) positive cells specific for self major histocompatiblility complex (MHC) molecules. This chapter will review the types of thymic parenchymal cells and their role in T-cell differentiation.

Before discussing the features of thymic parenchymal cells, it is first useful to describe the highlights of intrathymic T-cell development. To produce a repertoire of mature T cells, the thymus performs three major tasks. First, the thymus attracts a steady flow of small numbers of stem cells from the BM and induces these cells to proliferate and differentiate into immature thymocytes.[2] After entering the thymus, prothymocyte stem cells undergo 100-1000 fold expansion and begin to differentiate by rearranging TcR genes and expressing TcR, CD4 and CD8 molecules on the cell surface. Second, the thymus induces selective survival of thymocytes expressing TcR specific for the "self" MHC molecules expressed on cortical epithelial cells (EC).[3-8] This process, termed positive selection, rescues only a very small proportion (<5%) of thymocytes; the remaining cells die in situ, probably from some form of programmed cell death (apoptosis). Third, the thymus clonally deletes thymocytes that have overtly high affinity for self MHC molecules.[4-6,8] This process of negative selection ensures self tolerance

*This work as supported by grants CA 38355, AI 21487, CA 25803, AI 07244 from the United States Public Health Service. Dr. Surh is a Special Fellow of the Leukemia Society of Americas. Publication no.8194-IMM is from the Scripps Research Institute.

induction. With this brief description of thymic function, the remainder of this chapter deals with the microanatomy of the thymus from the perspective of αβ T-cell maturation. The thymic microenvironments involved in γδ T-cell generation is not discussed as information on this topic is very sparse. Detailed information on thymocyte differentiation and selection is given in other chapters.

ARCHITECTURE OF THE THYMUS

The thymus is a bilobed organ located in the upper part of the anterior mediastinum.[1] The thymus is large in infancy and grows progressively until the age of puberty. Thereafter, marked atrophy occurs and the thymus remains very small throughout adult life. Histologically, the thymus is divided into two distinctive compartments, the cortex and the medulla (Fig. 1a). The greater density of lymphoid cells in the cortex than the medulla makes these two compartments easily visible in sections. In addition to the cortex and medulla, the thymus can be further compartmentalized to include two additional areas: the subcapsulary region and the corticomedullary junction (CMJ). In these four thymic compartments, distinctive microenvironments composed of disease populations of stromals cells control the various steps involved in T-cell differentiation.

i) The *subcapsular region* contains the most immature population of thymocytes. These cells are double-negative (DN) for both CD4 and CD8 expression,[9,10] and act as precursor cells for the majority population of CD4+8+ cells in the deep cortex.[6] The DN population is the immediate progenitor of the BM-derived subset of prothymocytes which enter the thymus from the arterioles that line the CMJ.[11] The prevailing view is that prothymocytes migrate outward through the cortex to the subcapsular area. Here, DN cells proliferate extensively and start to differentiate. In mice, a subpopulation of differentiating DN cells can be detected in situ on the basis of interleukin (IL)-2 receptor α (IL-2Rα) expression; DN cells transiently express the IL-2Rα chain just prior to expression of both CD4 and CD8 molecules.[12] IL-2α+ cells are limited to the DN population and are present through-

out the cortex (Fig. 1b).[9] However, the majority of these cells are concentrated under the capsule. The wide distribution of IL-2Rα+ cells in the cortex might imply that DN cells migrate from the subcapsular region to the deep cortex prior to differentiation into DP cells. Alternatively, prothymocytes entering at the CMJ may begin to differentiate into IL-2α+ cells during migration toward the subcapsular region. Another distinct feature of the subcapsular region, and also of the adjacent outer cortex, is the presence of thymic nurse cells. These structures encapsulate 20-40 thymocytes and can be detected by scanning electron microscopy.[13]

ii) In the main body of the *cortex*, immature double-positive (DP) CD4+CD8+ thymocytes are densely packed (Fig. 1c) among a network of reticular EC (Fig. 2a). DP cells represent the majority of the lymphoid cells in the thymus. These cells typically express a low density of αβ TcR molecules and co-express CD3 molecules. Most DP thymocytes die in the cortex within a few days and one-third of this population is replaced by newly-generated DP cells each day.[14] As mentioned earlier, only a small proportion of DP thymocytes (<5%) is destined for positive selection and export to the periphery.

iii) The *corticomedullary junction* is enriched for BM-derived cells, especially dendritic cells (DC) and B cells.[15-17] These cells have antigen-presenting cell (APC) function. Their main duty is to screen newly-selected thymocytes entering from the cortex and clonally delete cells with overt (high) affinity for self MHC.[18-22] The cells that survive negative selection are single-positive (SP) for either CD4 or CD8 and express high levels of αβ TcR molecules. After leaving the CMJ, these cells move to the deeper region of the medulla.

iv) In the *medulla*, recently-generated SP thymocytes from the cortex and CMJ are exposed to additional BM-derived APC and also to a heterogeneous population of EC (Fig. 2).[13,23,24] This presumably ensures full self tolerance induction. SP thymocytes undergo progressive maturation in the medulla and upregulate a variety of cell surface molecules including CD44 (Fig. 1d) and high molecular weight isoforms of CD45.[25] SP cells remain in

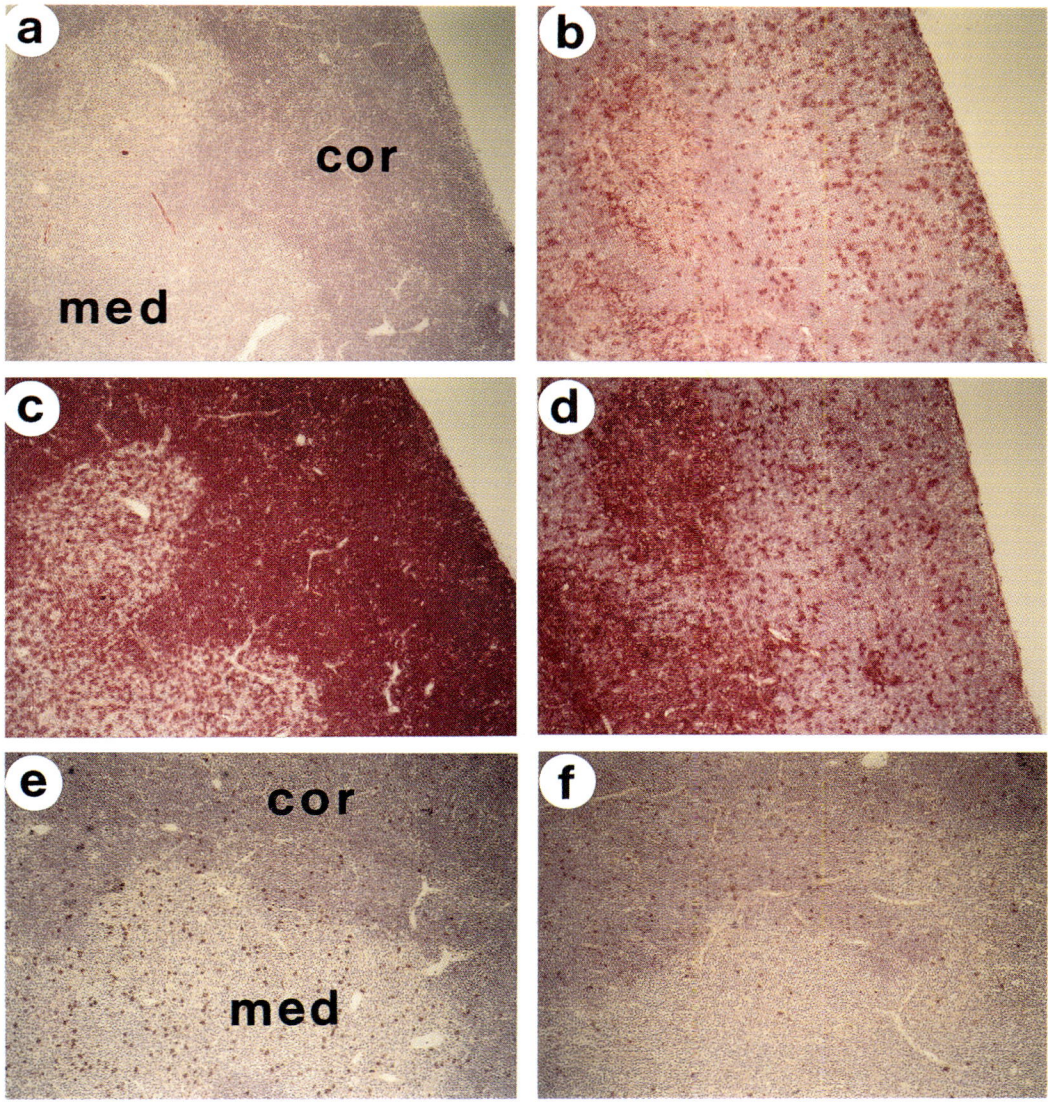

Fig. 1. Distribution of thymocyte subsets in normal adult thymus. Adjacent cryostat sections of a normal C57BL/ 6 (B6) thymus were stained for various differentiation markers using mAbs and enzyme-conjugated secondary reagents;[24] sections were counterstained with hematoxylin: (a) Background staining with only secondary reagents alone. (b) IL-2Rα: staining is restricted to a subset of CD4-8- thymocytes and is found predominately in the subcapsular region with scattered cells in the deep cortex (cor); weak diffuse staining in the medulla (med) is presumably due to dendritic cells. (c) CD8: staining is apparent on nearly all cells in the cortex, most of which are CD4+8+ cells; 25-30% of SP cells in the medulla are CD8+4-. (d) CD44 (Pgp-1): there is strong staining on SP cells in the medulla and scattered staining in the cortex; the CD44+ cells in the cortex are presumably either a subset of CD4-8- cells or recently generated SP cells. (e) Vβ3 in B6 thymus: this subset of αβ TcR+ cells is scattered throughout the cortex and medulla; the intensity of staining is higher in the medulla, indicative of higher TcR expression on mature SP cells. (f) Vβ3 in BALB/c thymus: stained cells are detectable in the cortex but are rare in the medulla; the paucity of Vβ3+ cells in the medulla reflects clonal deletion to the Mlsᶜ antigens expressed in the BALB/c strain. All sections were photographed at x100. Reproduced from the Journal of Experimental Medicine, 1992, 176:495-505, by copyright permission of the Rockefeller University Press.

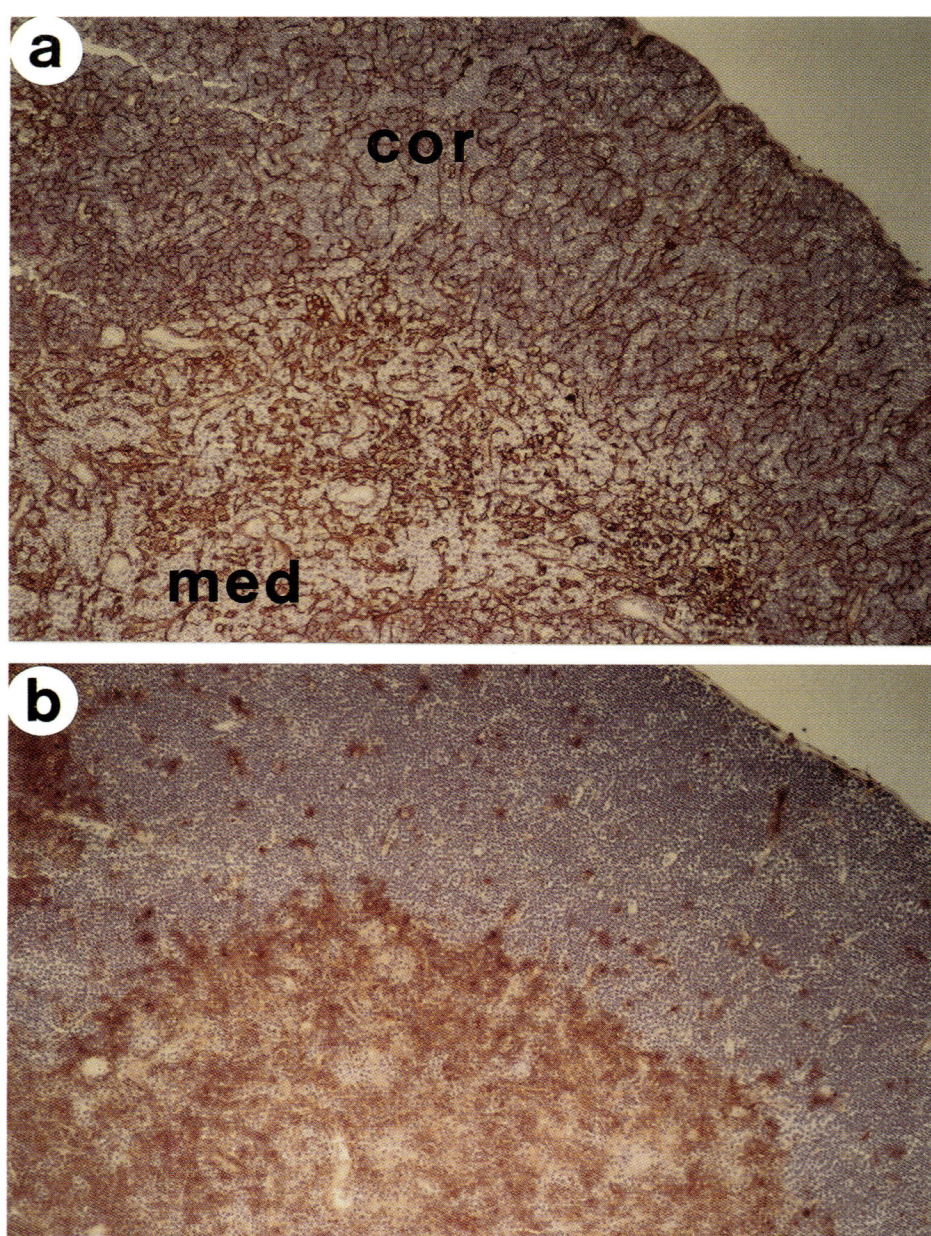

Fig. 2. Distribution of EC and MHC class II⁺ (I-E⁺) BM-derived cells in thymus of BM chimeras. Chimeras were prepared by exposing B6 (I-E⁻) mice to 1100 cGy and reconstituting these mice with BM cells from B10.A(5R) (I-E⁺) mice.[24] Thymuses from the chimeras were removed at 2 months post-reconstitution. The sections shown were counterstained with hematoxylin. (a) EC stained with anti-keratin antibody: reticular staining of EC is evident throughout the thymus, both in the cortex (cor) and medulla (med). (b) BM-derived cells stained with anti-I-E antibody: there is strong staining of the medulla, the stained cells being a mixture of donor BM-derived DC, MØ and B cells; a few I-E⁺ cells are scattered in the cortex; the identity of these cells is not clear. All sections were photographed at x100. Reproduced from the Journal of Experimental Medicine, 1992, 176:495-505, by copyright permission of the Rockefeller University Press.

the medulla for a variable period and then exit into the periphery.

ONTOGENY OF THE THYMUS

Cells from at least three embryonic origins congregate during ontogeny to differentiate into the nonhemopoietic structures of the thymus: the ectoderm of third branchial cleft, the endoderm of the third pharyngeal pouch and the neural crest mesectoderm.[26-28] A meticulous three-dimensional reconstructional study from serial sections of days 9-17 fetal thymuses has provided evidence that the embryonic ectodermal and endodermal cells contribute to the formation of the epithelial cells of the outer region (cortex) and the inner region (medulla) of the thymus, respectively.[27] In addition to ectodermal and endodermal cells, the neural crest mesectoderm colonizes the thymus and leads to the formation of thymic mesenchymal cells.[28] The embryonic cells from these origins congregate from gestation day 9, and, starting around day 11, the thymic lobes migrate in a caudal and medial direction, undergoing elongation during this process. By day 14, migration of the thymic anlage is complete and the two thymic lobes are juxtaposed in the anterior mediastinum. In athymic nude mice, thymic development appears to be abruptly terminated during gestation day 10-11 due to failure of cell contribution from the ectodermal branchial cleft.[29]

The embryonic fetal thymic anlage is first seeded with hemopoietic cells from the fetal liver between days 11-12.[30] The earliest evidence of T-cell differentiation in the thymus occurs at gestation day 14 with the rearrangement of TcR γ, δ and β chain genes.[31] The first surface TcR$^+$ cells to appear are DN $\gamma\delta^+$ cells on day 14.[32,33] $\alpha\beta$ TcR$^+$ cells require rearrangement of the β-chain locus for initiation of differentiation.[34] Expression of low levels of $\alpha\beta$ TcR, along with upregulation of CD4 and CD8, is first detectable on days 16-17.[35] SP thymocytes with high levels of $\alpha\beta$ TcR expression are not apparent until days 18-19. With regard to nonlymphoid hemopoietic cells, DC are detectable in the thymus as early as day 16

of gestation and macrophages (M∅) are present from around days 17-19.[36-38] B cell precursors are detectable from day 14 of gestation, but surface μ^+ B cells do not appear until just prior to birth at around day 18.[39]

The appearance of $\alpha\beta$ TcR$^+$ cells in the thymus is preceded by the expression of MHC molecules on EC.[24,40,41] Both class I and II molecules are clearly detectable on EC from around day 16, and MHC expression progressively increases to reach adult levels by the time of birth (days 20, 21) (Fig. 3). The kinetics of MHC expression thus appears to correlate with the maturation of thymocytes. Some of the MHC expression in the fetal thymus reflects staining of BM-derived APC,[42] but the precise identity of these cells and their kinetics of MHC expression have not been determined.

CELL TYPES IN THE ADULT THYMUS

The nonlymphoid component of adult thymus can be categorized into three large groups of cells: (1) mesenchyme-derived connective tissues and vessels, (2) a heterogeneous population of EC, and (3) BM-derived APCs. The features of these three types of thymic stromal cells are discussed below.

MESENCHYME-DERIVED CELLS

The thymus is encapsulated by loose connective tissue composed of fibroblasts and extracellular matrix.[43] In mouse thymus, the connective tissue penetrates the cortex, forming short septa which often contain blood vessels. In larger mammals the connective tissue septa penetrate deep into the thymus and divide the thymus into numerous lobules.

The vascularization of the thymus is unusual. Arterioles, which enter the thymus at the corticomedullary junction, give off capillaries which ascend into the cortex to the subcapsular area where they loop back toward the medulla.[44-46] The descending capillaries join to form larger capillary vessels and finally fuse into postcapillary venules at the CMJ or in the medulla. In some cases the capillaries exit the thymic parenchyma and enter the connective tissue of the capsule before reentering the cortex through the

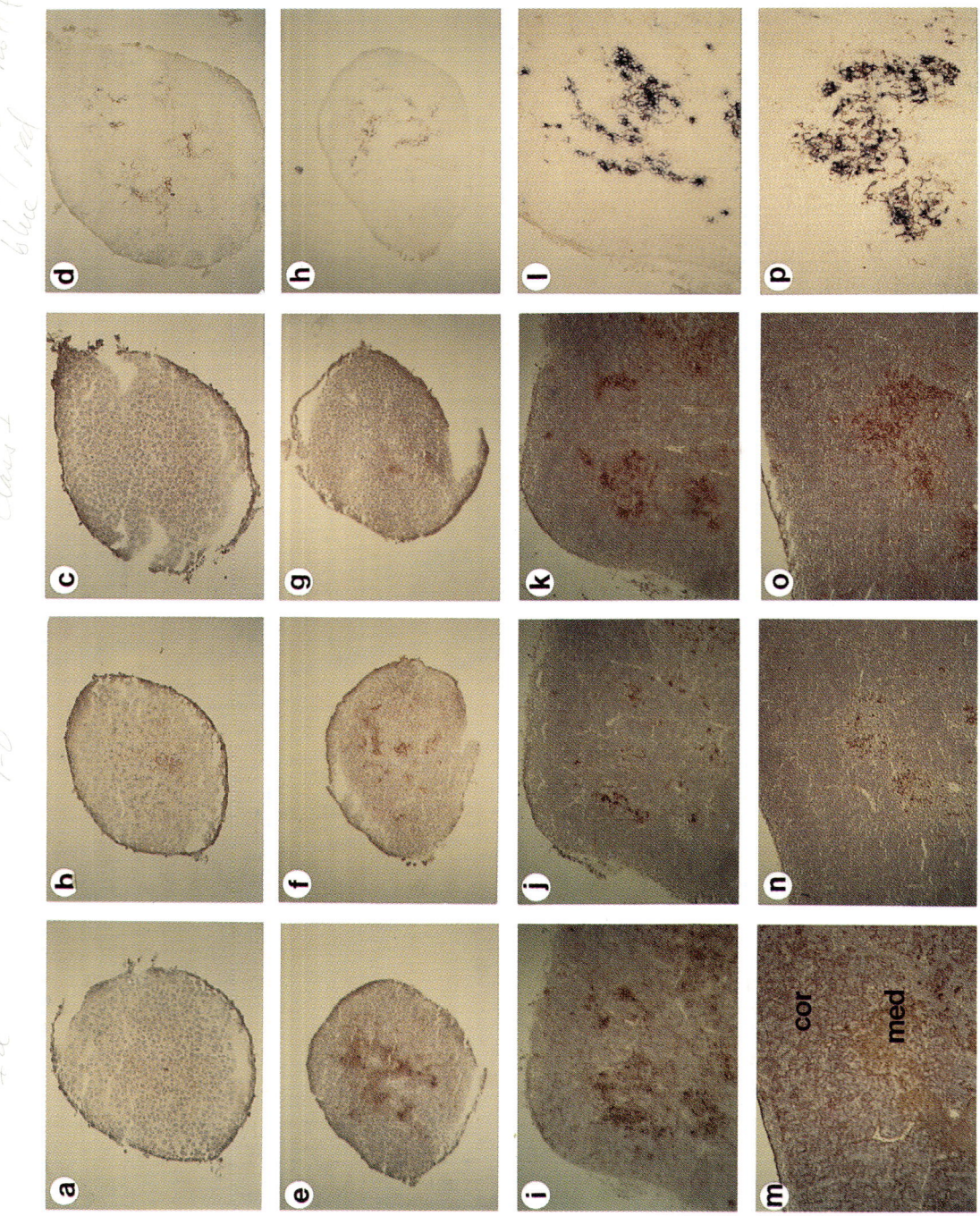

Fig. 3. Ontogeny of H-2 class I, class II, UEA-1, and I-O expression in the fetal thymus. Serial sections of BALB/c thymuses from day 14 fetus (a-d), day 16 fetus (e-h), newborn (i-l), and 10-day-old neonatal (m-p) mice were stained for the expression of Ia (I-A^d) (a, e, i, and m), I-O (b, f, j, and n), and class I (L^d) (c, g, k, and o) molecules, and counterstained with hematoxylin. Some of the sections were double stained for UEA-1 (in blue) vs. I-O (in red) (d, h, l, and p) as previously described;[24] these sections were not counterstained with hematoxylin. I-A and class I expression (a, e, i, and m; and c, g, k, and o) is not clearly evident until about day 16 of gestation; staining is first detectable in the medulla and remains low on cortical epithelium until the time of birth (I-A) or after birth (class I). By contrast, UEA-1 (d, h, l, and p) and I-O (d, h, l, and p; and b, f, j, and n) is apparent on small central aggregates of cells as early as day 14 of gestation. Expression of these two markers increases progressively during ontogeny and reaches adult levels only after birth. Before birth, both markers seem to be expressed on the same cells (d, h, and l). By 10 days after birth, a distinct population of UEA-1⁻ I-O⁺ cells is evident (p). All sections were photographed at magnification of 100, except a-d, and p which were taken x160. Reproduced from the Journal of Experimental Medicine, 1992, 176:611-616, by copyright permission of the Rockefeller University Press.

connective tissue septa. A small number of capillaries from the arterioles also directly enter the medulla and connect with the venules. It is suggested that progenitor cells from the bone marrow enter the thymus through small arterioles along the CMJ and then migrate to the subcapsular area.[11] As thymocytes mature, the cells travel toward the medulla and then exit the thymus through the postcapillary venules[47] or the efferent lymphatic vessels[48] in the medulla.

Although a few capillaries in the capsule are fenestrated, the capillaries in the cortex have endothelial cells which form impermeable tight junctions with each other.[44] These vessels are also surrounded by phagocytic macrophages to form a second barrier to circulating blood proteins. The impermeable endothelial junctions are not present in the arterioles and venules in the medulla. Thus, although the cells in the medulla are well exposed to circulating serum proteins, the differentiating thymocytes in the cortex are isolated from blood-borne proteins

by an effective blood-thymus barrier.[44] Interestingly, however, intraperitoneally injected antibodies[49] and silica particles[50] are able to penetrate the thymic capsule via lymphatic vessels and enter the cortex. The functional significance of this transcapsular route is unclear.

EPITHELIAL CELLS

Unlike other lymphoid organs, the thymus contains a dense network of EC, both in the cortex and medulla (Fig. 2a). Thymic EC (TEC) display considerable heterogeneity. Initially, ultrastructural studies indicated that TEC in the cortex are morphologically different from TEC in the medulla.[51,52] Electron microscopy (EM) defined the reticular nature of cortical TEC and revealed elongated processes of "pale" cytoplasm, due to scarcity of electron dense macromolecules. In contrast, the TEC in the medulla were found to be globular and voluminous with darker electron dense cytoplasm. Subsequent studies demonstrated further heterogeneity in TEC. For example, a meticulous EM study of the human thymus[53] revealed that TEC under the outer capsule are morphologically different from the major population of TEC in the deep cortex. TEC can now be morphologically classified into at least six different subsets.[53] Furthermore, most TEC, including those in the cortex, appeared to be at various stages of activation or differentiation. Interestingly, there is a subpopulation of undifferentiated immature TEC in the medulla, which suggests that most TEC may be continuously regenerated instead of being long-lived static cells.

TEC express keratin (Fig. 2a) and impressive evidence for heterogeneity in TEC populations has come from detailed analysis of cytokeratin expression.[54-56] Cytokeratins are a group of at least 19 intermediate cytoskeletal filament proteins with MW ranges of 40-68 Kd.[57] Cytokeratin expression depends on many factors, including the type of epithelium concerned and the stage of differentiation. Selective expression of only low MW keratin is indicative of simple undifferentiated epithelium whereas expression of high MW keratin subunits characterizes more differentiated epithelium.[57] Work from many labs has found that

TEC contain a number of different types of keratin proteins.[54-56,58] The patterns of keratin expression on the various subsets of TEC are complex. In general, the keratins expressed on cortical EC are low MW, which suggests that most of cortical EC fall under the category of simple epithelium. A more diverse pattern of keratin expression is observed in the medulla. In particular, some medullary EC express high MW keratins typical of complex epithelia such as keratinized stratified epithelium. In fact, in many species (but not mice) medullary EC form dense aggregates of keratinized epithelium termed Hassel's corpuscles.[59] Interestingly, in terms of keratin expression the EC in the subcapsulary region resemble medullary EC rather than the EC in the deep cortex.[54,55] Whether subcapsular and medullary EC have a common origin is unknown.

Although ultrastructural and cytokeratin composition studies have provided valuable information on the heterogeneity of TEC, the most direct evidence on TEC diversity has come from studies with mAbs. The first set of mAbs which showed reactivity to TEC were MHC specific.[60] Subsequently, many laboratories produced mAbs reactive to TEC of man, mouse and rat in the hope of clearly defining the subtypes of TEC and generating probes useful for studying TEC-associated molecules involved in thymocyte differentiation.[61,62] In addition, a few lectins were discovered which react with a subpopulation of medullary EC.[23] Collectively, mAbs and lectins have proved to be invaluable tools for classifying TEC into subsets according to their location within the thymus. Some of the reagents useful for studying TEC subsets in mice,

Table 1. Reagents for detecting thymic stromal cells

Reagents	Type, origin	Specificity	Reference
MHC-class II			
BP107	(mAb, mouse)	I-A$^{b(d)}$	121
10-2.16	(mAb, mouse)	I-A$^{k(r,f,s)}$	122
14-4-4S	(mAb, mouse)	I-E	123
K507	(purified Ab, rabbit)	I-O (β-chain)	65
Y-Ae	(mAb, mouse)	I-A^b/I-E$_\alpha$ peptide	124
MHC-class I			
12-2-2S	(mAb, mouse)	K^k	123
Y3	(mAb, mouse)	K^b	125
28-14-8S	(mAb, mouse)	D^{b}L$^{d(q)}$	126
30-5-7	(mAb, mouse)	L^d	127
Epithelial cells			
MD-1	(mAb, rat)	Medullary EC	66
Th-4	(mAb, mouse)	Medullary EC	128
UEA-1	(lectin)	Medullary EC	23
6C3	(mAb, rat)	Cortical EC	63
Antikeratin	(antiserum, rabbit)	pan cytokeratin	commercial (Dako)
Bone marrow-derived cells			
NLDC-145	(mAb, rat)	DC + cortical EC	15
F4/80	(mAb, rat)	MØ	129
7D4	(mAb, rat)	IL-2R$_\alpha$	130
1.M.7.8.1	(mAb, rat)	CD44	131
KJ25	(mAb, hamster)	TcR V$_\beta$ 3	132

along with other mAbs discussed in this chapter, are listed in Table 1.

Histology of Cortical Epithelial cells

In the cortex of the adult mouse thymus, reticular EC are readily visible with mAbs to MHC molecules:[24,60] anti-class II (I-A, I-E) mAbs produce strong staining (I-A in Fig. 4a), while the expression of class I (D, K, L) molecules is generally much weaker (D in Fig. 4c). The expression of MHC molecules in the cortex is apparent in all EC, including subcapsular EC, and cortical staining with anti-MHC mAbs resembles the staining pattern observed with anti-pancytokeratin antibody (Fig. 4f). Cortical EC are detectable with numerous other mAbs reactive with TEC,[61] such as the mAb 6C3 (Fig. 4d),[63] and NLDC-145, which also crossreacts with DC (Fig. 4g).[15] Most, if not all, of these non-MHC specific anti-cortical EC mAbs, including 6C3, recognize all the EC in the cortex with the exception of the subcapsular EC:[61] the subcapsular EC are recognized by many mAbs to subsets of medullary EC (see below). This suggests that, with the exception of subcapsular EC, the EC in the cortex are a fairly homogeneous population, and differ only in their level of activation (as detected in the ultrastructural studies discussed above).[53]

Histology of Medullary Epithelial Cells

The EC in the medulla are much more heterogeneous than cortical EC. Staining adult mouse thymus with anti-pancytokeratin antibody reveals that medullary EC are clearly detectable as a dense network of voluminous and semireticular cells with short cytoplasmic processes (Figs. 2a, 4f). Although early ultrastructural studies revealed that some EC in the medulla express both class I and II MHC molecules,[52,64] visualizing MHC expression on medullary EC by light microscopy is difficult because of dense staining of adjacent BM-derived cells (Fig.4a,c). However, clear staining of medullary EC is apparent with an antibody to a nonpolymorphic class II molecule, termed I-O.[24,65] This antibody detects B cells in peripheral lymphoid organs. In the thymus,

however, I-O expression defines a subpopulation of medullary EC with semireticular morphology (Fig. 4b).[24] Medullary EC can also be detected with many other TEC-specific mAbs, such as MD-1 which stains a population of fusiform cells (Fig.4i).[66] Many of these antibodies also react with EC under the capsule.[61] In addition to antibodies, two lectins were discovered that react with carbohydrate moieties expressed selectively on distinct subpopulations of EC in the medulla:[23] *Tetragonolobus purpureas* agglutinin (TPA) and *Ulex europeus* agglutinin 1 (UEA 1). TPA appears to recognizes the cells that form Hassel's corpuscles, whereas UEA-1 reacts with a reticular population of EC present throughout the medulla (Fig. 4e).

As mentioned above, MHC$^+$ EC in the thymic medulla are difficult to study by conventional histology because of the adjacent MHC$^+$ BM-derived cells. This problem can be avoided by preparing BM chimeras, e.g., by subjecting (MHC^a X MHC^b)F$_1$ mice to heavy irradiation followed by reconstitution with MHC^a BM cells. In these parent → F$_1$ chimeras, host BM-derived cells, including the APC in the thymus, are rapidly replaced by donor-derived cells. This means that MHC^b expression in the thymus is restricted to EC. With this approach, staining for MHC^b reveals scattered large clumps of densely stained EC in the medulla (Fig. 5).[24] These cells express both MHC class I (Fig.5i) and class II molecules (Fig. 5a), and co-express the ligand for the lectin UEA-1 (Fig. 5e). The finding that a population of MHC$^+$/UEA-1$^+$ EC exists in the medulla confirms a similar conclusion reached from an EM study by Farr and Anderson.[23] In contrast to conventional class I & II MHC molecules, nonpolymorphic I-O molecules are expressed on sheets of EC distributed evenly throughout the medulla (Fig. 5b). Double staining reveals that most of the I-O$^+$ cells do not express conventional MHC molecules; conversely, most of the MHC$^+$ cells are I-O$^-$ (Fig. 5f, g). These findings indicate the existence of two subpopulations of EC in the medulla distinguishable by their mutually exclusive expression of MHC and I-O molecules.[24] In contrast to the adult thymus,

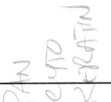

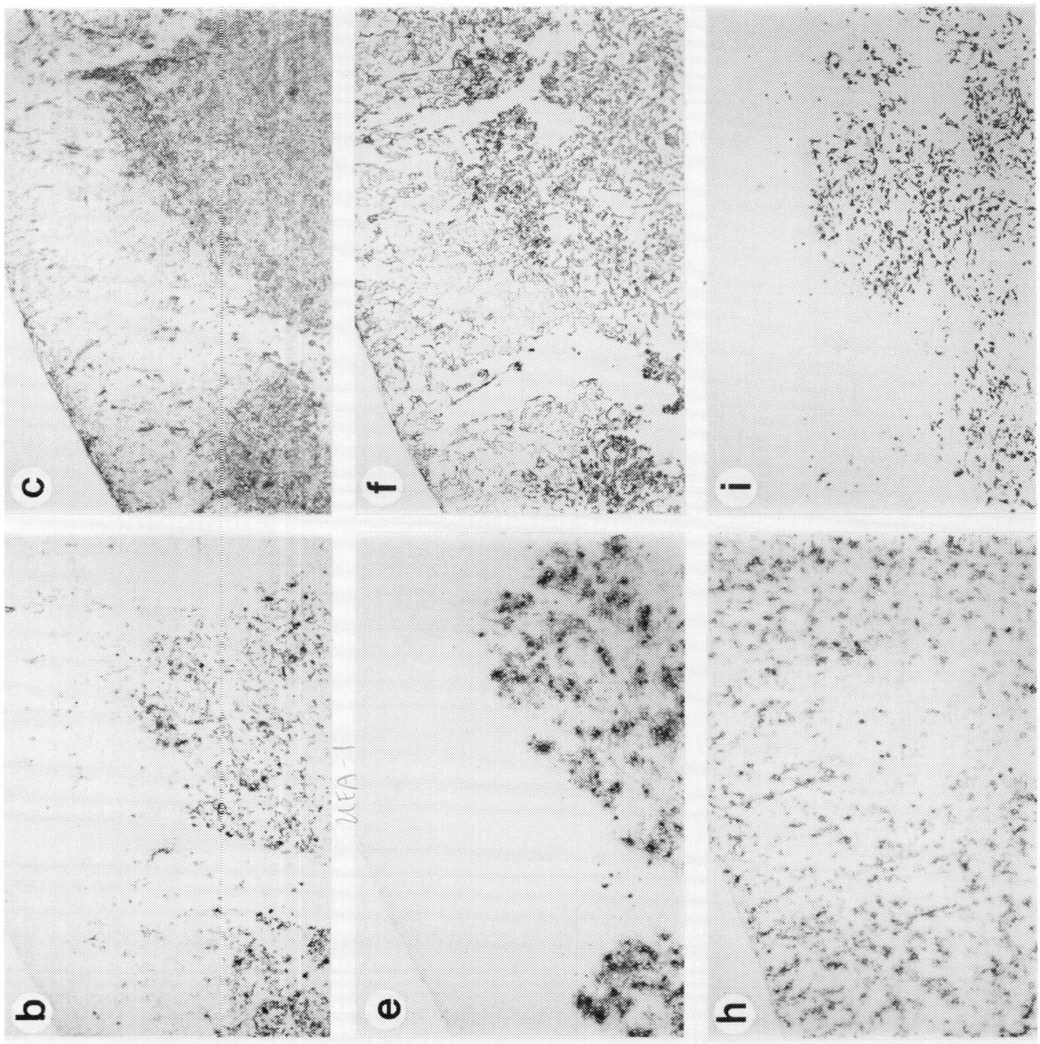

cor

med

a

b

c

d

e

f

g

h

i

Fig. 4. Normal adult thymus stained with some of the reagents listed in Table 1. Serial sections of a normal B6 (I-A^b) thymus were stained for the following markers. (a) I-A^b: there is confluent staining of BM-derived cells in the medulla (med) and reticular staining in the cortex (cor) typical of epithelial cells. (b) I-O: the medulla shows predominant staining of a network of stellate cells that resemble epithelial cells under higher power (see Fig. 5g): staining of the cortex is sparse. (c) K^b: as for I-A expression, there is strong staining of BM-derived cells in the medulla; reticular staining of cortical epithelium is weak but significant. (d) 6C3: staining is restricted to cortical epithelial cells. (e) UEA-1: staining is restricted to dense aggregates of epithelial cells the medulla; by electron microscopy, UEA-1 staining is restricted to epithelial cells.^23 (f) Pancytokeratin: staining is evident on the network of epithelial cells present in both the cortex and medulla. (g) NLDC-145: there is strong staining of cortical epithelial cells and weaker staining in the medulla, presumably of DC. (h) F4/ 80: scattered punctate staining of both cortex and medulla, indicative of MØ. (i) MD-1: staining of a lattice of stellate epithelial cells in the medulla. Eosinophils scattered in the medulla (which possess endogenous peroxidase activity) are depicted with arrows (see d and g). All sections were photographed at x100. Reproduced from the Journal of Experimental Medicine, 1992, 176:495-505, by copyright permission of the Rockefeller University Press.

most medullary EC in the early fetal thymus are double positive for MHC and I-O (Fig. 3d, h, l). This finding suggests that the MHC$^+$I-O$^-$ and MHC$^-$I-O$^+$ subsets may differentiate from MHC$^+$I-O$^+$ progenitors.

Double staining for MHC and I-O indicates that the MHC$^+$ I-O$^-$ and MHC$^-$ I-O$^+$ subsets account for the majority of the EC in the medulla. However, in comparison to the cytokeratin staining pattern, a small proportion of medullary EC are MHC$^-$I-O$^-$. These cells, some of which stain with the MD-1 antibody, may represent a third subset of medullary EC. Alternatively, the MHC$^-$I-O$^-$ cells might be immature precursors of the MHC$^+$ and I-O$^+$ subsets (or precursors of MHC$^+$I-O$^+$ intermediates). It should be emphasized that information on the heterogeneity of medullary EC is still in its infancy, and much additional information will be needed to determine the lineage relationship of the various medullary EC subsets.

BONE MARROW-DERIVED CELLS

Although the thymus anlage consists initially of an aggregate of EC, the thymus rapidly becomes infiltrated with hemopoietic cells and these cells soon account for the bulk of thymic tissue. In addition to large numbers of immature T cells, the thymus contains a spectrum of other hemopoietic cells including macrophages (MØ), DC, and B cells plus small numbers of NK cells, eosinophils and basophils. MØ, DC and B cells have APC function and these cells play a crucial role in negative selection.[5,22] Whether NK cells and granulocytes play a role in thymocyte differentiation is unknown.

The population of thymic MØ is heterogeneous in terms of morphology, maturation stages and expression of MHC molecules. In rats, heterogeneity in thymic MØ can be depicted with a set of mAbs that recognize subsets of MØ; the functional difference between these subsets has not been studied.[67,68] In mice, nearly all thymic MØ are detectable with the mAb F4/80 (Fig. 4h).[69] MØ are scattered throughout the cortex and medulla and also line blood vessels and the connective tissue of the thymic capsule. Most of the MØ in the cortex are negative for MHC class II expression, and under EM examination have abundant phagolysosomes; these structures contain digested remnants of thymocytes, and resemble tingible-body MØ found in the germinal centers of spleen and LN.[70] The main function of cortical MØ may be to phagocytose the massive numbers of DP cells that die in the cortex, presumably from apoptosis. This idea is supported by the finding that, unlike low density thymocytes (DP blasts, SP and DN cells), high-density DP thymocytes are selectively taken up by peritoneal MØ in vitro and completely digested within several hours.[71] Phagocytic MØ are also found in the medulla, but are less apparent in the corticomedullary junction where immature monocytes predominate.[72] Another population of MØ, distinguishable by their expression of MHC class II molecules, is reported to be present in both the cortex and medulla.[73] However, class II$^+$ MØ are sparse in the cortex and are difficult to study in the medulla because of close intermingling class II$^+$ DC.

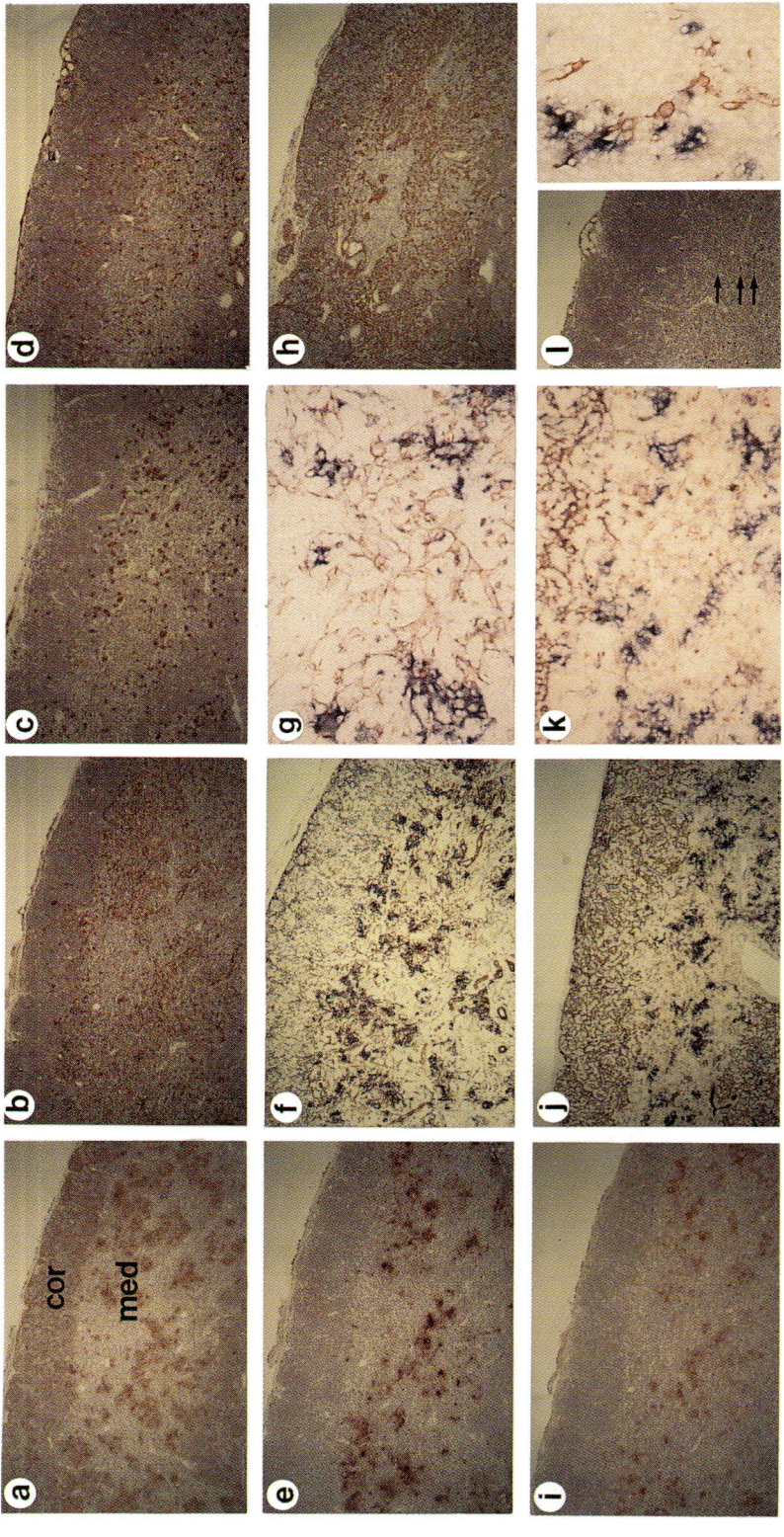

Fig. 5. Host H-2 expression in thymic medulla of a long-term parent → F1 BM chimera prepared with supralethal irradiation. Chimeras were prepared by exposing (B6 x CBA/Ca) F₁ (H-2ᵇ x H-2ᵏ) to 1300 cGy and reconstituting these mice with T-depleted B6 BM cells.¹³³ Thymuses were removed at 6 months post reconstitution and stained for the expression of the following molecules using one- or two-color staining procedures. (a) I-Aᵏ (host I-A): patches of dense staining are prominent in the medulla (med); there is also reticular staining of epithelial cells in the cortex (cor). (b) I-O: a lattice of stained cells is spread throughout most of the medulla; in accordance with previous findings⁶⁵ there is crossreactive staining of some of the blood vessels. (c) B220: scattered stained cells (presumably B cells) are evident in the cortical-medullary junction. (d) F4/80: scattered stained cells (presumably MØ) are visible in both the cortex and medulla. (e) UEA-1: the clumped staining in the medulla resembles the medullary staining for I-Aᵏ. (f) Two-color staining for I-Aᵏ (blue) and I-O (red): the cortex shows only blue (I-Aᵏ) staining whereas the medulla shows both blue and red (I-O) staining. (g) Higher power (x400) view of f: a network of red-stained (I-O⁺) cells is seen with most of these cells showing little or no blue staining; blue-stained (I-Aᵏ) cells are more scattered; some of the blue-stained cells show little or no red staining whereas other cells appear to show both colors (although it is unclear whether the double staining is real or reflects intertwining of the processes of adjacent cells). (h) Cytokeratin: dense staining of epithelial cells in both cortex and medulla. (i) Kᵏ (host class I): the clumped staining in the medulla resembles the staining patterns for UEA-1 and I-Aᵏ. (j) Two-color staining for I-Aᵏ (blue) and NLDC-145 (red): double staining (which yields a brown color) is prominent in the cortex (indicative of NLDC⁺ I-A⁺ cortical epithelium) but not in the medulla. (k) High-power (x250) view of j (corticomedullary region): distinct populations of blue-only (I-Aᵏ medullary epithelium) and red-only (donor-derived DC) cells are evident; double-stained (brown) cells are very rare in the medulla but are easily seen in the cortex (top). (l, left) Background staining with an irrelevant antibody (anti-Lᵈ) reveals endogenous peroxidase-containing cells scattered in the medulla (arrows). (l, right) High power (x400) view of C.B-17 SCID thymus stained for UEA-1 (blue) and I-O (red), separate populations of UEA-1⁺ and I-O⁺ epithelial cells are clearly apparent with almost no double-positive cells. Except for the double-stained sections, cell sections were counterstained with hematoxylin. Except for g, k, and l (right), all sections were photographed at x100. Reproduced from the Journal of Experimental Medicine, 1992, 176:495-505, by copyright permission of the Rockefeller University Press.

In contrast to the ubiquitous distribution of MØ, thymic DC are present only in the CMJ and medulla. DC show strong expression of both MHC class I and II molecules and, together with MHC⁺ EC, account for the confluent MHC staining observed in the medulla. In the mouse, DC are detectable with the mAb NLDC-145, which also stains cortical EC (Fig. 4g).[15] Morphologically, the majority of DC in the thymus lack phagolysosomes or other cytoplasmic organelles typical of phagocytic cells.[70] Instead, the DC contain pale cytoplasmic processes, relatively free of organelles, that interdigitate with surrounding thymocytes. In addition, many DC contain Birbeck granules typical of epidermal Langerhans cells.[74] Even though thymic DC are clearly BM-derived,[75] the exact origin of thymic DC cells is still unclear. In particular it is not known whether these cells enter the thymus as fully-differentiated DC from the spleen, BM and skin or differentiate in the thymus from a precursor cell. There are reports that thymic DC possess some of the phenotypic and functional characteristics of epidermal Langerhans cells, DC in the lung and a subpopulation of splenic DC,[76-78] implying that thymic DC have migrated from peripheral sources. However, others have found that thymic DC differ from splenic DC by expressing a set of markers usually found only on T cells, including Thy-1, CD2, CD4 and CD8αβ.[79] Evidence that DC can differentiate from thymic stem cells has come from studies involving intrathymic injection of a small subset of thymic CD4ˡᵒ cells. These cells, which have stem cell activity,[80] give rise not only to thymocytes but also to DC.[81] This finding strongly suggests that at least a proportion of thymic DC are generated in situ rather than migrating from the periphery as fully mature cells. Continuous in situ generation of DC in the thymus may account for the relatively fast turnover rate of thymic DC.[82] Thymic MØ turn over more slowly and these cells appear not to be generated in situ.

Thymic B cells constitute less than 0.5% of total lymphocytes in the normal adult thymus and are localized predominantly in the CMJ (Fig. 4c); in some cases, especially

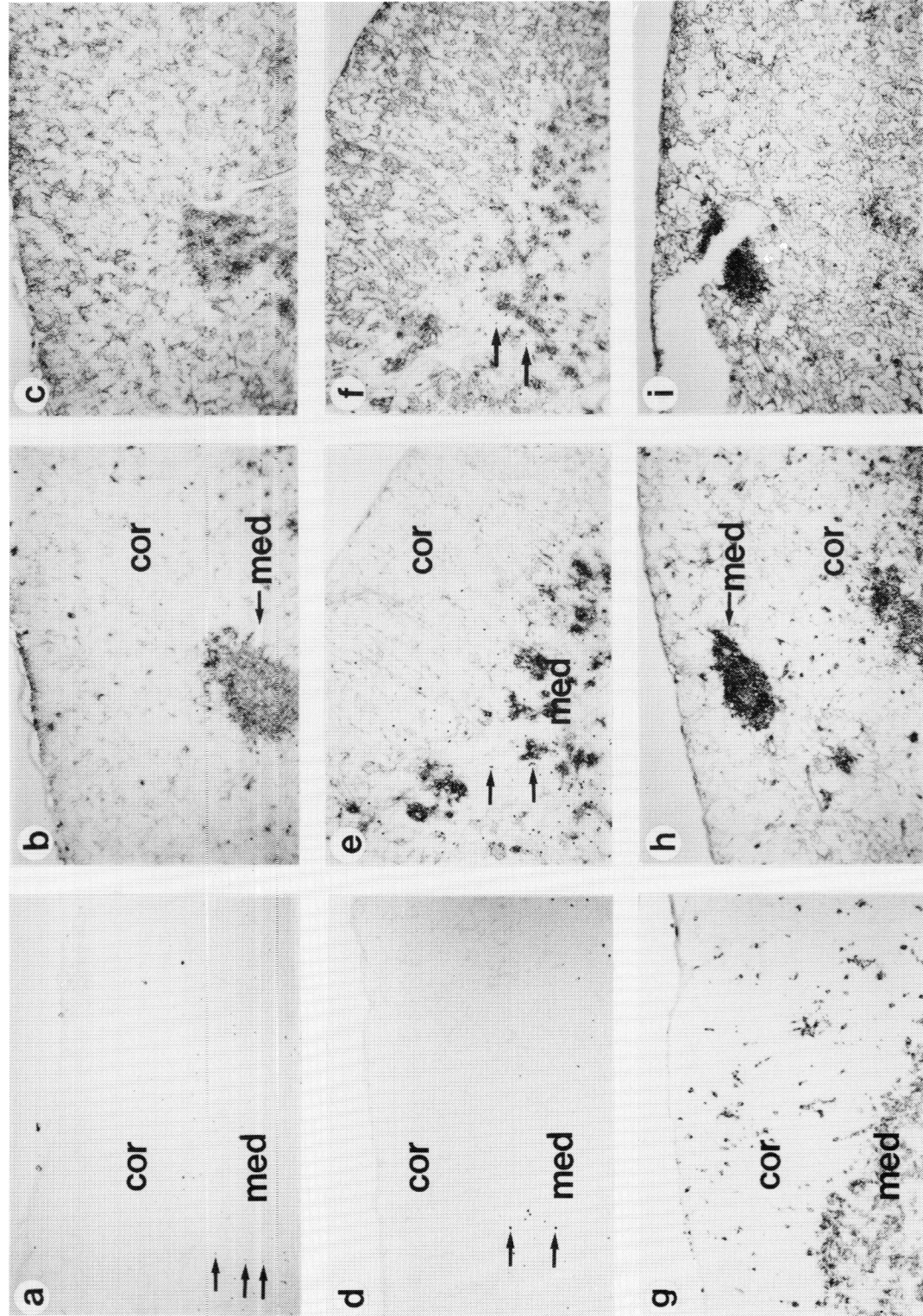

Fig. 6. Y-Ae expression on TEC. The Y-Ae epitope is a complex of I-E peptide bound to I-A^b molecules and requires joint expression of I-E and I-A^b molecules on the same cell.[109] Serial sections of thymus from various strains, including the 36-5 (I-E only on TEC) and 107-1 (normal I-E expression) transgenic lines (both I-A^b), were stained: counterstaining with hematoxylin was omitted. (a) Y-Ae staining of a control Y-Ae⁻ CBA/J (H-2^k) (I-A^k, I-E) thymus: no staining is evident except for faint background staining of blood vessels; small dark granular staining is due to endogenous peroxidase-positive cells (arrows) (also prominent in d-f). (b) Y-Ae staining of Y-Ae⁺ B10.A(5R) (I-A^b, I-E⁺) thymus: there is strong staining throughout the medulla (med) and on scattered cells (presumably MØ) in the cortex (cor): there is also very weak but significant staining of cortical EC (compare with a and d). (c) I-E staining of 5R thymus: typical confluent staining of the medulla and reticular staining of the cortex is seen. (d) Y-Ae⁻ B6 (I-A^b, I-E⁻) thymus: no staining except for weak background staining of blood vessels and on cells with endogenous peroxidase activity. (e) Y-Ae expression in 36-5 (I-A^b, I-E only on TEC) thymus: there is strong staining on clumps of cells in the medulla, and weak staining of EC in the cortex. (f) I-E expression in 36-5 thymus: staining of cortical epithelium is much stronger than for Y-Ae (compare with e), whereas staining of the medulla is similar. (g) Y-Ae expression in thymus from B10.A(5R) BM → 1,100-rad B6 BM chimera: there is strong confluent staining of BM-derived cells in the medulla and punctate staining of scattered cells (probably MØ) in the cortex; there is no staining of cortical EC. (h) Y-Ae staining of 107-1 (I-A^b, I-E) thymus: there is strong confluent staining of the medulla and of scattered cells (presumably MØ) in the cortex; there is also appreciable staining of the cortical EC (note that the 107-1 transgenic mouse has a higher copy number of I-E genes than normal I-E⁺ mice).[124] (i) I-E expression in 107-1 thymus: there is strong staining of both cortex and medulla (compare with h). All sections were photographed at x100.

in certain autoimmune diseases, thymic B cell numbers can increase dramatically.[83] Unlike splenic B cells, the majority of thymic B cells are CD5⁺.[17] CD5⁺ B cells tend to secrete autoantibodies, but whether these cells are a separate lineage is still controversial.[84] Although the functional role of thymic B cells is unclear, these cells may contribute to tolerance induction of thymocytes to B cell specific antigens. In this regard there is evidence that full tolerance

induction of thymocytes to endogenous superantigens, e.g., Mls^c antigens, requires the presence of B cells.[85-86] Since B cells are very rare in the cortex, superantigen-induced clonal deletion of T cells in largely restricted to the medulla (illustrated in Fig. 1f for deletion of Vβ3⁺ T cells).

FUNCTIONS OF THE THYMIC EPITHELIAL CELLS

Two major functions are ascribed to TEC: 1) induction of thymocyte differentiation and 2) positive selection of self MHC-restricted T cells. The requirement for TEC in thymocyte differentiation is best illustrated by the lack of thymic T-cell development in nude mice, and the ability to restore thymopoiesis in these mice by engraftment of thymuses depleted of BM-derived cells.[87] However, the cellular interactions and soluble factors that guide thymocyte differentiation are still poorly understood. Nonetheless it is clear that MHC expression on TEC is not required during the early stages of differentiation. This is apparent from the finding that "knockout" mice lacking both class I and II MHC molecules possess normal numbers of DP thymocytes.[88]

TEC play a decisive role in positive selection. As mentioned earlier, positive selection is the process by which the thymus selects T cells restricted to self MHC molecules.[3,89,90] In contrast to DP cells, the production of SP thymocytes requires contact with MHC molecules; MHC class II molecules control the production of CD4 SP cells and class I molecules control CD8 SP cells. This is illustrated by the finding that β2m-knockout mice deficient in class I expression produce CD4 cells but fail to generate CD8 cells;[91,92] conversely, class II-deficient mice produce CD8 cells but not CD4 cells.[93,94] Based on studies with BM-chimeras[89,90,95] and grafting studies with APC-depleted thymuses,[3] it is clear that positive selection is largely under the control of TEC rather than BM-derived cells. Direct evidence that cortical EC control positive selection has come from studies on transgenic mice expressing MHC class II molecules in defined sites in the thymus. The key finding is that selective expression of class II on cortical EC is sufficient to

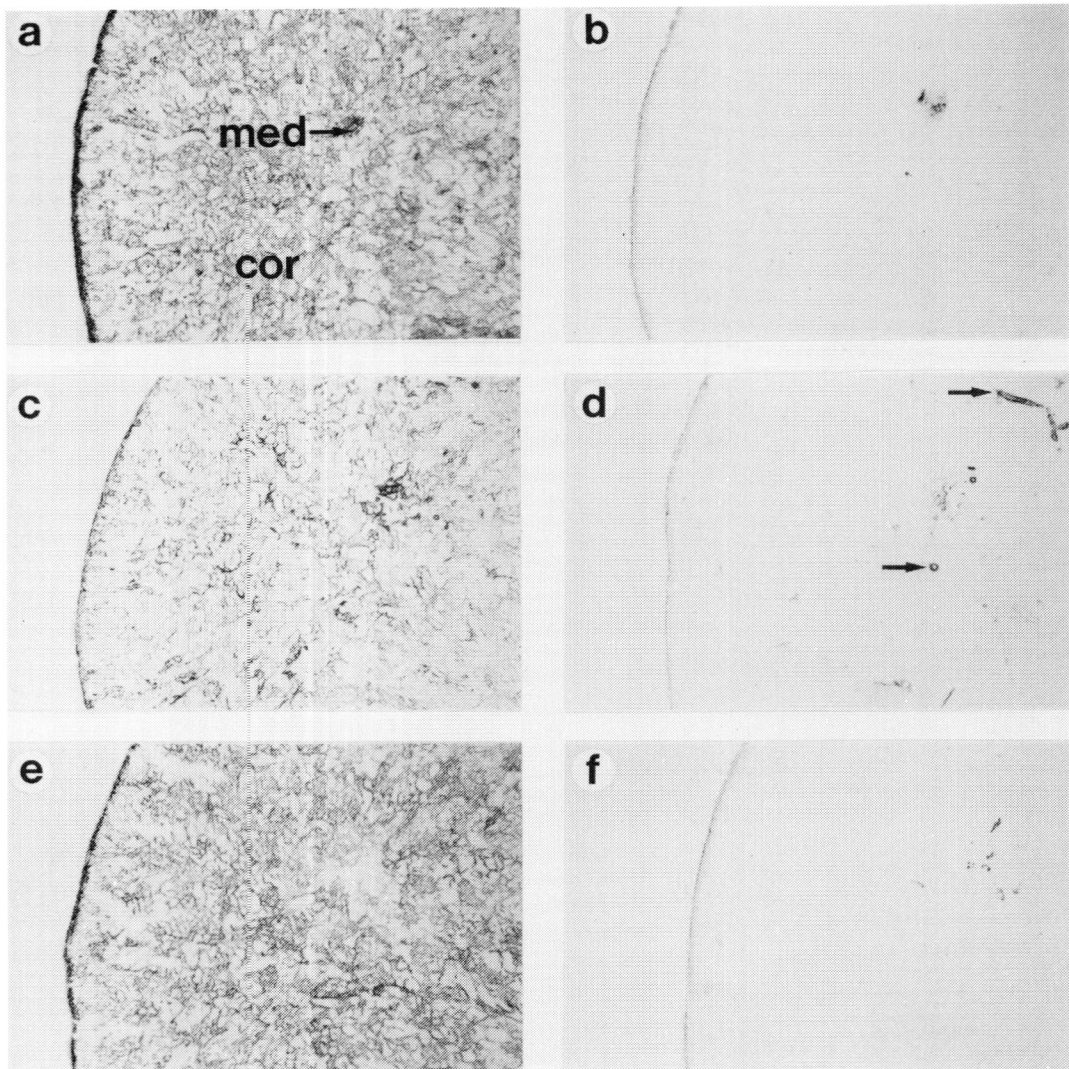

Fig. 7. Atrophy of medullary EC subsets in mice treated with cyclosporin (CsA). Young BALB/c mice were given a low dose of irradiation (600 cGy) and then injected daily for 3 weeks with CsA (10 mg dissolved in olive oil given by intraperitoneal injection).[134] Sections of thymus were stained with various reagents; counterstaining with hematoxylin was omitted. Staining for I-A^d (a), keratin (c) and 6C3 (e) reveals a uniform pattern of reticular staining throughout the thymus, indicating a marked overrepresentation of cortical tissue with virtually no medulla. Staining for UEA-1 (b), I-O (d) and MD-1 (f) reveals only occasional small clusters of medullary EC. All sections were photographed at x100.

generate large numbers of CD4 cells whereas class II expression restricted to medullary EC generates very few CD4 cells.[96] More recently it has been found that positive selection of CD4 cells fails to occur in irradiated class II-deficient mice reconstituted with normal BM cells, i.e., a situation in which class II molecules are expressed strongly on thymic APC but not on TEC.[97] Collectively, these various studies provide strong evidence that positive selection of CD4 cells is controlled by cortical EC and not by BM-derived APC or medullary EC.

Cortical EC are also primarily responsible for positive selection of CD8 cells. For CD8 cells, however, it seems that BM-derived cells are able to induce a low level of positive selection, at least under experimental conditions. This is apparent from the finding that reconstituting β2m-knockout (class I deficient) mice with normal BM-cells generates small numbers of CD8 cells that are restricted to the MHC molecules expressed on the injected BM-derived cells.[98] Why BM-derived cells induce low-level positive selection of CD8 but not CD4 cells is unknown, but it might be related to the fact that the BM-derived cells in the cortex, i.e., MØ and thymocytes express varying levels of class I but show only very limited expression of class II molecules. Class I expression on these BM-derived cells in the cortex might be capable of inducing a minor degree of positive selection, perhaps with the aid of differentiation signals from the adjacent cortical EC.[98]

In contrast to cortical EC, much less is understood about the function of EC in the medulla. Since the EC in the medulla are quite heterogeneous, it is likely that each subpopulation of medullary EC performs a separate task. The MHC+/I-O− subpopulation of medullary EC expresses typical class I and II molecules at the same level as BM-derived cells, and these MHC+ EC probably make a substantial contribution to tolerance induction. Initial studies on tolerance induction in the thymus led to the conclusion that tolerance is primarily under the control of BM-derived cells. Subsequently, however, many groups have concluded that TEC, especially medullary EC, do contribute to tolerance.[99-102,103,104] Unlike BM-derived APC, however, TEC generally induce only partial tolerance. Tolerance induced by TEC is more pronounced in vivo than in vitro assays and it is quite likely that tolerance is restricted to high-affinity T cells.[104] The alternative possibility is that TEC are intrinsically strongly tolerogenic but express a more limited array of self peptides than BM-derived cells.[105]

The inability of TEC to induce complete tolerance may be related to the limited capacity of TEC to function as APC. It has been known for several years that cortical EC are a poor source of APC for stimulating mature T cells. This may reflect that cortical EC fail to provide costimulatory signals and/or are deficient in processing antigens.[106,107]

In contrast, medullary EC have quite strong APC function. These cells appear to be capable of antigen presentation and T-cell activation since EC lines with the phenotype of medullary EC are able to present soluble foreign antigens to T-cell clones and activate these cells.[108] Whether the APC function of these EC lines is as efficient as professional APC, however, is not clear. Nevertheless, it is of interest that medullary EC resemble BM-derived cells in expressing B7, a costimulatory molecule that interacts with the CD28 molecules on T cells (personal communication from Degermann, S and Lo, D). B7 expression on medullary EC is quite strong and may contribute to the tolerogenicity of these cells.

In addition to presentation of foreign antigens, medullary EC appear to resemble BM-derived cells in terms of presentation of certain self antigens. This is apparent from studies on the expression of the Y-Ae epitope, a complex of I-Eα peptide bound to I-A^b molecules.[24,109] In the thymus of I-E+I-A^{b+} mice, the Y-Ae epitope is strongly expressed on the MHC+ subset of medullary epithelial cells; Y-Ae is also expressed on cortical EC but at a much lower level (Fig. 6).[24] These findings suggest that the range of self antigens (peptides) expressed on TEC and BM-derived cells might be quite similar. If so, the inability of TEC to induce full tolerance of T cells probably reflects a lack of certain cell surface accessory molecules.

The role the I-O+/MHC− subset of medullary EC in T-cell development is obscure. The function of I-O molecules is unknown and the peculiar tissue distribution of these molecules (medullary EC and B cells) has yet to be explained.[65] It is notable that I-O molecules are highly conserved throughout the mammalian species, and that the genes for both I-O α and β chains are localized adjacent to the genes for the peptide transporters and the proteosome subunits.[110] These features imply that I-O molecules might play an important role in T-cell function.

The fact that medullary EC have unique properties and exist in the thymus as a conspicuous population suggests that medullary EC must have a vital role in some aspect of

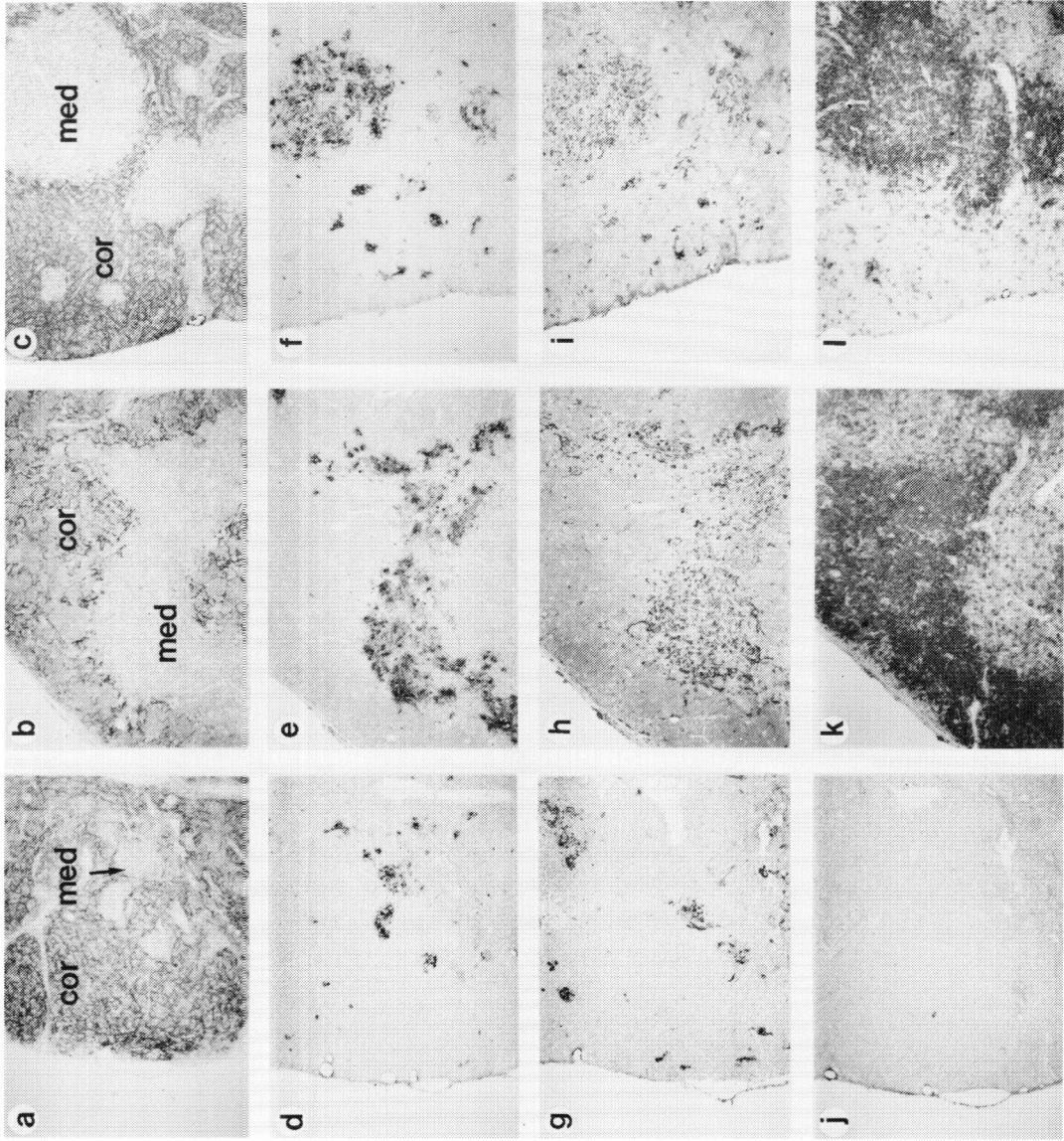

thymocyte maturation. Interestingly, however, the reverse might be true. In this respect, recent evidence suggests that the development of a full network of EC in the medulla requires the presence of mature SP T cells. Thus, in situations where SP populations of thymocytes are sparse, e.g., in SCID mice and normal mice treated with cyclosporin (CsA) or total lymphoid irradiation, the medulla is dramatically reduced in size and medullary EC are almost absent (Figs. 7, 8).[111-114] This atrophy of the medulla and medullary EC is reversible. Thus,

restoring thymopoiesis to the SCID thymus by reconstitution with normal BM cells leads to full regeneration of the medulla (Fig. 8).[111,112] Evidence that the development of the medulla requires the presence of mature T cells comes from the finding that the medulla of the SCID thymus can be selectively regenerated by giving repeated intravenous injections of large numbers of mature T cells (Fig. 8);[112] these cells reach the SCID thymus because, unlike the thymus of normal mice, the SCID thymus is permeable to circulating T cells. Further

Fig. 8. T cell control of the growth/expansion of medullary EC in SCID mice. Serial sections were stained; sections were lightly counterstained with hematoxylin. (a) 6C3 expression in normal SCID thymus. There is strong reticular staining of EC in the collapsed cortex. Unstained (medullary) areas are sparse. (b) 6C3 expression in the thymus of SCID mouse reconstituted with normal BALB/c BM. Staining pattern resembles the normal thymus with reticular staining of cortical epithelium and large unstained areas of medulla. (c) 6C3 expression in thymus of SCID mouse given multiple injections of BALB/c lymph node (LN) T cells from birth (total of 2.2 X 10^8 T cells over 4-5 weeks).[112] Cortex is condensed and shows strong staining. Unstained areas of medulla are prominent. (d) UEA-1 expression in normal SCID thymus. Only sparse aggregates of stained cells are evident. Stained areas correspond to the area of 6C3 medulla (compare with a). (e) UEA-1 expression in thymus of BM → SCID mouse. Staining of the medulla is much more extensive than in the normal SCID thymus (compare with d). (f) UEA-1 staining of LN T cells → SCID mice. As in BM → SCID mice, staining of the medulla is much more extensive than in the normal SCID thymus. (g) I-O expression in normal SCID thymus. Only sparse aggregates of stained cells are evident. (h) I-O expression in thymus of BM → SCID mouse. There is extensive staining of the medulla. (i) I-O expression in thymus of LN T → SCID mouse. There is extensive staining of the medulla. (j) CD8 expression in normal SCID thymus. No staining is evident. (k) CD8 expression in thymus of BM → SCID mouse. There is strong staining of the medula (presumably of CD4+8+ cells), and only scattered staining of the cortex (presumably of CD4-8+ cells). (l) CD8 expression in thymus of LN → SCID mouse. In marked contrast to BM → SCID mice, there is only scattered staining of the cortex (presumably indicating a paucity of CD4+8+ cells) and strong staining of the medulla (immigrant CD4-8+ cells). All sections were photographed at x100.

evidence that mature T cells guide the differentiation of medullary EC is provided by the finding that the lack of mature T cells in p56^lck knockout mice is associated with marked atrophy of the medulla.[115] Moreover, in a certain TcR transgenic line, which for some unknown reasons possesses unusually high numbers of mature T cells in the thymus, the medulla is greatly enlarged with an expanded network of EC.[116] The critical questions of how and why mature T cells regulate medullary EC growth is unknown, although it is possible that placing the size of the medulla under T-cell control optimizes negative selection in the medulla.[112]

FUTURE DIRECTIONS

Despite the significant strides made in understanding positive and negative selection in the thymus, the molecular mechanisms controlling these selection processes are yet to be elucidated. In particular, very little is known about the various soluble factors and cell surface molecules which are presumed to control the interaction of T cells with TEC. To a large extent, the paucity of information on this topic is a reflection of the lack of suitable in vitro system for studying thymic selection with isolated populations of EC. Thus although investigators have established numerous lines of thymic EC, most of these cell lines have proved to be incapable of supporting thymocyte differentiation in vitro. This might reflect that a functional thymic microenvironment requires contributions from several types of EC in a three-dimensional structure. Alternatively, the cell lines tested may have lost their functional capacity during in vitro culture, although it is of interest that some TEC lines are able to induce positive selection when injected intrathymically.[117,118] Recently, an ingenious method for inducing positive selection in vitro has been established by Jenkinson et al.[119] These workers cultured a population of TcR- DP thymocytes with freshly-prepared heterogeneous populations of TEC on millipore filters and showed that mature SP cells developed within 4 days.[119] This method presumably allows immature T cells to interact with TEC in a three-dimensional network. Using this system, the same group has since found evidence that contact with purified TEC alone is not sufficient to induce differentiation of TcR- DN precursor thymocytes into DP cells; this early step of thymocyte development seems to require cell contact with both TEC and mesenchyme-derived cells such as fibroblasts.[120] The system developed by Jenkinson et al clearly has great potential for revealing the various steps involved in thymocyte differentiation.

SUMMARY

As the primary organ for generation of T cells, the thymus is equipped with a dense network of EC and BM-derived APC. These parenchymal cells provide the appropriate microenvironments required to induce differentiation of prothymocytes and selection of self MHC-restricted thymocytes. The EC in the thymus are extremely complex and heterogeneous in terms of their surface markers, morphology, and keratin composition. Cortical EC control positive selection of T cells and express MHC class I and II molecules; this population of EC is fairly homogeneous in morphology and has characteristics of simple epithelium. The EC in the medulla are much more diverse and can be divided into at least two populations according to their mutually exclusive expression of conventional MHC class I and II molecules verses I-O molecules. The MHC$^+$ subset of EC contributes to negative selection (tolerance induction) in the thymus, but the function of I-O$^+$ EC is unknown. Interestingly, the growth and full differentiation of both subsets of medullary EC is dependent on the presence of mature T cells. Like EC, the BM-derived APC in the thymus are heterogeneous and comprise a mixture of DC, MØ and B cells; how these cells enter the thymus is not well understood. The primary function of the BM-derived APC in the thymus is to induce negative selection of T cells to self antigens. In addition, some of these cells, especially MØ, may play an important role in clearing the large numbers of T cells that die in the thymus. Obtaining definitive information on the roles of TEC and BM-derived APC will hinge on developing methods for studying thymocyte differentiation initiated and controlled by defined populations of stromal cells.

REFERENCES

1. Miller JFAP, Osoba D. Current concepts of the immunological function of the thymus. Physiol Rev 1967; 47:437-520.
2. Shortman K, Egerton M, Sprangrude GJ et al. The generation and fate of thymocytes. Sem Immunol 1990; 2:3-12.
3. Lo D, Sprent, J. Identity of cells that imprint H-2-restricted T-cell specificity in the thymus. Nature 1985; 319:672-675.
4. Adkins B, Mueller C, Okada CY et al. Early events in T-cell maturation. Ann Rev Immunol 1987; 5:325-365.
5. Sprent J, Lo D, Gao EK et al. T-cell selection in the thymus. Immunol Rev 1988; 101:173-190.
6. Fowlkes BJ, Pardoll DM. Molecular and cellular events of T-cell development. Adv Immunol 1989; 44:207-264.
7. Benoist C, Mathis D. Positive selection of the T-cell repertoire: where and when does it occur? Cell 1989; 58:1027-1033.
8. von Boehmer H. Developmental biology of T cells in T-cell receptor transgenic mice. Annu Rev Immunol 1990; 8:531-556.
9. Ceredig R, Lowenthal JW, Nabholz M et al. Expression of interleukin-2 receptors as a differentiation marker on intrathymic stem cells. Nature 1985; 314:98-100.
10. Raulet DH. Expression and function of interleukin-2 receptors on immature thymocytes. Nature 1985; 314:101-103.
11. Hirokawa K, Utsuyama M, Sado T. Immunohistological analysis of immigration of thymocyte-precursors into the thymus: evidence for immigration of peripheral T cells into the thymic medulla. Cell Immunol 1989; 119:160-170.
12. Shimonkevitz RP, Husmann LA, Bevan MJ et al. Transient expression of IL-2 receptor precedes the differentiation of immature thymocytes. Nature 1987; 329:157-159.
13. van Ewijk W. Cell surface topography of thymic microenvironments. Lab Invest 1988; 59:579-590.
14. Egerton M, Scollay R, Shortman K. Kinetics of mature T-cell development in the thymus. Proc Natl Acad Sci 1990; 87:2579-2582.
15. Kraal G, Breel M, Janse M et al. Langerhans' cells, veiled cells, and interdigitating cells in the mouse recognized by a monoclonal antibody. J Exp Med 1986; 163:981-997.
16. Breel M, Mebius RE, Kraal, G. Dendritic cells of the mouse recognized by two monoclonal antibodies. Eur J Immunol 1987; 17:1555-1559.
17. Miyama-Inaba M, Kuma SI, Inaba K et al. Unusual phenotype of B cells in the thymus of normal mice. J Exp Med 1988; 168:

811-816.

18. Lo D, Ron Y, Sprent J. Induction of MHC-restricted specificity and tolerance in the thymus. Immunol Res 1986; 5:221-232.

19. Kappler JW, Roehm N, Marrack P. T-cell tolerance by clonal elimination in the thymus. Cell 1987; 49:273-280.

20. MacDonald HR, Howe RC, Pedrazzini T et al. T-cell lineages, repertoire selection and tolerance induction. Immunol Rev 1988; 104:157-182.

21. Matzinger P, Guerder S. Does T-cell tolerance require a dedicated antigen-presenting cell? Nature 1989; 338:74-76.

22. Jenkinson EJ, Owen JJT. T-cell differentiation in thymus organ cultures. Sem Immunol 1990; 2:51-58.

23. Farr AG, Anderson SK. Epithelial heterogeneity in the murine thymus: fucose-specific lectins bind medullary epithelial cells. J Immunol 1985; 134: 2971-2977.

24. Surh CD, Gao EK, Kosaka H et al. Two subsets of epithelial cells in the thymic medulla. J Exp Med 1992; 176:495-505.

25. Wallace VA, Fung-Leung WP, Timms E et al. CD45RA and CD45RB^high expression induced by thymic selection events. J Exp Med 1992; 176:1657-1663.

26. Auerbach R. Morphogenetic interactions in the development of the mouse thymus gland. Dev Biol 1960; 2:271-284.

27. Cordier AC, Haumont SM. Development of thymus, parathyroids, and ultimo-branchial bodies in NMRI and nude mice. Am J Anat 1980; 157:227-263.

28. Le Douarin N, Jotereau FV. Tracing of cells of the avian thymus through embryonic life in interspecific chimeras. J Exp Med 1975; 142:17-40.

29. Cordier AC, Heremans JF. Nude mouse embryo: ectodermal nature of the primordial thymic defect. Scand J Immunol 1975; 4:193-196.

30. Owen JJT, Ritter MA. Tissue interaction in the development of thymus lymphocytes. J Exp Med 1969; 129:431-437.

31. Born W, Rathbun G, Tucker P et al. Synchronized rearrangement of T-cell γ and β chain genes in fetal thymocyte development. Science 1986; 234:479-482.

32. Bluestone JA, Pardoll D, Sharrow SO et al. Characterization of thymocytes with CD3 associated T-cell receptor structures. Nature 1987; 326:82-84.

33. Havran WL, Allison JP. Developmentally ordered appearance of thymocytes expressing different T-cell antigen receptors. Nature 1988; 335:443-445.

34. Mombaerts P, Clarke AR, Rudnicki MA et al. Mutations in T-cell antigen receptor genes α and β block thymocyte development at different stages. Nature 1992; 360:225-231.

35. Roehm N, Herron L, Cambier J et al. The major histocompatibility complex-restricted antigen receptor on T cells: distribution of thymus and peripheral T cells. Cell 1984; 38:577-584.

36. Duijvestijn AM, Sminia T, Kohler YG et al. Ontogeny of the rat thymus microenvironment: development of the interdigitating cell and macrophage populations. Dev Comp Immunol 1984; 8:451-460.

37. Kraal G, Avis L, Wijffels J et al. Different epitopes on the dendritic cell-associated NLDC-145 molecule during ontogeny. Immunobiol 1990; 181:388-397.

38. Sminia T, van Asselt AA, Van de Ende MB et al. Rat thymus macrophages: an immunohistochemical study on fetal, neonatal and adult thymus. Thymus 1986; 8:141-150.

39. Nango KI, Inaba M, Inaba K et al. Ontogeny of thymic B cells in normal mice. Cell Immunol 1991; 133:109-115.

40. Jenkinson EJ, van Ewijk W, Owen JJT. Major histocompatibility complex antigen expression on the epithelium of the developing thymus in normal and nude mice. J Exp Med 1981; 153:280-292.

41. van Vliet E, Jenkinson EJ, Kingston R et al. Stromal cell types in the developing thymus of the normal and nude mouse embryo. Eur J Immunol 1985; 15:675-681.

42. Lu C, Beller DI, Unanue ER. During ontogeny, Ia-bearing accessory cells are found early in the thymus but late in the spleen. Proc Natl Acad Sci 1980; 77:1597-1601.

43. van Vliet E, Mels M, van Ewijk W. Monoclonal antibodies to stromal cell types of the mouse thymus. Eur J Immunol 1984; 14:524-529.

44. Raviola E, Karnovsky MJ. Evidence for a blood-thymus barrier using electron-opaque

tracers. J Exp Med 1972; 136:466-498.

45. Clark SL Jr. The thymus in mice of strain 129/J studied with the electron microscope. Am J Anat 1963; 112:1-33.

46. Weiss L. Electron microscopic observations on the vascular barrier in the cortex of the thymus of the mouse. Anat Rec 1963; 145:413-438.

47. Saint-Marie G, Leblond CP. Cytological features and cellular migration in the cortex and medulla of thymus in the young adult rat. Blood 1964; 23:275-299.

48. Yamashita A, Miyasaka M, Trnka Z. Early post-thymic T cells: studies on lymphocytes in the lymph coming from the thymus of sheep. In: B. Morris and M. Miyasaka, eds. Immunology of the sheep. Editiones <Roche>, Basle, Switzerland, 1985: 162-180.

49. Nieuwenhuis P, Stet RJM, Wagenaar JPA et al. The transcapsular route: a new way for (self-) antigens to by-pass the blood-thymus barrier? Immunol Today 1988; 12:372-375.

50. Eggli P, Schaffner T, Gerber H et al. Accessibility of thymic cortical lymphocytes to particles translocated from the peritoneal cavity to parathymic lymph nodes. Thymus 1986; 8:129-139.

51. Mandel T. Differentiation of epithelial cells in the mouse thymus. Z Zellforsch 1970; 106:498-515.

52. Farr AG, Nakane PK. Cells bearing Ia antigens in the murine thymus: an ultra-structural study. Am J Path 1983; 111: 88-96.

53. van de Wijngaert FP, Kendall MD, Schuurman HJ et al. Heterogeneity of epithelial cells in the human thymus: an ultrastructural study. Cell Tissue Res 1984; 237:227-237.

54. Laster AJ, Itoh T, Palker TJ et al. The human thymic microenvironment: thymic epithelium contains specific keratins associated with early and late stages of epidermal keratinocyte maturation. Differentiation 1986; 31:67-77.

55. Nicolas JF, Reano A, Kaiserlian D et al. Epithelial cell heterogeneity in the guinea pig thymus: immunohistochemical characterization of four thymic epithelial subsets defined by monoclonal anti-keratin anti-

bodies. Eur J Immunol 1986; 16:457-464.

56. Savino W, Darenne M. Developmental studies on expression of monoclonal antibody-defined cytokeratins by thymic epithelial cells from normal and autoimmune mice. J Histochem Cytochem 1988; 36:1123-1129.

57. Moll R, Franke WW, Schiller DL et al. The catalog of human cytokeratins: patterns of expression in normal epithelia, tumors, and cultured cells. Cell 1982; 31:11-24.

58. Farr AG, Braddy S. Patterns of keratin expression in the murine thymus. Anat Rec 1989; 224:374-378.

59. Haynes BF. The human thymic micro-environment. Adv Immunol 1984; 36:87-142.

60. Rouse RV, van Ewijk W, Jones PP et al. Expression of MHC antigens by mouse thymic dendritic cells. J Immunol 1979; 122:2508-2515.

61. Brekelmans P, van Ewijk W. Phenotypic characterization of murine thymic micro-environments. Sem Immunol 1990; 2:13-24.

62. Kampinga J, Berges S, Boyd RL et al. Thymic epithelial antibodies:immunohisto-chemical analysis and introduction of nomenclature. Thymus 1989; 13:165-173.

63. Adkins B, Tidmarsh GF, Weissman. Normal thymic cortical epithelial cells developmentally regulate the expression of a B-lineage transformation-associated antigen. Immunogen 1988; 27:180-186.

64. van Ewijk W, Rouse RV, Weissman I. Distribution of H-2 microenvironments in the mouse thymus. J Histo Cyto 1980; 28:1089-1099.

65. Karlsson L, Surh CD, Sprent J et al. A novel class II MHC molecules with un-usual tissue distribution. Nature 1991; 351: 485-488.

66. Rouse RV, Bolin LM, Bender JR et al. Monoclonal antibodies reactive with subsets of mouse and human thymic epithelial cells. J Histo Cyto, 1988; 36:1511-1517.

67. Dijkstra CD, Dopp EA, Joling P et al. The heterogeneity of mononuclear phagocytes in lymphoid organs: distinct macrophage subpopulations in the rat recognized by monoclonal antibodies ED1, ED2 and ED3. Immunology 1985; 54:589-599.

68. Colic M, Popovic LJ, Gasic S et al.

Immunohistochemical characterization of rat thymic non-lymphoid cells: II. Macrophages and granulocytes defined by monoclonal antibodies. Immunology 1990; 69:416-422.

69. Hume DA, Robinson AP, Macpherson GG et al. The mononuclear phagocyte system of the mouse defined by immunohistochemical localization of antigen F4/80: relationship between macrophages, Langerhans cells, reticular cell, and dendritic cells in lymphoid and hematopoietic organs. J Exp Med 1983; 158:1522-1536.

70. Duijvestijn AM, Hoefsmit, ECM. Ultrastructure of the rat thymus: the microenvironment of T-lymphoctye maturation. Cell Tissue Res 1981; 218:279-292.

71. Inaba K, Inaba M, Knashi T et al. Macrophages phagocytose thymic lymphocytes with productively rearranged T-cell receptor α and β genes. J Exp Med 1988; 168:2279-2294.

72. Milicevic NM, Milicevic Z, Colic M et al. Ultrastructural study of macrophages in the rat thymus, with special reference to the cortico-medullary zone. J Anat 1987; 150:89-98.

73. Beller DI, Unanue, ER. Thymic macrophages modulate one stage of T-cell differentiation in vitro. J Immunol 1978; 121:1861-1864.

74. Birbeck MS, Breathnach AS, Everall JD. An electron microscopic study of basal melanocytes and high-level clear cells (Langerhans cells) in vitiligo. J Invest Derm 1961; 37:51-64.

75. Barclay AN, Mayrhofer G. Bone marrow origin of Ia-positive cells in the medulla of rat thymus. J Exp Med 1981; 153:1666-1671.

76. Crowley M, Inaba K, Witmer-Pack M et al. The cell surface of mouse dendritic cells: FACS analysis fo dendritic cells from different tissues including thymus. Cell Immunol 1989; 118:108-125.

77. Pollard AM, Lipscomb MF. Characterization of murine lung dendritic cells: similarities to Langerhans cells and thymic dendritic cells. J Exp Med 1990; 172:159-167.

78. Ardavin C, Shortman K. Cell surface marker analysis of mouse thymic dendritic cells. Eur J Immunol 1992;

22:859-862.

79. Vremec D, Zorbas M, Scollay R et al. The surface phenotype of dendritic cells purified from mouse thymus and spleen: investigation of the CD8 expression by a subpopulation of dendritic cells. J Exp Med 1992; 176:47-58.

80. Wu L, Scollay R, Egerton M et al. CD4 expressed on earliest T-lineage precursor cells in the adult murine thymus. Nature 1991; 349:71-74.

81. Ardavin C, Wu L, Li CL et al. Thymic dendritic cells and T cells develop simultaneously in the thymus from a common precursor population. Nature 1993; 362: 761-763.

82. Kampinga J, Nieuwenhuis P, Roser B et al. Differences in turnover between thymic medullary dendritic cells and a subset of cortical macrophages. J Immunol 1990; 145:1659-1663.

83. Watanabe K, Tanaka R, Nishimura T et al. I-E-restricted monoclonal expansion of B lymphocytes in the thymus of NOD mouse. Int Immunol 1991; 3:839-842.

84. Kearney JF. CD5+ B-cell networks. Curr Opin Immunol 1993; 5:223-226.

85. Inaba M, Inaba K, Hosono M et al. Distinct mechanisms of neonatal tolerance induced by dendritic cells and thymic B cells. J Exp Med 1991; 173:549-559.

86. Webb S, Sprent J. Factors controlling the reactivity of immature and mature T cells to Mls^a antigens in vivo. Immunol Rev 1993; 131:169-188.

87. Hong R, Schulte-Wissermann H, Jarrett-Toth E et al. Transplantation of cultured thymic fragments. II. Results in nude mice. J Exp Med 1979; 149:398-415.

88. Chan SH, Cosgrove D, Waltzinger C et al. Another veiw of the selective model of thymocytes selection. Cell 1993; 73:225-236.

89. Zinkernagel RM, Callahan GN, Klein J et al. Cytotoxic T cells learn specificity for self H-2 during differentiation in the thymus. Nature 1979; 271:251-253.

90. Fink PJ, Bevan MJ. H-2 antigens of the thymus determine lymphocyte specificity. J Exp Med 1978; 148:766-775.

91. Zijlstra M, Bix M, Simister NE et al. β2-microglobulin deficient mice lack CD4-8+ cytotoxic T cells. Nature 1990; 344:742-746.

92. Koller BH, Marrack P, Kappler JW et al. Normal development of mice deficient in β2M, MHC class I proteins and CD8+ T cells. Science 1990; 248:1227-1230.

93. Cosgrove D, Gray D, Dierich A et al. Mice lacking MHC class II molecules. Cell 1991; 66:1051-1066.

94. Grusby MJ, Johnson RS, Papaioannou VE et al. Depletion of CD4+ T cells in major histocompatibility complex class II-deficient mice. Science 1991; 20:1417-1420.

95. Ron Y, Lo D, Sprent J. T-cell specificity in twice-irradiated F$_1$→parent bone marrow chimeras: failure to detect a role for immigrant marrow-derived cells in imprinting intrathymic H-2 restriction. J Immunol 1986; 137:1764-1771.

96. Cosgrove D, Chan SH, Waltzinger C et al. The thymic compartment responsible for positive selection of CD4+ T cells. Int Immunol 1992; 4:707-710.

97. Markowitz JS, Auchincloss HJ, Grusby MJ et al. Class II-positive hematopoietic cells cannot mediate positive selection of CD4+ T lymphocytes in class II-deficient mice. Proc Natl Acad Sci 1993; 90:2779-2783.

98. Bix M, Raulet D. Inefficient positive selection of T cells directed by haematopoietic cells. Nature 1992; 359:330-333.

99. Salaun J, Bandeira A, Khazaal I et al. Thymic epithelium tolerizes for histocompatability antigens. Science 1990; 247:1471-1474.

100. Hoffman MW, Allison J, Miller JFAP. Tolerance induction by thymic medullary epithelium. Proc Natl Acad Sci 1992; 89:2526-2530.

101. Schonrich G, Momburg F, Hammerling GJ et al. Anergy induced by thymic medullary epithelium. Eur J Immunol 1992; 22:1687-1691.

102. Burkly LC, Degermann S, Longley J et al. Clonal deletion of Vβ5+ T cells by transgenic I-E restricted to thymic medullary epithelium. J Immunol 1993; 151:3954-3960.

103. Houssaint E, Flajnik, M. The role of thymic epithelium in the acquisition of tolerance. Immunol Today 1990; 11:357-360.

104. Sprent J, Kosaka H, Gao EK et al. Intrathymic and extrathymic tolerance in bone marrow chimeras. Immunol Rev 1993; 133:151-176.

105. Bonomo A, Matzinger P. Thymus epithelium induces tissue-specific tolerance. J Exp Med 1993; 177:1153-1164.

106. Lorenz RG, Allen PM. Thymic cortical epithelial cells lack full capacity for antigen presentation. Nature 1989; 340:557-559.

107. Ransom J, Wu R, Fischer M et al. Antigen presenting ability of thymic macrophages and epithelial cells: evidence for defects in the antigen processing function of thymic epithelial cells. Cell Immunol 1991; 134:180-190.

108. Mizuochi T, Kasai M, Kokuho T et al. Medullary but not cortical thymic epithelial cells present soluble antigens to helper T cells. J Exp Med 1992; 175:1601-1605.

109. Rudensky AY, Rath S, Preston-Hurlburt P et al. On the complexity of self. Nature 1991; 353:660-662.

110. Karlsson L, Peterson, PA. The α chain gene of H-2O has an unexpected location in the major histocompatibility complex. J Exp Med 1992; 176:477-483.

111. Shores EW, van Ewijk W, A S. Reorganization and restoration of thymic medullary epithelial cells in T-cell receptor-negative SCID mice: evidence that receptor-bearing lymphocytes influence maturation of the thymic microenvironment. Eur J Immunol 1991; 21:1657-1661.

112. Surh CD, Ernst B, Sprent J. Growth of epithelial cells in the thymic medulla is under the control of mature T cells. J Exp Med 1992; 176:611-616.

113. Schuurman HJ, van Loveren H, Rozing J et al. Cyclosporin and the rat thymus. An immunohistochemical study. Thymus 1990; 16:235-254.

114. Adkins B, Gandour D, Strober S et al. Total lymphoid irradiation leads to transient depletion of the mouse thymic medulla and persistent abnormalities among medullary stromal cells. J Immunol 1988; 140:3373-3379.

115. Molina TJ, Kishihara K, Siderovski DP et al. Profound block in thymocyte development in mice lacking p56^{lck}. Nature 1992; 357:161-164.

116. Ferrick DA, Chan A, Rahemtulla A et al. Expression of a T-cell receptor γ-chain (Vγ1.1Jγ4Cγ4) transgene in mice influences T-cell receptor ontogeny and thymic architecture during development. J Immunol 1990; 145:20-27.

117. Vukmanovic S, Grandea III AG, Faas SJ et al. Positive selection of T-lymphocytes induced by intrathymic injection of a thymic epithelial cell line. Nature 1992; 359:729-732.

118. Hugo P, Kappler JW, Godfrey DI et al. A cell line that can induce thymocyte positive selection. Nature 1992; 360:679-682.

119. Jenkinson EJ, Anderson G, Owen JJT. Studies on T-cell maturation on defined thymic stromal cell populations in vitro. J Exp Med 1992; 176:845-853.

120. Anderson G, Jenkinson EJ, Moore NC et al. MHC class II-positive epithelium and mesenchyme cells are both required for T-cell development in the thymus. Nature 1993; 362:70-73.

121. Symington FW, Sprent J. A monoclonal antibody detecting an Ia specificity mapping in the I-A or I-E subregion. Immunogenetics 1981; 14:53-61.

122. Oi VT, Jones PP, Goding JW et al. Properties of monoclonal antibodies to mouse Ig allotypes, H-2, and Ia antigens. Curr Topic Microbiol Immunol 1978; 81:115-129.

123. Ozato K, Mayer N, Sachs DH. Hybridoma cell lines secreting monoclonal antibodies to mouse H-2 and Ia antigens. J Immunol 1980; 124:533-540.

124. Murphy DB, Lo D, Rath S et al. A novel MHC class II epitope expressed in thymic medulla but not cortex. Nature 1989; 338:765-768.

125. Hammerling GH, Rusch E, Tada N et al. Localization of allodeterminants on H-2K^b antigens determined with monoclonal antibodies and H-2 mutant mice. Proc Natl Acad Sci 1982; 79:4737-4741.

126. Ozato K, Sachs DH. Monoclonal antibodies to mouse MHC antigens. III. Hybridoma antibodies reacting to antigens of the H-2^b haplotype reveal genetic control of isotype expression. J Immunol 1981; 126:317-321.

127. Ozato K, Hansen TH, Sachs, DH. Monoclonal antibodies to mouse MHC antigens. II. Antibodies to the H-2L^d antigen, the products of a third polymorpic locus of the mouse major histocompatibility complex. J Immunol 1980; 125:2473-2477.

128. Hirokawa K, Utsuyama M, Moriizumi E et al. Analysis of the thymic microenvironment by monoclonal antibodies with special reference to thymic nurse cells. Thymus 1986; 8:349-360.

129. Austyn JM, Gordon S. F4/80, a monoclonal antibody directed specifically against the mouse macrophages. Eur J Immunol 1981; 11:805-815.

130. Malek TR, Robb RJ, Shevach EM. Identification and initial characterization of a rat monoclonal antibody reactive with the murine interleukin 2 receptor-ligand complex. Proc Natl Acad Sci 1983; 80:5694-5698.

131. Trowbridge IS, Lesley J, Schulte R et al. Biochemical characterization and cellular distribution of a polymorphic, murine cell-surface glycoprotein expressed on lymphoid cells. Immunogenetics 1982; 15:299-312.

132. Pullen A, Marrack P, Kappler J. The T-cell repertoire is heavily influenced by tolerance to polymorphic self-antigens. Nature 1988; 335:796-801.

133. Gao EK, Lo D, Sprent J. Strong T-cell tolerance in parent → F$_1$ bone marrow chimeras prepared with supralethal irradiation: evidence for clonal deletion and anergy. J Exp Med 1990; 171:1101-1121.

134. Gao, EK, Lo, D, Cheney, R et al. Abnormal differentiation of thymocytes in mice treated with cyclosporin A. Nature 1988; 336:176-179.

Phenotypic and Functional Stages in the Intrathymic Development of TcR αβ Thymocytes

Janko Nikolić-Žugić

The thymus has been recognized as the key site of T-cell development for over three decades (reviewed in 1 and 2). During a good part of the first two decades of thymology, this retrosternal organ of mixed embryonic origin has been viewed as a black box that occasionally allows a glimpse into its interior through the use of innovative experiments. The main revolution in dissecting phenotypic and functional stages of thymocyte development began with the advent of multicolor flow cytometry and the availability of monoclonal antibodies against defined membrane molecules. At present, thymologists can conclude with great satisfaction that this revolution has resulted in a near-complete illumination of the phenotypic steps in the intrathymic development of the main T-cell lineage bearing αβ T-cell receptors. (Inasmuch as the mouse provides the best defined model for studying T-cell development, this text, unless specifically stated, will be devoted to murine T-cell development.)

The most popular and perhaps the most useful phenotypic division of thymocytes was made in the late seventies and is based on the surface expression of accessory CD8 and CD4 molecules.[3] Unlike peripheral T cells that generally express these molecules in a mutually exclusive fashion, thymocytes express all possible combinations of CD8 and CD4. At the time of their initial analysis of the expression of CD8 and CD4 on human thymocytes, Reinherz and Schlossman put forward a logical hypothesis: the most numerous, immature CD8+CD4+ (double-positive, DP) cells must be the precursors of the mature CD8+CD4- and CD8-CD4- single-positive (SP) thymocytes.[3] However, it has long been known that the production of T cells in the thymus exceeds by far the thymic output;[4] and studies by Shortman, Scollay and their colleagues[5,6] indicated that an overwhelming majority of DP thymocytes die in the thymus, raising the possibility that DP cells are a dead-end population. Initial experiments involving adoptive transfer of DP cells indeed failed to document a precursor role for these cells. Moreover, elegant experiments by Fowlkes and her coworkers[7] demonstrated that a numerically minor, and therefore largely neglected, population of CD8⁻CD4⁻ double-negative (DN) thymocytes contains precursors of all other thymocyte subsets. Soon thereafter it became clear that considerable heterogeneity exists within each of the four populations defined by CD8/4 expression. (This important point is unfortunately still overlooked in the primary literature by authors who use only CD8 and CD4 to subdivide thymocytes.) Since then, studies using in vivo transfers of thymocyte subsets, in vivo metabolic labeling of thymocytes followed by kinetic studies of progeny of labeled thymocytes and in vitro cultivation of isolated fetal thymic lobes have been successfully employed to solve most questions regarding the major developmental pathway of T-cell receptor (TcR) αβ thymocytes (reviewed in 8 and 9). At this point, we shall take a chronological journey through the thymus and look at the phenotypic changes that follow the major TcR αβ pathway of development, starting with the first cells that colonize the thymus.

EARLY PRECURSORS

The murine thymic rudiment becomes colonized around day 11 (the seventh week in the human) of intrauterine development, and T-cell precursors continue to migrate into the thymus throughout the life of a mammal.[10] The first cells to colonize the thymus originate from the yolk sac.[11,12] The source of thymic immigrants changes to fetal liver and, probably even before birth, shifts for the rest of life to the bone marrow.[10,11] These immigrants originate from totipotential stem cells, and, in the adult, share a number of markers with their precursors.[13,14] It is unclear how restricted is the developmental potential of the first wave of cells that colonizes the thymus. The most discriminating experiments in that regard were recently published by Shortman's group.[15-17] These authors have identified the phenotype of the earliest adult thymic immigrant as Sca-1⁺Sca-2⁺CD44⁺Thy-1ˡᵒ HSAˡᵒCD8⁻4ⁱⁿᵗTcR⁻ (Fig. 1). Such a precursor is quite restricted in its developmental potential[15] and can at best be described as a lymphoid precursor. Indeed,

this cell mainly generates thymocytes and, under specific conditions, can generate B but no other lineages.[16] It was recently reported that this population also contains precursors of thymic dendritic cells,[17] but the conclusion that dendritic cells and T cells have a common intrathymic precursor was not unequivocally supported by the design of the experiments. Namely, the number of cells injected intrathymically in these experiments was too abundant (10⁴) to discriminate between the coexistence of T and dendritic precursors within the same population and a genuine common precursor. Proof for either alternative has to be sought at a clonal level.

There is now sound evidence that CD4ˡᵒ T-cell precursors spend some time in the thymus without ostensibly changing their phenotype or proliferating. After this initial lag phase, the first phenotypic changes on such cells were thought to involve a downregulation of CD4 and an upregulation of Thy-1 and HSA expression. However, recent experiments from Zlotnik's laboratory have recharted some of the earliest developmental steps.[18] Using the expression of *c-kit* to dissect the early developmental stages, these authors have demonstrated that the expression of CD4 persists in cells that have already upregulated Thy-1 and HSA. Such cells are *c-kit* positive, and, as described in Chapter 4, antibodies against this kinase can abrogate the development of the earliest precursors in fetal thymic organ culture (FTOC).[19] (The mechanism of antibody action in this case is not clear, because mice harboring a dominant-negative mutation of *c-kit* appear to have normal T-cell numbers and function [P. Besmer, personal communication].) The germline status of the T-cell receptor genes in these cells fits well with the idea that they do not differ from the earliest precursors.[18,19]

EXPRESSION OF CD25 AND THE ONSET OF TcR β REARRANGEMENT

The next change in T-cell development is marked by the downregulation of CD4, followed by the onset of CD25[20-22] expression (Fig. 1), the cells still being positive for *c-kit*. These cells are best described as CD8⁻

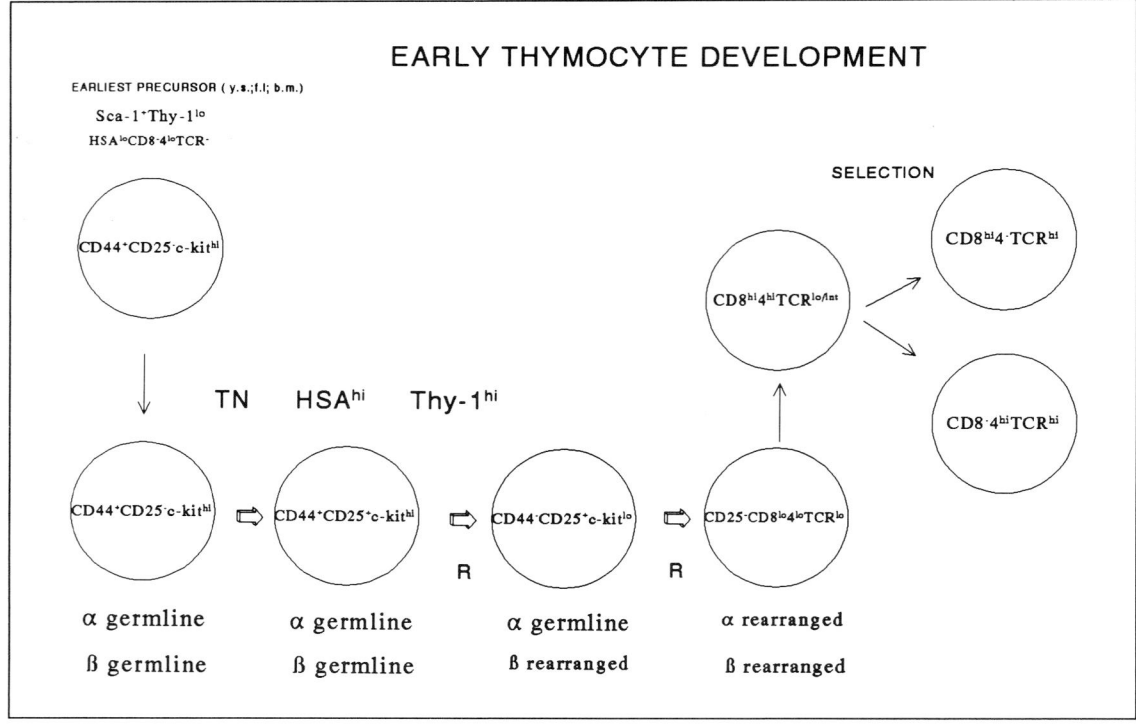

Fig. 1. Early thymocyte development. Additional markers were omitted in the figure for the sake of clarity. See text for further detail.

CD4⁻TcR⁻ triple-negative (TN). Transient expression of CD25 (IL-2 receptor α subunit; p55) that occurs on these cells marks an important point in early thymocyte development.[23,24] The functional relevance of this receptor on TN thymocytes has been controversial since its discovery. Namely, whereas some experiments suggested an important function of CD25 and its interaction with IL-2 in T-cell development,[25-28] other studies failed to detect any functional relevance of CD25.[29-31] Perhaps most intriguingly, mice with disrupted IL-2 genes do not show any aberrations in intrathymic T-cell development.[32] It is certainly possible that another factor substitutes for IL-2 and interacts with CD25 in this case, or that perhaps another unknown molecule pairs with the β, γ or βγ chains of the IL-2R to yield a novel structure that transmits important signals to developing thymocytes. Such modular organization exists in other molecular systems, e.g., signal-transducing

ζ/ε and FcR subunits, transcription factors, etc. But it is equally possible that this particular receptor happens to be a byproduct of the activation of early precursors, and that its expression is not necessary for further development. Little is known of thymocyte expression of the other two chains (β and γ) that together with CD25 form a high affinity IL-2 receptor. However, thymocyte development is severely compromised in the X-linked severe combined immunodeficiency in man and the molecular basis of this disease is a nonsense mutation in IL-2R γ chain.[33] As discussed by Taniguchi and Minami,[34] it is difficult to reconcile these results with apparently normal thymocyte development in IL-2 "knockout" mice, unless one postulates that other ligands may interact with the IL-2R chains. Regardless of this ongoing controversy, CD25 has been a very useful marker for subdividing early thymocytes and it is from this standpoint that I shall use it in this chapter.

CD25 is expressed at high levels on two TN subsets: CD44$^+$CD25$^+$ (Fig. 1) and CD44$^{-/lo}$CD25$^+$. The work of Godfrey et al[18,19] demonstrates the germline status of the TcR β locus in CD44$^+$CD25$^+$c-kit$^+$ TN cells. By contrast, rearrangement is essentially complete in all cells that are CD44^{lo}CD25^{hi} *c-kit*^{lo}.[18] During this time, the α locus remains in the configuration[35,36] and will not rearrange until the next step in differentiation. Therefore, downregulation of c-kit and CD44 coincides with a complete rearrangement of the TcR β chain genes. It is still unknown what triggers the recombination at the β locus.

A functional β rearrangement is both necessary and sufficient for the abrogation of further recombination at the β locus. Studies of Krimpenfort et al[37] have elegantly demonstrated a requirement for the protein product of the rearranged β gene in this process. These authors have introduced a rearranged TcR β transgene carrying a major deletion of almost the entire V$_β$, the entire D$_β$ and the 5' portion of the J$_β$ region. Such a transgene completely abrogated (allelically excluded) the rearrangement of endogenous β genes. However, a frameshift mutation in this construct that results in a sterile transcript abrogated the ability of the construct to mediate allelic exclusion.[37,38] It is at present unclear whether TcR β protein has to be expressed at the membrane for allelic exclusion to occur.

Recent work has shown that in certain nonphysiological situations,[39-42] as well as in fetal day 16 thymocytes,[43] β chain can reach the surface of thymocytes and be expressed in the form of ββ homodimers, associated in a nonconventional way with the components of the CD3 complex. There is a lot of speculation about the potential significance of this complex for the transition of early thymocytes into intermediate thymocytes. The best experimental evidence that β chain rearrangement and/or transcription is important for this transition comes from mice carrying a targeted disruption of TcR β genes.[41] In these animals thymocyte development is arrested at the CD25$^+$ stage, and these cells are unable to progress to the DP stage.

Interestingly, the same phenomenology is observed in mice unable to rearrange their TcR genes due to natural (SCID) or introduced (RAG-1 and RAG-2)[44] mutations that affect recombinatorial machinery. In either case, the introduction of a rearranged β chain transgene corrected the defect, and allowed progression to the DP stage.[42,45]

A similar arrest occurs in mice deficient for the protein-tyrosine kinase Lck.[46,47] Indeed, an experimentally induced disruption of the *lck* gene[46] and the introduction of a dominant-negative mutant[47] of *lck* have the same consequence: arrest in thymocyte maturation at the CD25$^+$ TN stage (that normally rearranges TcR β, but not α, locus). By contrast, even modest overexpression of a constitutively active form of *lck* (F505*lck*)[48] results in arrest of V$_β$ recombination at the D-J stage (no V-D joining)[49] resulting in phenotypic arrest at a pre-DP (TcR^{lo}HSA^{hi}SP) or DP stage. TcR α joining is not affected. This effect does not depend on the association of Lck with CD4 and CD8, because these molecules are not yet expressed and because a mutation in F505Lck that abrogates the association with CD4 and CD8 still interrupts the rearrangement.[50] Although we shall discuss these results in greater detail in the last chapter, they strongly suggest that normal Lck function is required for early development and rearrangement, but that this enzyme probably does not signal the initiation of β rearrangement.

It is unclear whether the rearrangement, transcription, translation or surface expression of β chain carries critical information allowing the cell to turn on the expression of accessory molecules and undergo other phenotypic changes. (Curiously, rearrangement of TcR δ, but not α or γ locus, also seems to be able to mediate similar effects.[41]) Several authors have hypothesized that T-cell development may be analogous to B cell development, where the immunoglobulin heavy chain gets expressed at the surface in the complex with a surrogate light chain.[41-45] Interactions between such a receptor and an unknown ligand then propel a cell to the next stage of development. There is at present no evidence for the existence of ββ homodimers* on normal adult thymocytes; however, the existence of ββ dimers has been demonstrated by the densitometric analysis of TcRβ and TcRα precipitates[43] from day 16 fetal thymocytes, although it remains to be established how many cells in such a setting express αβ versus ββ receptors, and do these receptors coexist on the same cell.

It is my bias that the recognition of extracellular ligands by the surface β chain is not critical for further development of early thymocytes. This is based on Krimpenfort's experiments,[37,38] where a heavily truncated TcR β still led the thymocytes to the DP stage, and one needs a vivid imagination to envision how such a receptor could bind any physiologically relevant ligand. Another argument against an obligatory role for the recognition by β chain comes from studies using TcR transgenic mice.[51] In that system, we found no evidence for the existence of ββ homodimers on transgenic equivalents of CD25⁺TN and CD25⁻TL cells, based on staining with transgene-specific anti-TcRα and anti-TcRβ antibodies. Whenever the cells were positive for TcR β, they also expressed the α protein. In the absence of adequate TcR α-specific antibodies that could be used for surface staining and signaling experiments in normal thymocytes, the issue of the relevance of ββ versus αβ receptors will remain unresolved.

Other markers used to dissect the stages of TN development include CD2 and the FcγR II/III.[52] Although this subdivision has its merits in fetal thymocytes, in the adult it is far less precise than the one based on CD44, CD25 and *c-kit*.

---

* Most recent experiments from von Boehmer's laboratory (H. von Boehmer, personal communication) have revealed the β chain is in fact coupled to a novel protein, p33, and not to another β chain. Therefore, ββ homodimers mentioned throughout the text are really β/p33 dimers, and p33 could be responsible for signaling.

EARLY INTERMEDIATE CD8^{lo}CD4^{lo}TCR^{lo} THYMOCYTES: TCR α REARRANGEMENT

The most profound changes in the biology of thymocytes occur with the downregulation of CD25 (Fig. 1). These changes transform a prothymocyte into a typical cortical thymocyte over the course of 10-12 hours. CD8 and CD4 molecules are expressed at the cell surface in very low levels[53,54] and the cells still score DN by direct flow cytometry. However, a discrete shift in mean fluorescence reveals low expression of accessory molecules,[54,55] and CD8 and CD4 mRNA can be detected in their cytoplasm.[55] Low levels of CD8 and CD4 can be used to separate these cells from real DN cells by panning.[53,54] CD8^{lo}CD4^{lo} cells are the first subset to rearrange the TcR α locus.[56,35] The rearrangement is a complete one (V-J), and the cells begin to express the full length message for α chain (V-J-C) and low levels of the TcR at the surface, based on the staining with anti-TcR β mAb.[56,57] It is difficult to discriminate whether all CD8^{lo}CD4^{lo} cells express this molecule owing to the low intensity of TcR β staining, but based on fluorescence shifts we estimate that at least 70% of these cells do.[56] I therefore refer to these cells as CD8^{lo}CD4^{lo}TcR^{lo}—triple-low (TL).

As discussed above, it is possible that some of these cells, as well as some of their DP progeny, express ββ homodimers. But it appears unclear why a cell that had already rearranged its TcR α genes would need to express a ββ homodimer as opposed to the ab heterodimer, especially since only the latter can be used for intrathymic selection. The expression of ββ homodimers would make sense if the TcR α rearrangement was unsuccessful and/or if ββ homodimers indeed do transmit developmentally important signals. However, β rearrangement is not a prerequisite for rearrangement. It is widely believed—based on experiments using TcR transgenic mice—that rearranged β genes or their products efficiently shut down further recombination at the β locus.[44,58-60] This leads to stringent allelic exclusion of β genes and it is rare to see more than one rearranged and functional β gene per cell. On the other hand, α rearrangement appears to proceed for some time despite successful rearrangement of other α genes, most likely until the cell is positively selected or dies. Accumulating evidence indeed implicates negative regulation of the TcR α rearrangement via the TcR already expressed at the cell surface.[61-63]

It has long been known that some DN thymocytes can become CD8[+] or DP after overnight culture in the absence of thymic epithelium.[64-66] This phenomenon was fully explained when we[54,56] and others[67,68] demonstrated that the only population of DN cells capable of converting to DP in vitro are the TL cells. Thus an unknown signal, allowing the initial activation of CD8 and CD4 gene transcription leads to an initially low expression of these molecules at the protein level (TL stage), followed by an upregulation of their expression and the transition to DP cells. This signal clearly depends on intact thymic microenvironment because of the following findings: (i) the immediate precursors of CD25[-]TL cells are CD25[+]TN, and these cells cannot become DP in vitro[54,67] and (ii) when allowed to develop in an irradiated thymus, CD25[+]TN cells complete their differentiation by becoming CD25[-]TL and then DP.[53,68] The nature of the intrathymic signal that mediates this transition is not known. One possibility is that TcR β genes rearranged at CD25[+]TN stage become

expressed as ββ homodimers. Upon recognizing an unknown ligand, ββ dimers would transmit a signal to the cell to activate and subsequently upregulate CD8 and CD4 expression. It is also possible that a rearranged β chain mediates its regulatory effects intracellularly, without being expressed at the surface, e.g., via the induction of a non-TcR membrane molecule or a transcription factor that could catalyze the entire process. Finally, the signal could be completely independent of the β chain and act by actually inducing the recombination of the β chain, the expression of which would in turn regulate the DN → DP transition.

Which factors control the expression of the rearranged TcR at the membrane? We investigated this issue in anti-(H-Y+D[b]) TcR transgenic mice.[51] In this strain, α and β transgenes are controlled by their natural endogenous transcriptional elements. The fact that they are rearranged allowed us to ask whether rearrangement could be a limiting factor for the surface expression of TcR. Contrary to earlier reports that the transgene is "prematurely" expressed on DN cells,[69,70] we found rearranged transgenes to be subject to strict developmental control of membrane expression, very much like the endogenous TcR genes. The transgenes are expressed only after the cell begins to downregulate CD25 (Table 1),[51] similar to the situation encountered in normal development.

Table 1. Coordinate expression of transgenic TcR α and β chains follows the downregulation of CD25

DN subset	% Tg TcR$_\alpha$[+] cells	% Tg TcR$_\beta$[+] cells
CD25[hi]	8.7	9.5
CD25[lo/int]	38.6	37.5
CD25[-]	> 90	> 90

Female transgenic α(H-Y + D[b]) thymocytes were treated with mAb and complement to prepare DN cells, and the surviving thymocytes analyzed for the surface expression of transgenic TcR proteins and CD25 by flow cytometry. Absolute numbers of CD25[+] cells/thymus were reduced to one third of normal controls.[51]

Thus, the decisive control of TcR expression must be exerted at the transcriptional or post-transcriptional level(s).

TL cells also clearly express, or are in the process of upregulating, a number of other markers expressed on DP thymocytes. Among these are CD2 and CD28. A subset of TL cells (about 16%, S. Andjelíc, unpublished results) expresses CD69, an early activation antigen recently associated with positive selection, as well as Fas, an apoptosis-related membrane molecule.[71,72] We could also detect mRNA for another activation/costimulatory antigen, CTLA-4. The expression of CTLA-4 was restricted almost exclusively to the TL cells. The expression of CD69 and CTLA-4 probably correlates with the fact that TL cells are the most actively cycling cells in the murine thymus.[73] Even more importantly, the layout of cellular signaling machinery changes drastically during the transition from CD25$^+$TN to CD25$^-$TL cells and begins to resemble that of DP cells, as will be discussed in the last chapter.

INTERMEDIATE DP THYMOCYTES— THE STAGE OF SELECTION

TL cells will become DP by one of the following three routes (Fig. 2). They can upregulate both molecules simultaneously and become DP directly. Alternatively, they can upregulate one accessory molecule ahead of the other, giving rise to CD8^{hi}CD4^{lo}TcR^{lo} or CD8^{lo}CD4^{hi}TcR^{lo} cells. The latter cells can readily be distinguished from post-selectional maturing single-positive (SP) thymocytes by low TcR[74] and high HSA[75] levels. These cells cannot be induced to proliferate by any stimulation, and can spontaneously become DP in vitro. It is not clear what is the mechanism for preferential upregulation of one or the other accessory molecule, but this phenomenon is somewhat strain-related in mice.[76-78] From the standpoint of intrathymic selection (as discussed in Chapter 7) the upregulation of one of the accessory molecules may allow a thymocyte to be selected before it reaches DP stage. A transition between immature SP and DP thymocytes occurs over a few hours both in vivo and in vitro.[54,68,77,79]

DP cells are by far the most dominant thymocyte subset. The majority of these cells express low levels of TcR. But 3-5% DP thymocytes express high levels of this molecule and are therefore considered to be a subset that has just undergone positive selection.[80-84] However, even if this is correct, more recent results indicate that additional intrathymic processing is required for final maturation. For example, Petrie et al have demonstrated that TcR^{hi}DP cells from *bcl-2* transgenic mice can differentiate into either CD8$^+$ or CD4$^+$ SP cells in vivo, but only to CD8$^+$ SP cells in vitro.[85] It is not clear what proportion of DP thymocytes expresses TcR αβ heterodimers (all points of previous discussion on αβ versus ββ receptors are valid here as well), but a minimal estimate is 70%. This value may be misleading in light of a continuous rearrangement of TcRα chain genes at the DP stage[63] (Fig. 2). With regard to other molecules, DP thymocytes express high levels of HSA, Fas and PNA and about half of them expresses CD69. As mentioned before, this antigen is thought to be associated with positive selection.[80] But inasmuch as very few DP thymocytes may undergo positive selection, this antigen is hardly diagnostic of positive selection.

An overwhelming majority of DP cells are morphologically small but a fraction is blastoid, and these cells presumably represent a few precursors that have acquired high levels of CD8 and CD4 before they ended the last round of division.[82,83] It is generally believed that selection operates on resting, noncycling cells, and that it does not involve cell proliferation.[81,83] For these reasons, and owing to the high death rate of DP thymocytes, it was difficult to prove that these cells actually produce SP progeny. Finally, transfer experiments and labeling studies have demonstrated indirectly[53] and later directly[84] that DP cells do yield SP progeny, albeit with low efficacy. Initial experiments used large, blastoid DP cells for transfer,[84] although more recent transfer experiments demonstrated that resting DP cells can also mature into SP thymocytes (Lundberg K and Shortman K, in preparation). These authors have also noticed that CD4^{hi}8-3^{hi} cells differentiate

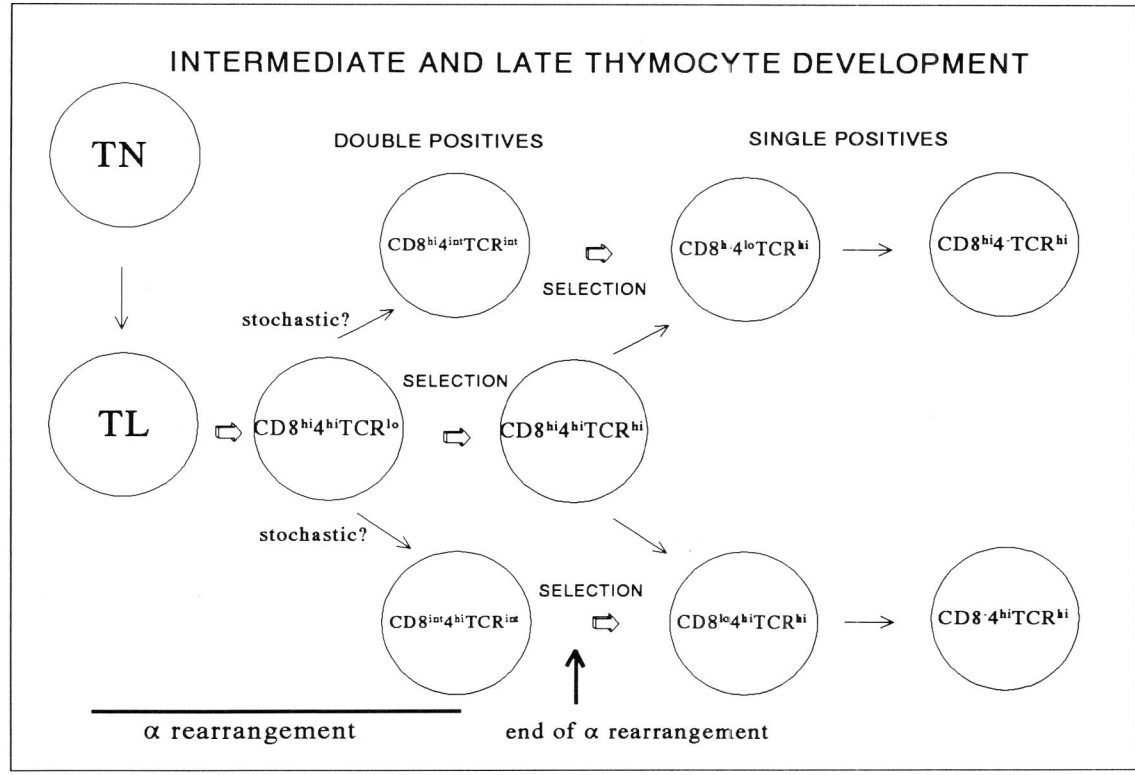

Fig. 2. Intermediate and late thymocyte development. Possible sites of selection (both positive and negative), of stochastic phenotype changes and of the end of TcR α rearrangement are indicated. "Double positives" and "single positives" refer to cells that fit within the corresponding quadrants by flow cytometric analysis.

much faster from small DP precursors than CD4-8^{hi}3^{hi} cells, that seem to be retained at a DP CD3^{hi} stage. The reason for this difference is unknown at present. The transition between TL and DP cells takes about 8–12 hours, and that between DP and SP about two to three days.[81-83] DP cells therefore include precursors that just became DP, DP cells undergoing positive selection, DP cells dying due to lack of positive selection, DP cells undergoing negative selection, and DP cells that have passed positive selection and are about to turn off one of the accessory molecules, and become SP.

LATE INTERMEDIATES AND THE FINAL MATURATION

The transition between DP and SP cells is gradual. The intensity of expression of several markers changes in a predictable fashion, and

that has allowed the isolation of intermediate stages in this process. Using multicolor flow cytometry, Guidos and co-workers identified cells that bear high levels of one accessory molecule and intermediate levels of the other, and showed that these cells express TcR levels lower than these in mature T cells but higher than DP thymocytes.[84] These cells, according to the authors, have undergone positive selection but not mouse mammary tumor virus (MMTV)- mediated negative selection. A similar subset was detected by Crompton et al in TcR Tg mice maintained on a nonselectional MHC background, and was characterized as cortisone-sensitive and not deleted by MMTV products (an indication of relative immaturity), but could, upon transfer into athymic recipients, yield TcR^{hi} progeny.[86] Consistent with a post-positive selection status of such cells, another group of authors, working in normal mice, has observed that they bear high levels of the early activation antigen CD69 (RN Germain, personal communication). Surprisingly, that group has failed to demonstrate any function or precursor capacity for these cells, raising the possibility that these cells are destined to die. These controversial results are not resolved at present, but our recent observations may provide some clues to reconcile them.

For a long time, SP cells have been regarded as thymic equivalents of mature, immunocompetent peripheral T cells. However, we[87] and others[88,89] have delineated two major subsets of mature $CD4^+TcR^{hi}$ SP thymocytes, the more numerous of which is not completely mature. Using the expression of CD8, HSA and Qa-2, $CD4^+TcR^{hi}$, SP thymocytes can be divided into $CD8^{lo}HSA^{int}Qa-2^-$ and $CD8^-HSA^{lo/-}Qa-2^{lo/int}$ cells.[87,88] The former subset makes up 70% of all $CD4^+$ SP thymocytes and cannot respond to immobilized anti-TcR mAb in the presence of cytokines, nor to allogeneic cells in the absence of IL-2. The latter subset (30% of $CD4^+$ SP thymocytes) is phenotypically fully mature, and functionally equivalent to splenic $CD8^-CD4^+HSA^-Qa-2^+$ cells. Acquisition of CD44, a late activation marker, most likely occurs in both subsets. Analogous subsets exist in the $CD8^+$ SP lineage.[89]

A logical hypothesis stemming from these discoveries is that the less mature cells represent direct descendants of DP cells, and that they mature into truly single-positive cells in the thymus or the periphery. However, our recent experiments show that $CD8^{lo}CD4^+$ cells cannot mediate a lethal graft-versus-host disease (GvHd), nor can they survive in the peripheral lymphoid organs of syngeneic nude animals (R. Dyall and J. N-Zugic, manuscript in preparation). These cells react to TcR crosslinking by a high degree of apoptotic cell death and can only survive and yield peripheral progeny if reintroduced into the thymic microenvironment. Given that these cells have undergone changes thought to be associated with positive selection (upregulation of TcR) and negative selection (MMTV-mediated

deletion of reactive V_β TcR), it appears that late contact with the thymic environment is necessary for the final maturation of thymocytes. This result is in agreement with Germain's observations on late intermediates (see above), and with recent data implying a degree of stochasticity in CD8/4 exclusion, as will be discussed in detail in Chapters 5 and 6. The final maturation would consequently need to occur, at least in part, in the thymus.

The signals for migration from the thymus are poorly understood, but could be mediated by cell-matrix interactions. Indeed, some integrins, including VLA molecules, are developmentally regulated such that their expression decreases as the thymocyte matures.[90] Daily output from the thymus is estimated at $1-2 \times 10^6$ cells/day in young adult mice.[6,82] The remaining thymocytes will die by one of the processes discussed in the last chapter.

MINOR αβ DIFFERENTIATION PATHWAY

In addition to the main αβ lineage pathway described above, a distinct lineage that produces $CD8^-CD4^-TcR^{int}$ cells exists in the thymuses of adult mice. This lineage is poorly characterized, but it is certain that it does not undergo conventional processes of positive and negative selection. The cells of this lineage were originally discovered by Budd et al,[91] and were initially thought to contain precursors of DP thymocytes and other T cells. However, their late appearance (not detectable until 3 wk of adult life), an unusually high (up to 70%) frequency of expression of $V_\beta8$ TcR and a good degree of immunocompetence were not consistent with this idea.[36,91,92]

Initial studies on these cells indicated that they arise as a consequence of the downregulation of accessory molecules in potentially autoreactive DP thymocytes. Such a mechanism was documented as an alternative way of functionally tolerizing autoreactive cells in several transgenic models. However, the evidence for the DP origin of these cells is indirect, and is based on the methylation patterns of the CD8 gene.[94] Cells of this phenotype were recently generated in vitro by Suda and Zlotnik from CD25⁺HSA⁺ precursors (by αCD3 and IL-7 stimulation) without passing via the DP stage. The same authors showed that these DN cells in vivo undergo a phenotypic change in a sequence: HSA⁺CD44⁻ → HSA⁻CD44⁻ → HSA⁻CD44⁺, and that this sequence also pertains to γδ DN cells.[95] Further experiments using intrathymic transfer and/or cell labeling are required to resolve the origin of these cells.

In vivo repopulation experiments have shown that mature, peripheral DN cells can be generated from thymic DN precursors,[96] and, more precisely, from purified CD25⁺DN cells (J. Nikolic-Zugic, unpublished observations). Based on these and other experiments, it seems probable that mature αβ-bearing DN cells can branch off from the main lineage at, or near, the CD25⁺ DN stage. The β locus rearrangement begins not earlier than the CD44ˡᵒCD25⁺ stage,[18] and the separation of αβ and γδ lineages can happen at or near that point.[57] However, the separation of these lineages probably can occur at other stages as well. Some of the most informative experiments along these lines were those by Tonegawa's group, demonstrating that some γδ cells do pass via the DP stage, and that disruption of the δ locus leads to disappearance of the DP γδ⁺ cells.[41] Signals and molecules guiding its development are, however, poorly understood.

TcRαβⁱⁿᵗDN thymocytes and T cells similar to the ones described above accumulate in at least two nonphysiological situations: in TcR transgenic mice and in mice carrying a homozygous *lpr* mutation. Every TcR transgenic (Tg) mouse strain generated so far has turned out to have an accumulation of mature, nonprecursor receptor-bearing DN thymocytes that may make up to 15-20% of total thymocytes.[70,92-99] These cells are of the HSA⁺CD44ˡᵒ phenotype and were initially thought to be a precursor population that prematurely expresses the TcR. They are present during early ontogeny, irrespective of the presence of selecting MHC molecules that are critical for the generation of mature TcR Tg⁺ single-positive cells. We have recently directly demonstrated that these cells can only yield peripheral DN cells but

not phenotypically different thymic progeny.[51] It is conceivable that thymic HSA⁺TcRⁱⁿᵗDN cells in TcR transgenic mice could be analogous to the cells of the same phenotype discovered by Suda and Zlotnik in normal animals.[95] But it is equally possible that the transgenic and normal subsets belong to different lineages, given their very different ontogenic appearance. It remains to be elucidated how the transgene mediates the accumulation at this particular developmental stage.

One of the murine models of the human systemic lupus erythematosus (SLE) is the *lpr* mutation (rev. in 100). This mutation is associated with an enormous accumulation of peripheral T cells of the TcRⁱⁿᵗDN phenotype. *lpr* DN cells express various non-T-cell markers (most notably B220⁺), are refractory to most stimuli and accumulate with age, in particular after two months of life. The *lpr* mutation is a retrotransposon-induced frameshift defect in the coding region of the Fas gene,[101,102] whose product seems to be one of the molecules that signals cell death to the host cells.[103,104] The role of Fas in regulating cell survival during thymic selection and/or peripheral immune response is very likely.[105,106] In normal mice, this antigen is expressed in the greatest quantities on DP cells and is gradually lost in SP thymocytes. In the periphery, it is mainly absent but can be induced by cell activation. Small numbers of B220⁺DN T cells (up to 10% of all DN thymocytes) can be detected in *lpr* thymuses prior to the accumulation of these cells in the periphery. How the Fas defect results in the generation of DN cells and whether the DN cells are culprits in autoimmunity is not clear at present. Further, we do not know the relationship of *lpr* cells to DN cells in normal mice.

Some results indicate that a TcRⁱⁿᵗDN subset can be produced in the gut of the normal mice by an extrathymic pathway.[103] Skewed expression of Vβ fragments as well as other data have suggested that thymic αβⁱⁿᵗDN cells could be selected by a superantigen-like ligand, since conventional negative and positive selection do not operate on these cells.[107-109] Virtually nothing is known on the physiological function of these cells. In summary, these cells could be an evolutionary aberration or a subset with a novel and specialized function.

PHENOTYPIC STAGES IN FETAL THYMIC DEVELOPMENT

The development of the first wave of fetal thymocytes is synchronous and it recapitulates most of the features of adult thymocyte development. However, certain important differences do exist and should be borne in mind.[110-113] For example, fetal TN cells are larger than the adult ones, and fetal DN cells contain neither HSA⁻ nor Thy-1⁻ subsets that accumulate with age,[110] probably due to inefficient production of these cells by a minor differentiation pathway(s). As the first wave of precursors colonizes the thymus, it contains precursors not only of T cells, but most likely of the non-T residents of the thymus that are of hematopoietic origin. This first wave of immigrants appears to undergo very few changes in the first two days of their intrathymic life, except for the development of some TcRγδ⁺ cells. However, studies of early fetal thymocyte development are hampered by two technical problems. It is physically very difficult to extract a day 11-13 fetal thymus, and even if one succeeds, the number of organs necessary to obtain cells for analysis is prohibitively high.

Branching of NK cells and T cells occurs in the fetus on days 13-14. At that point, most fetal thymocytes express FcγRII/III and can, under the appropriate conditions, almost clonaly become NK cells. Therefore, it seems likely that T and NK cells share the same precursor, at least during fetal development. The exact branching point in the adult has not yet been precisely defined.

It is assumed that the sequence of marker acquisition is similar in the fetus and the adult.[112] On day 14 a thymic lobe contains about 10^4 cells, and these express high levels of Thy-1, HSA and CD44. In fact, four subsets of thymic TN cells are already distinguishable based on the expression of CD44 and CD25, with almost 75% of cells expressing CD25.[112,114] Some of the most mature among these are expected to rearrange TcRβ genes. Initial studies have, however, placed this re-

arrangement as late as days 16-16.5.[115] It is likely that this result would be challenged with the use of more sensitive techniques.

In the search for fetal TL cells we recently demonstrated that these cells can be detected in low numbers around day 15, that they dominate the thymus on day 15.5 and that their relative representation progressively decreases thereafter.[114] Like the adult TL cells, they can become DP in vitro and their α chain genes are rearranged and transcribed. Since the first C_α transcripts can be detected on day 15[114]—contrary to the original mRNA analysis that placed this expression at day 17[115]—it is likely that TcR β genes also undergo rearrangement and are transcribed earlier, i.e., on day 14. Unlike adult TL cells that are CD25⁻(80-90%) or CD25ˡᵒ (10-20%) and CD44ˡᵒ, the majority of fetal TL homologues express CD25, and some even express CD44.[114] As discussed before, one reason for this discrepancy may lie in homeostatic differences between the fetal and the adult thymus. Adult DN thymocytes encounter a "full" thymus that probably slows down the progression of newly arrived cells through each developmental stage. By contrast, the fetal thymus is "empty," and no "steady-state" constraints are imposed on the time that the first wave of precursors will spend at each stage. Another difference between the development of adult thymocytes and the first wave of fetal precursors may be in the turnover of membrane molecules (slower in the latter population). Finally, the cellular composition of the thymic stroma differs markedly between the adult and the fetus.

Although we call fetal cells TL, the existence of TcR αβ heterodimers at the surface of these cells has not been conclusively documented, despite the fact that surface staining does reveal low expression of TcRβ. In fact, a recent report has documented the existence of ββ homodimers on day 16 thymocytes.[43] It remains to be seen whether this is another peculiarity of fetal development. Overall TcR expression on fetal and even newborn thymocytes is quite low, for unknown reasons. CD2 is expressed at the same time, or later than CD25 in the mouse, but probably at an earlier corresponding stage in the human thymus. Along with FcγRII/III, CD2 was used to delineate fetal TN cells in a similar manner as CD44 and CD25. According to this division, FcγRII/III⁺CD2⁻ cells correspond to a pre-TcR rearrangement stadium (probably CD44⁺CD25⁻ᵒʳ ⁺). Next, these cells gain CD2, and begin the rearrangement of the β locus, to finally become FcγRII/III⁻CD2⁺ before becoming DP. The precise correlation of the last two stages to CD44/CD25 defined stages remains to be established. Due to the lack of or low expression of FcγRII/III on adult TN cells, the value of this division is restricted to the fetal development.

In most mouse strains, CD8 is expressed at intermediate high levels before CD4 around days 16-16.5.[65,111] First DP cells are detectable immediately thereafter, and the first SP cells as of days 17.5-19. Lymphokine-secreting and cytotoxic functions can be demonstrated around that time,[65] but the breadth of the TcR repertoire of these cells has not been established. As noticed for CD25 and CD44 during early fetal development, a large extent of "bleeding" of some molecules into the next phenotypic stage is evident at the level of fetal and newborn SP cells. Most notably, almost all fetal and early newborn CD4⁺ SP cells express low levels of CD8 (J. Nikolic-Zugic, unpublished results). The converse is apparently true for CD8⁺ SP cells. Lymphokine secretion patterns are unique for the SP cells in the fetus.[116] One study has also described that recent thymic emigrants in the fetus/newborn bear HSA and perhaps other markers of thymocytes.[117] Furthermore, some signaling functions (or a lack thereof) are characteristic for fetal development,[118] and the fetal and even newborn thymus cannot impart tolerance to a number of antigens.[119,120] One reason for this may be a lack of expression of certain autoantigens during fetal life.[120] Another reason may be the absence of mature deleting epithelium and/or hematopoietic cells from the fetal thymus.[121]

FUTURE DIRECTIONS

Phenotypic dissection of the intrathymic development of αβ T cells has progressed to the point at which there is a good consensus about the stages of major αβ developmental pathway. An orderly sequence of acquisition of membrane molecules correlates with the maturational status of thymocytes. Gaps in our knowledge still exist concerning a few points regarding the minor pathway(s) and the fetal development. Of course, with the discovery of each new molecule, studies of its distribution on thymocyte subsets will add new information and might help delineate finer substages of development. But the early pioneering work that chartered the intrathymic developmental pathway is over, and most of the excitement has now shifted to the investigation of functional, molecular and intracellular mechanisms that bring about thymic maturation and selection. Of course, these studies will be greatly facilitated by a well charted map of the phenotypic territory.

SUMMARY

The earliest precursors of αβ-bearing T cells enter the thymus bearing very few molecules that mark their mature progeny. In the course of their initial maturation, these cells undergo tremendous proliferation, extensive phenotypic changes and somatic recombination at the TcR locus. All these changes generate a dominant population of thymocytes that bears CD8, CD4 and low levels of the TcR. Upon successful completion of intrathymic selection, these cells will be transformed into single-positive thymocytes that bear high levels of TcR and that are ready to populate peripheral lymphoid tissues. In addition to this major pathway of αβ T-cell development in the thymus, a minor, and still poorly defined pathway leads to production of a mature DN subset of T cells. Fetal development follows the rules established in the adult, with some notable exceptions regarding the cell size, makeup and function.

REFERENCES

1. Davies AJ. The tale of T cells. Immunol Today 1993; 14:137-140.
2. Miller JFAP. Experimental thymology has come of age. Thymus 1979; 1:3.

3. Reinherz EL, Kung PC, Goldstein, G.et al. Discrete stages of intrathymic differentiation: analysis of normal thymocytes and leukemic lymphoblasts of T-cell lineage. Proc Natl Acad Sci USA 1980; 77:1588.

4. Metcalf D. Cold Spring Harbor Symp Quant Biol 1967; 32:583.

5. McPhee D, Pye J, Shortman K. The differentiation of T-lymphocytes. V. Edvidence for intrathymic death of most thymocytes. Thymus 1979; 1:151.

6. Scollay R, Butcher E, Weissman I. Thymus migration: quantitative studies on the rate of migration of cells from the thymus to the periphery in mice. Eur J Immunol 1980; 10:1231.

7. Fowlkes BJ, Edison L, Mathieson BJ et al. Early T lymphocytes: differentiation in vivo of adult intrathymic precursor cells. J Exp Med 1985; 162:802.

8. Nikolic-Zugic J. Phenotypic and functional stages in thymocyte development. Immunol Today 1991; 12:65.

9. Shortman K. Cellular aspects of early T-cell development. Curr Opinion Immunol 1992; 4:140.

10. Owen JJT, Ritter M. Tissue interactions in the development of the thymus lymphocytes. J Exp Med 1969; 129:431.

11. Metcalf D, Moore MAS. Embryonic aspects of haemopoiesis. In: Neuberger A, Tatum EL, eds. Frontiers of Biology, Vol 24. Amsterdam, London: North-Holland Publishing Co., 1971; 24:195.

12. Palacios R, Imhof B. At day 8 to 8.5 of mouse development the yolk sac, not the embryo proper, has lymphoid precursor potential in vivo and in vitro. Proc Natl Acad Sci USA 1993; 90:6581-6586.

13. Spangrude GJ, Heimfeld S, Weissman IL. Purification and characterization of mouse hematopoietic stem cells. Science 1988; 241:58-62.

14. Lesley J, Hyman R, Schulte R. Evidence that the Pgp-1 glycoprotein is expressed on thymust-homing progenitor cells in the thymus. Cell Immunol 1985; 91:397.

15. Wu L, Scollay R, Egerton M et al. CD4 expressed on earliest T-lineage precursor cells in the adult murine thymus. Nature 1991; 349:71.

16. Wu L, Antica M, Johnson GR et al. Developmental potential of the earliest precursor cells from the adult mouse thymus. J Exp Med 1991; 174:1617-1627.

17. Ardavin C, Wu L, Chung-Leung L et al. Thymic dendritic cells and T cells develop simultaneously in the thymus from a common precursor population. Nature 1993; 362:761-763.

18. Godfrey DL, Kennedy J, Suda T et al. A developmental pathway involving four phenotypically and functionally distinct subsets of CD3⁻CD4⁻CD8⁻ triple-negative adult mouse thymocytes defined by CD44 and CD25 expression. J Immunol 1993: 150:4244-4252.

19. Godfrey DI, Zlotnik A, Suda T. Phenotypic and functional characterization of c-kit expression during intrathymic T-cell development. J Immunol 1992; 149:2281.

20. Raulet DH. Expression and function of interleukin-2 receptors on immature thymocytes. Nature 1985; 314:101.

21. Ceredig R, Lowenthal JW, Nabholz M et al. Expression of interleukin-2 receptors as a differentiation marker on intrathymic stem cells. Nature 1985; 314:98.

22. Habu S, Okumura S, Diamantstein T et al. Expression of interleukin-2 receptor on murine fetal thymocytes. Eur J Immunol 1985; 15:456.

23. Shimonkevitz RP, Husmann LA, Bevan MJ et al. Transient expression of IL-2 receptor precedes the differentiation of immature thymocytes. Nature 1987; 329:157.

24. Lesley J, Schulte R, Hyman R. Kinetics of thymus repopulation by intrathymic progenitors after intravenous injection: Evidence for successive repopulation by an IL-2R⁺,Pgp-1⁻ and by an IL-2R⁻,Pgp-1⁺ progenitor. Cell Immunol 1988; 117:378.

25. Jenkinson EJ, Kingston R, Owen JJT. Importance of IL-2 receptors in intra-thymic generation of cells expressing T-cell receptors. Nature 1987; 329:160.

26. Tentori L, Longo DL, Zuniga-Pflucker JC et al. Essential role of the interleukin 2-interleukin 2 receptor pathway in thymocyte maturation in vivo. J Exp Med 1988; 168:1741-1747.

27. Hardt C, Diamantstein T, Wagner H.

Developmentally controlled expression of IL-2 receptors and of sensitivity ti IL-2 in a subset of embryonic thymocytes. J Immunol 1985; 134:3891-3894.

28. Zuniga-Pflucker JC, Smith KA, Tentori L et al. Are the IL-2 receptors expressed in the murine fetal thymus functional? Devel Immunol 1990; 1:59-66.

29. von Boehmer H, Crisanti A, Kieselow P et al. Absence of growth by most receptor-expressing fetal thymocytes in the presence of interleukin-2. Nature 1985; 314:539.

30. Ceredig R. Proliferation in vitro and interleukin production by 14 day fetal and adult Lyt2⁻L3T4⁻ mouse thymocytes. J Immunol 1986; 137:2260.

31. Lowenthal JW, Howe RC, Ceredig R et al. Functional status of interleukin 2 receptors expressed by immature (Lyt2⁻L3T4⁻ thymocytes. J Immunol 1986; 137:2579.

32. Schorle H, Holtschke T, Hunig T et al. Development and function of T cells in mice rendered interleukin-2 deficient by gene targeting. Nature 1991; 352:621-624.

33. Noguchi M, Yi H, Rosenblatt HM et al. Interleukin-2 receptor γ chain mutation results in X-linked sever combined immunodeficiency in humans. Cell 1993; 73:147-157.

34. Taniguchi T, Minami Y. The IL-2/IL-2 receptor system: a current overview. Cell 1993; 73:5-8.

35. Pearse M, Wu L, Egerton M et al. A murine early thymocyte developmental sequence is marked by transient expression of the interleukin 2 receptor. Proc Natl Acad Sci USA 1989; 86:1614.

36. Crispe IN, Moore MW, Husmann LA et al. Differentiation protential of subsets of CD4⁻8⁻ thymocytes. Nature 1987; 329:336.

37. Krimpenfort P, Ossendorp F, Borst J et al. T-cell depletion in transgenic mice carrying a mutant gene for TcR-β. Nature 1989; 341:742-746.

38. Ossendorp F, Jacobs H, van der Horst G et al. T-cell receptor-αβ lacking the β-chain V domain can be expressed at the cell surface but prohibits T-cell maturation. J Immunol 1992; 148:3714-3722.

39. Kishi H, Borgulya P, Scott B et al. Surface expression of the β T-cell receptor (TcR) chain in the absence of other TcR or CD3 proteins on immature T cells. EMBO J 1991; 10:93-100.

40. Groettrup M, Baron A, Griffiths G et al. T-cell receptor (TcR) β chain homodimers on the surface of immature but not mature α, γ, δ chain deficient T-cell lines. EMBO J 1992; 11:2735-2740.

41. Mombaerts P, Clarke AR, Rudnicki MA et al. Mutations in T-cell antigen receptor genes α and β block thymocyte development at different stages. Nature 1992; 360:225-231.

42. Scott B, Bluthmann H, Teh HS et al. The generation of mature T cells requires interaction of the αβT-cell receptor with major histocompatibility antigens. Nature 1989; 338:591-593.

43. Groettrup M, von Boehmer H. T-cell receptor β chain dimers on immature thymocytes from normal mice. Eur J Immunol 1993; 23:1393-1396.

44. Alt FW, Oltz EM, Young F et al. VDJ recombination. Immunol Today 1992; 13:306-314.

45. Shinkai Y, Koyasu S, Nakayama K et al. Restoration of T-cell development in RAG-2-deficient mice by functional TcR transgenes. Science 1993; 259:822-825.

46. Molina TJ, Kishihara K, Siderovski DP et al. Profound block in thymocyte development in mice lacking p56ᵏᵏ. Nature 1992; 357:161.

47. Levin SD, Anderson SJ, Forbush KA et al. A dominant-negative transgene defines a role for p56ˡᶜᵏ in thymopoiesis. EMBO J 1993; 4:1671.

48. Abraham KM, Levin SD, Marth JD et al. Thymic tumorigenesis induced by overexpression of p56ˡᶜᵏ. Proc Natl Acad Sci USA 1991; 88:3977.

49. Anderson SJ, Abraham KM, Nakayama T et al. Inhibition of T-cell receptor β-chain gene rearrangement by overexpression of the non-receptor protein tyrosine kinase p56ˡᶜᵏ. EMBO J 1992; 11:4877.

50. Levin SD, Abraham, KM, Anderson SJ et al. The protein tyrosine p56ˡᶜᵏ regulates thymocyte development independently of its interaction with CD4 and CD8 coreceptors. J Exp Med 1993; 178:245-255.

51. Nikolic-Zugic J, Andjelic S, Teh H-S et al.

Influence of T-cell receptor (TcR) $\alpha\beta$ transgenes on early T-cell development. Eur J Immunol 1993; 23:1699-1704.

52. Rodewald H-R, Awad K, Moingeon P et al. FcγRII/III and CD2 expression mark distinct subpopulations of immature CD4⁻ CD8⁻ murine thymocytes: in vivo developmental kinetics and T-cell receptor β chain rearrangement status. J Exp Med 1993; 177:1079-1092.

53. Nikolic-Zugic J, Bevan MJ. Thymocytes expressing CD8 differentiate into CD4⁺ cells following intrathymic injection. Proc Natl Acad Sci USA 1988; 85:8633.

54. Nikolic-Zugic J, Moore MW, Bevan MJ. Characterization of the subset of immature thymocytes which can undergo rapid in vitro differentiation. Eur J Immunol 1989; 19:649.

55. Petrie HT, Pearse M, Scollay R et al. Development of immature thymocytes: initiation of CD3, CD4, and CD8 acquisition parallels down-regulation of the interleukin-2-receptor α-chain. Eur J Immunol 1990; 20:2813.

56. Nikolic-Zugic J, Moore MW. T-cell receptor expression on immature thymocytes with in vivo and in vitro precursor potential. Eur J Immunol 1989; 19:1957.

57. Petrie HT, Scollay R, Shortman K. Commitment to the T-cell receptor α/β or γ lineages can occur just prior to the onset of CD4 and CD8 expression among immature thymocytes. Eur J Immunol 1992; 22:2185-2188.

58. Uematsu Y, Ryser S, Dembic Z et al. In transgenic mice the introduced functional T-cell receptor β gene prevents expression of endogenous β genes. Cell 1988; 52:831-841.

59. Bluthmann H, Kisielow P, Uematsu Y et al. T-cell-specific deletion of T-cell receptor transgenes allows functional rearrangement of endogenous α- and β-genes. Nature 1988; 334:156-159.

60. Malissen M, Trucy J, Jouvin-Marche E et al. Regulation of TcR α and β gene allelic exclusion during T-cell development. Immunol Today 1992; 13:315-322.

61. Turka LA, Schatz DG, Oettinger MA et al. Thymocyte expression of RAG-1 and RAG-2: termination by T-cell receptor cross-linking. Science 1991; 253:778-781.

62. Brandle C, Muller C, Rulicke T et al. Engagement of the T-cell receptor during positive selection in the thymus down-regulates RAG-1 expression. Proc Natl Acad Sci USA 1992; 89:9529-9533.

63. Petrie HT, Livak F Schatz DG et al. Multiple rearrangements in T-cell receptor α chain genes maximize the production of useful thymocytes. J Exp Med 1993; 178:615-622.

64. Ceredig R, Sekaly RP, MacDonald HR. Differentiation in vitro of Lyt2⁺ thymocytes from embryonic Lyt-2 precursors. Nature 1983; 303:248.

65. Kisielow P, Leisserson W, von Boehmer H. Differentiation of thymocytes in fetal organ culture: analysis of phenotypic changes accompanying the appearance of cytolytic and interleukin 2-producing cells. J Immunol 1984; 133:1117.

66. Fowlkes BJ, Mathieson BJ. Differentiation in vitro of an adult precursor thymocyte. In: Regulation of the Immune System. Alan R. Liss, Inc., 1984:275.

67. Wilson A, Petrie HT, Scollay R et al. The acquisition of CD4 and CD8 during the differentiation of early thymocytes in short-term culture. Int Immunol 1989; 1:605.

68. Petrie HT, Hugo P, Scollay R et al. Lineage relationships and developmental kinetics of immature thymocytes: CD3, CD4, and CD8 acquisition in vivo and in vitro. J Exp Med 1990; 172:1583.

69. Teh HS, Kishi H, Scott B et al. Early deletion and late positive selection of T cells expressing a male-specific receptor in T-cell receptor transgenic mice. Devel Immunol 1990; 1:1-10.

70. Berg LJ, Fazekas de St Groth B, Pullen AM et al. Phenotypic differences between $\alpha\beta$ versus β T-cell receptor trangenic mice undergoing negative selection. Nature 1989; 340:559-562.

71. Drappa J, Brot N, Elkon K. The Fas protein is expressed at high levels on double positive thymocytes and activated mature T cells in normal but not MRL/lpr mice. Proc Natl Acad Sci USA 1993; 90:10340.

72. Andjelic S, Drappa J, Lacy E et al. The

onset of Fas expression parallels the acquisition of CD8 and CD4 in fetal and adult αβ thymocytes. 1994; 6 (in press).

73. Scollay R, Wilson A, D'Amico A et al. Developmental status and reconstitution protential of subpopulations of murine thymocytes. Immunol. Reviews 1988; 104:81.

74. Bluestone JA, Pardoll DM, Sharrow SO et al. Characterization of murine thymocytes with CD3-associated T-cell receptor structure. Nature 1987; 326:82.

75. Crispe IN, Bevan MJ. Expression and functional significance of the J11d marker on mouse thymocytes. J Immunol 1987; 138:2013.

76. Matsumoto K, Yoshikai Y, Matsuzaki G et al. A novel CD3-J11d+ subset of CD4+CD8- cells repopulating the thymus in radiation bone marrow chimeras. Eur J Immunol 1989; 19:1203.

77. MacDonald HR, Budd RC, Howe RC. A CD3- subset of CD4-8+ thymocytes: a rapidly cycling intermediate in the generation of CD4+8+ cells. Eur J Immunol 1988; 18:519.

78. Hugo P, Petrie HT. Multiple routes for late intrathymic precursors to generate CD4+CD8+ thymocytes. In: Advances in Molecular and Cell Biology, vol 5. JAI Press Inc., 1992:37-53.

79. Guidos CJ, Weissman IL, Adkins B. Intrathymic maturation of murine T lymphocytes from CD8+ precursors. Proc Natl Acad Sci USA 1989; 86:7542-7546.

80. Swat W, Dessing M, Baron A. et al. Phenotypic changes accompanying positive selection of CD4+CD8+ thymocytes. Eur J Immunol 1992; 22:2367.

81. Shortman K, Vremec D, Egerton M. The kinetics of T-cell antigen receptor expression by subgroups of CD4+8+ thymocytes: delineation of CD4+8+3²+ thymocytes as post-selection intermediates leading to mature T cells. J Exp Med 1991; 173:323.

82. Egerton M, Scollay R. Shortman K. Kinetics of mature T-cell development in the thymus. Proc Natl Acad Sci USA 1990; 87:2579-2582.

83. Penit C. Positive selection is an early event in thymocyte differentiation: high TcR expression by cycling immature thymocytes precedes final maturation by several days. Int Immunol 1990; 2:630-638.

84. Guidos CJ, Danska JS, Fathman CG et al. T-cell receptor-mediated negative selection of autoreactive T lymphocyte precursors occurs after commitment to the CD4 or CD8 lineage. J Exp Med 1990; 172:835.

85. Petrie HT, Strasser A, Harris AW et al. CD4+8- and CD4-8+ mature thymocytes require different post-selection processing for final development. J Immunol 1993; 151:1273-1279.

86. Crompton T, Ohashi P, Schneider SD et al. A cortisone sensitive CD3low subset of CD4+CD8- thymocytes represents an intermediate stage in intrathymic repertoire selection. Int Immunol 1992; 4:153-161.

87. Nikolic-Zugic J, Bevan MJ. Functional and phenotypic delineation of two subsets of CD4 single positive cells in the adult murine thymus. Int Immunol 1990; 1:135.

88. Ramsdell F, Jenkins M, Dinh Q et al. The majority of CD4+8- thymocytes are functionally immature. J Immunol 1991; 147:1779-1785.

89. Fowlkes BJ, Pardoll DM. Molecular and cellular events of T-cell development. Adv Immunol 1989; 44:287.

90. Wadsworth S, Halvorson MJ, Chang AC et al. Multiple changes in VLA protein glycosylation, expression, and function occur during mouse T-cell ontogeny. J Immunol 1993; 150:847-857.

91. Budd RC, Miescher GC, Howe RC et al. Developmentally regulated expression of T-cell receptor β chain variable domains in immature thymocytes. J Exp Med 1987; 166:577.

92. Fowlkes BJ, Kruisbeek, AM, Ton-That H et al. A novel population of T-cell receptor αβ-bearing thymocytes which predominantly expresses a single Vβ gene family. Nature 1987; 329:251.

93. Howe RC, MacDonald RH. Heterogeneity of immature (Lyt2-L3T4-) thymocytes. Identification of four major phenotypically distinct subsets differing in cell cycle status and in vitro activation requirement. J Immunol 1988; 140:1047.

94. Wu L, Pearse M, Egerton M et al. CD4-

CD8⁻ thymocytes that express the T-cell receptor may have previously expressed CD8. Int Immunol 1990; 2:51-56.

95. Suda T, Zlotnik A. Origin, differentiation, and repertoire selection of CD3⁺CD4⁻CD8⁻ thymocytes bearing either αβ or γδ T-cell receptors. J Immunol 1993; 150:447.

96. Guidos CJ, Weissman IL, Adkins B. Developmental potential of CD4⁻8⁻ thymocytes: peripheral progeny include mature CD4⁻8⁻ T cells bearing αβ T-cell receptor. J Immunol 1989; 142:3773-3780.

97. Kisielow P, Bluthmann H, Staerz UD et al. Tolerance in T-cell receptor transgenic mice involves deletion of nonmature CD4⁺8⁺ thymocytes. Nature 1988; 333:742.

98. Teh HS, Kisielow P, Scott B et al. Thymic major histocompatibility complex antigens and the αβ T-cell receptor determine the CD4/CD8 phenotype of T cells. Nature 1988; 335:229.

99. Kaye J, Hsu M-L, Sauron M-E et al. Selective development of CD4⁺ T cells in transgenic mice expressing a class II MHC-restricted antigen receptor. Nature 1989; 341:746-749.

100. Cohen PL, Eisenberg RA. The *lpr* and *gld* genes in systemic autoimmunity: life and death in the *Fas* lane. Immunol Today 1992; 13:427.

101. Adachi M, Watanabe-Fukunaga R, Nagata S. Aberrant transcription caused by the insertion of an early transposable element in an intron of the Fas antigen gene of lpr mice. Proc Natl Acad Sci USA 1993; 90:1756.

102. Chu JL, Drappa J, Parnassa A et al. The defect in Fas mRNA expression in MRL/lpr mice is associated with insertion of the retrotransposon, ETn. J Exp Med 1993; 178:723-730.

103. Itoh N, Yonehara S, Ishii A et al. The polypeptide encoded by the cDNA for human cell surface antigen Fas can mediate apoptosis. Cell 1991; 66:233.

104. Watanabe-Fukunaga R, Brannan CI, Itoh N et al. The cDNA structure, expression, and chromosomal assignment of the mouse Fas antigen. J Immunol 1992; 148:1274.

105. Zhou T, Bluethmann H, Eldrige J et al.

106. Russell JH, Rush B, Weaver C et al. Mature T cells of autoimmune lpr/lpr mice have a defect in antigen-stimulated suicide. Proc Natl Acad Sci USA 1993; 90:4409.

107. Russell JH, Meleedy-Rey P, McCulley DE et al. Evidence for CD8-independent T-cell maturation in transgenic mice. J. Immunol. 1990; 144:3318.

108. Huang L, Crispe IN. Distinctive selection mechanisms govern the T-cell receptor repertoire of peripheral CD4⁻CD8⁻ α/β T cells. J Exp Med 1992; 176:699-706.

109. von Boehmer H, Kirberg J, Rocha B. An unusual lineage of α/β cells that contains autoreactive cells. J Exp Med 1991; 174:1001-1008.

110. Scollay R. Differences in HLy2⁻L3T4⁻ thymocytes from foetal and adult murine thymus. Immunol Letters 1987; 15:171-177.

111. Husmann LA, Shimonkevitz RP, Crispe IN et al. Thymocyte subpopulations during early fetal development in the BALB/c mouse. J Immunol 1988; 141:736.

112. Havran WL, Allison JP. Developmentally ordered appearance of thymocytes expressing different T-cell antigen receptors. Nature 1988; 335:443.

113. Rodewald HR, Moingeon P, Lucich JL et al. A population of early fetal thymocytes expressing FcγRII/III contains precursors of T lymphocytes and NK cells. Cell 1992; 69:139.

114. Andjelic S, Jain N, Nikolic-Zugic J. Ontogeny of fetal CD8ˡᵒ4ˡᵒ thymocytes: expression of CD44, CD25 and early expression of TcR α mRNA. Eur J Immunol 1993; 23:2109-2115.

115. Snodgrass HR, Dembic Z, Steinmetz M et al. Expression of T-cell antigen receptor genes during fetal development in the thymus. Nature 1985; 315:232.

116. Bendelac A, Schwartz RH. CD4⁺ and CD8⁺ T cells acquire specific lymphokine secretion potentials during thymic maturation. Nature 1991; 353:68-71.

117. Kelly K, Scollay R. Analysis of recent thymic emigrants with subset- and maturity-related markers. Int Immunol 1990; 2:419.

118. Finkel TH, Cambier JC, Kubo RT et al. The

Origin of CD4⁻CD8⁻B220⁺ T cells in MRL-lpr/lpr mice. J Immuno 1993; 150:3651.

thymus has two functionally distinct populations of immature αβ⁺ cells: one population is deleted by ligation of αβ TcR. Cell 1989; 58:1047.

119. Smith H, Chen I-M, Kubo R et al. Neonatal thymectomy results in a repertoire enriched in T cells deleted in adult thymus. Science 1989; 245:749-752.

120. MacDonald HR, Lees RK. Programmed death of autoreactive thymocytes. Nature 1990; 343:642-644.

121. Boyd RL, Tucek CL, Godfrey DL et al. The thymic microenvironment. Immunol Today 1993; 14:445-462.

CHAPTER 4

CYTOKINES IN THE FETAL THYMUS

Simon R. Carding

Tannishtha

Generation of the T-cell repertoire begins during fetal development. It involves a complex and incompletely understood series of events that is initiated by the colonization of the thymus by fetal liver-derived stem cells. These cells then undergo a program of proliferation and differentiation to give rise to functionally competent T cells. Using monoclonal antibodies specific for various T-cell differentiation antigens, primarily CD4 and CD8, discrete and progressive stages through which developing T cells pass in the developing thymus have been identified (Fig. 1 and Chapter 3). The application of several molecular technologies has further defined the stages of T-cell development in which genes encoding components of the T-cell receptor (TcR) are rearranged, transcribed and expressed on the surface of developing T cells. More recently the application of genetically-engineered (transgenic) animals in which most or all of the peripheral T cells express the same TcR to studies of thymic selection have identified the stages at which T cells undergo positive and negative selection (reviewed in ref. 1).

Despite all of these advances in our understanding of T-cell development we still know very little about how thymocyte progression from one developmental stage to another is regulated. It has been proposed that the cellular elements of the thymic stroma are able to influence and possibly regulate the proliferation and differentiation of developing T cells through direct cell-cell contact or by the developmentally regulated production of soluble growth and differentiation factors. During the past 10 years a large number of in vitro and animal studies have provided indirect and direct

The authors would like to thank all the members of the Carding laboratory for their invaluable advice and assistance in assembling this manuscript. Dr. Carding is the recipient of a Junior Faculty Research Award from the American Cancer Society and portions of the work described here were supported by this award and by a University of Pennsylvania Research Foundation Award.

evidence for the effect of distinct cytokines on the proliferation and development of thymocytes at different stages of their intrathymic development (reviewed in 2). Here we will describe how the thymus is formed and subsequently colonized by T-cell progenitor cells and discuss the studies that provide direct evidence for the production and utilization of cytokines within the fetal thymus during T-cell development. We will also describe the results from our own studies and those of others in which the cellular source of cytokine production and utilization within the fetal thymus has been established. In addition, we will outline how the cytokine and cytokine receptor transgenic mice have been used to address the function of cytokines in T-cell development. Finally, we will discuss the issues that remain to be addressed concerning the involvement of cytokines in T-cell development and how more recently developed cellular and molecular procedures can be usefully applied to these studies.

ONTOGENY OF THE THYMUS

In mammals (by necessity mice have been the most extensively investigated species) the structural basis of the thymus first appears in the pharyngeal region in which the thymic endodermal epithelial cells are derived from the ventral parts of the third, and perhaps the fourth, pharyngeal pouch. On the eleventh day of gestation the ectoderm of the third branchial cleft proliferates and migrates to make contact with the endoderm of the third pouch to form the epithelial thymic analgen,

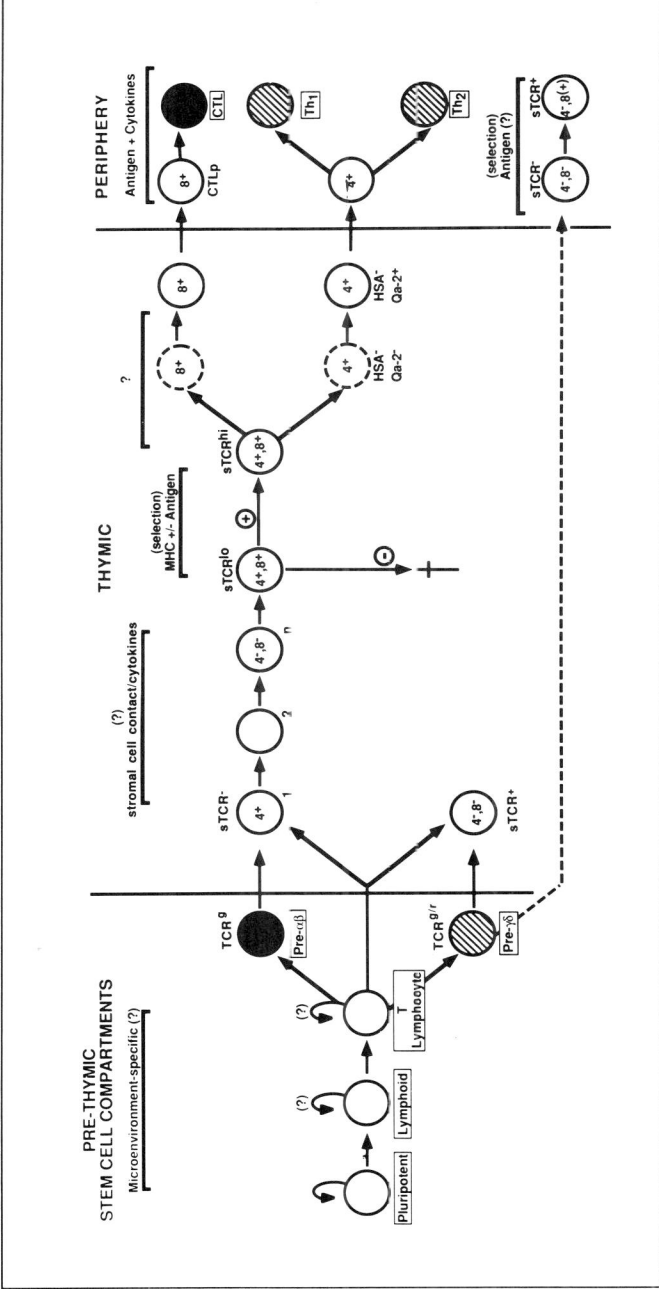

Fig. 1. Schematic representation of T-cell ontogeny during mammalian embryogenesis. It is apparent that our understanding of the mechanisms regulating any of the prethymic and thymic stages of T-cell development is minimal. An intrathymic stem cell's (CD4⁺CD8⁺, surface TcR [sTcR⁺]) progression through stages of proliferation (1,2,n), differentiation (CD4⁺0⁺) and positive (+) and negative (-) selection may be regulated through the production and response to different cytokines and through interactions with different thymic stromal cell populations.

which at this time is devoid of lymphocytes. Another important structural contribution to the developing thymus is made by stromal cells derived from the pharyngeal arch mesenchyme. These cells give rise to both the capsule that encases the thymus after it separates from the pharyngeal region around day 12 of gestation and the septa which penetrate into the body of the thymus to generate the many lobules characteristic of the adult thymus.

Thus by days 12 to 13 of mouse gestation the structural elements of the thymic rudiments on either side of the pharyngeal complex consist of an inner epithelial component with mesenchymal-derived central cleft and thin outer capsule. As development progresses the cleft is eliminated and the two rudiments migrate caudally until by days 17-18 they are in an anterior mediastinal position above the heart. It is during this migration that the mesenchymal septa begin to divide up the thymus into distinct lobules. Bone marrow-derived macrophages can be first detected immunohistochemically in the developing thymus by day 14 of gestation.[3] Using a similar approach dendritic cells can only be detected in the thymus around birth.[4] By day 18 cortex and medulla can be histologically distinguished. A similar pattern of thymus formation seems to occur in humans.[5]

One obvious but often neglected point is that the ontogeny of the thymus is synchronized with the development of the organism. It is likely, therefore, that there is some input from other developing systems, for example the neuroendocrine system, that may influence how and when in embryogenesis the thymus and indeed the immune system in general develops. The possibility that the nervous and endocrine systems are able to interact with and to modulate the activity of the immune system is the focus of several newly emerging areas of research.

PRE-T-CELL GENERATION AND THEIR COLONIZATION OF THE THYMUS

In the embryo the earliest identified site of cells capable of colonizing the thymus appears to be the mesenchymal blood islands

in the yolk sac.[6] Later in embryogenesis thymic precursors also appear in the fetal liver.[7] There is some evidence to suggest that exposure to secondary hematopoietic sites such as the liver may be necessary before yolk sac-derived cells can colonize the thymus.[8] It is not known whether cytokines play a role in the development of these pre-T cells in these extrathymic hematopoietic tissues. However, studies demonstrating that the proliferation and differentiation of pluripotent stem cells into lineage-specific precursors in vivo in adult animals[9] and in vitro in soft agarose can be affected by the exogenous addition of single or multiple cytokines[10,11] suggest that they may play an important role in influencing the fate of hematopoietic stem cells in vivo during fetal development.

Lymphoid cells characterized by their heavily basophilic cytoplasm[7,12] are first detected in the mouse thymic rudiment in close contact with the basement membrane at day 11 of gestation. At the time when migration into the thymus is initiated, the rudiment is not vascularized, implying that blood-born stem cells must leave adjacent vessels and traverse the surrounding mesenchyme before penetrating into the epithelial region of the thymus. At the present time the actual mechanism(s) of stem cell migration to the thymus is unknown. The involvement of chemotactic factors is, however, implied by the ability of populations of cells from fetal liver explants to migrate through porous nitrocellulose membranes[13-15] or agar[16] into adjacent thymus rudiments. Indeed, several factors that may influence chemotaxis have been identified[17] including a soluble form of β_2-microglobulin.[18] Even if chemotactic factors are involved in T-cell homing, it would appear unlikely that a diffuse gradient could operate within the blood stream causing the initial migration of blood-borne stem cells from vessels in the vicinity of the thymus. It has been proposed, therefore, that the first stages of thymic homing may be dependent upon the adhesion of stem cells to specific sites (receptors) on the endothelium of the vessels in the pre-thymic region, in a manner similar to that occurring between circulating peripheral lymphocytes and the endothelial cells of adult lymph nodes.[19] Once in the thymus the further development of the T-cell precursors comes under the influence of the thymic environment (Fig. 1).

CYTOKINE PRODUCTION IN THE FETAL THYMUS

There are two cellular components which can contribute to cytokine production within the fetal thymus; thymocytes themselves and the thymic stroma comprised of epithelial cells and bone marrow-derived macrophages and interdigitating dendritic cells. The relative composition of these varies throughout development (see previous section).

THYMOCYTES AS A SOURCE OF CYTOKINES

The cytokine producing-potential of fetal thymocytes within the fetal thymus has been demonstrated by studies in which fetal thymocytes, in isolation from the thymus, have been shown to secrete a variety of cytokines (including interleukin [IL] 1-7, interferon-γ [IFN-γ], tumor necrosis factor [TNF] and transforming growth factor-β [TGF-β]) after stimulation with either plant-derived mitogens (PHA and Con A) or phorbol esters and divalent cation-ionophores (reviewed in ref. .2). Whether or not these cytokines can be, and are, constitutively produced by these cells within the fetal thymus has not been possible to demonstrate directly using cytokine-specific indicator cell lines (cytokine bioassays) or conventional RNA-hybridization assays, e.g., Northern blotting, which are relatively insensitive and require prohibitively large numbers of cells. However, the application of more sophisticated and very sensitive molecular techniques such as the polymerase chain reaction (PCR) assay and in situ hybridization has not only resulted in the identification of the cytokines that are produced but also the temporal and spatial patterns of their expression in the fetal thymus during T-cell ontogeny (Table 1). For example, our own in situ hybridization studies of cytokine production during T-cell development in the fetal thymus have directly demonstrated that at defined periods of T-cell ontogeny a large number of thymocytes selectively express the genes

encoding IL-2 and IL-4.[2,20]

One potential problem in interpreting the results from molecular studies such as these in which mRNA production is detected is that it may not necessarily be indicative of the production of biologically active protein. However, Rothenberg and coworkers[21] have very recently demonstrated that during fetal thymic development, cytoplasmic IL-2 protein can be detected immunohistochemically in thymocytes at day 15 of gestation. Later in gestation, the number of IL-2-producing thymocytes decreases dramatically; a temporal pattern of protein production consistent with that of IL-2-mRNA expression that we and others have described in the fetal thymus (Table 1). Rothenberg[21] also found that the the IL-2-producing thymocytes in day 15 fetal thymuses are localized within one area of the thymus, in the periphery of the subcapsular region of the thymus. This region is thought to contain T-cell precursor populations that have only recently entered the thymus. To date similar studies of the spatial and temporal production of other cytokine proteins in the fetal thymus have not been attempted.

Thus, all of these studies of IL-2 production within the fetal thymus demonstrate that IL-2 is produced within discrete areas of the thymus at defined periods of T-cell development, presumably in response to developmental signals which provide the means for regulating or promoting the stage-specific development of distinct thymocyte populations. It will be of obvious interest to determine if the spatial pattern of production of other cytokines such as IL-4 are overlapping or are distinct from that of IL-2.

STROMAL CELL PRODUCTION OF CYTOKINES

Epithelial cells make up the largest cell population of the thymic stroma. However, these cells display considerable morphological and molecular heterogeniety[22] which presumably allows the formation of different microenvironments within the thymus. Based upon thymic staining patterns of a large panel of antibodies reactive with thymic epithelial cells, at least four distinct subpopulations can be distinguished.[23] The

Table 1. Constitutive production of cytokines by developing T cells in the fetal thymus

Cytokine		References
IL-1	Anti-IL-1 antibody inhibits T-cell development.	81
IL-2	60-80% d15 cells mRNA⁺	20
	50-55% d15 cells mRNA⁺	43
	mRNA⁺ cells in subcapsule at d14	21
	protein production in d15 thymi sections	
IL-4	30-40% d15 cells mRNA⁺	20
IL-7	Increasing numbers of mRNA⁺ cells between d12 and d15. Protein detected between d16 and d20	82
IFN-γ	3-5% d20 cells mRNA⁺	20
TNFα	mRNA detected in thymuses at d15 and d20.	83
	Increasing number mRNA⁺ cells between d15 and d20.	82
SCF	mRNA detected in d14 thymus.	82

SCF, stem cell factor.

functional significance of these phenotypically distinct populations of thymic epithelial cells is not known. Although it is now widely accepted that the stromal cells of the thymus provide "educational signals" which influence the development of T cells, the nature of these "signals" is not known. It is possible that stromal (epithelial) cell-derived cytokines and other soluble factors[24] may be able to serve, at least in part, as these thymic "educational signals".

Supernatants from thymic epithelial cell cultures derived from the mouse and human thymus have been shown by several group of investigators to contain a variety of cytokines (discussed in ref. 2). Interestingly, many of these cytokines (including IL-1, IL-3, IL-6, IL-7, TNF and several CSFs) have been shown to be produced by the cell lines in the absence of "deliberately-added" mitogens although the possibility that factors present in the culture media (sera) may be responsible for the induction of their production cannot be excluded. Our own in vivo studies have demonstrated the constitutive production of several cytokines by stromal cells in situ in the fetal thymus. These findings suggest that some of the in vitro grown cell lines may have equivalent cell populations in vivo. In these studies, we have used in situ hybridization to detect cytokine-specific gene expression within isolated populations of fetal thymic stromal cells (Fig. 2).

Disaggregated populations of thymocyte-depleted thymuses isolated from embryos at different stages of gestation were found to contain cells expressing IL-1α, IL-1β, IL-3 and IL-6. In additional experiments we have been unable to detect expression of several other cytokine encoding genes including IL-2, IL-4, IL-5, granulocyte macrophage colony stimulating factor [GM-CSF], IFN-γ and TNF, in fetal thymic stromal cells. However, studies of others have provided evidence for the production of cytokine protein by thymic stromal cells; immunohistochemical studies using monoclonal anti-cytokine antibodies and thymic tissue sections have shown that human fetal thymic epithelial cells produce IL-1 and G-CSF.[25]

Our subsequent analysis of highly enriched thymic epithelial cell preparations have shown that the IL-1β mRNA expression detected in the more heterogenous stromal cell preparations (Fig. 2) is restricted to bone marrow-derived cells and IL-1α restricted to a population(s) of epithelial cells (S.R. Carding, E.J. Jenkinson and J.J.T. Owen, unpublished observations). It is possible that cytokine production by thymocytes and stromal cells within the fetal thymus is coordinately regulated as a result of selective thymocyte-stromal cell interactions. For example, the appearance of IL-1α and IL-1β in the developing thymus may be a consequence of the sequential contact of thymocytes with bone marrow-derived stromal cells and

epithelial cell populations during their development. Indeed, analysis of thymic microenvironments after thymic reconstitution in chimeric mice has indicated that the earliest discernable interaction of thymocytes and stromal cells occurs with major histocompatability complex (MHC) class II⁻ cortical epithelial cells and class II⁺ dendritic cells.[26] As a consequence of such interactions, stromal cells may produce cytokines which thymocytes utilize directly as growth factors. Alternatively, stromal cell-derived cytokines may be responsible for inducing the production of distinct cytokines by thymocytes themselves. For example the production of IL-2 and/or IL-4 by fetal thymocytes may be dependant upon the production of IL-1 by stromal cells. This may explain an observation by Rothenberg and colleagues[27] demonstrating that exogenously-added IL-1 can

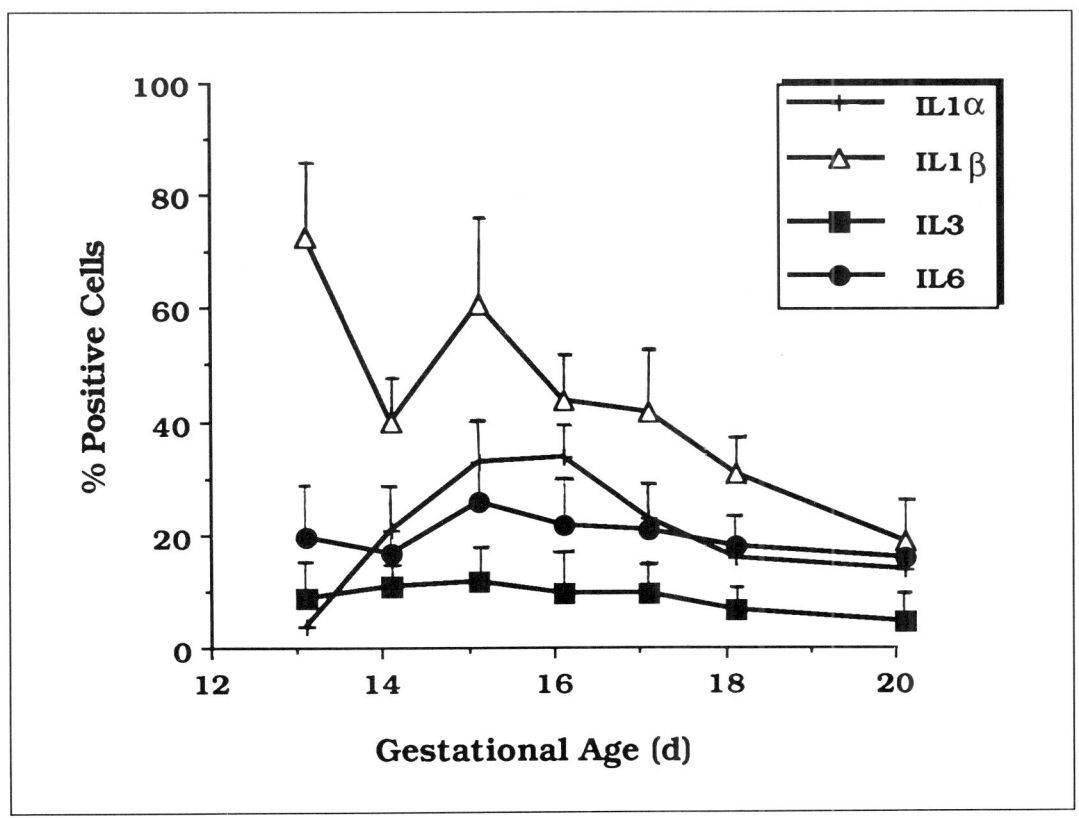

Fig. 2. Cytokine gene expression by thymic stromal cells throughout fetal thymic development. Cytokine specific mRNA was detected in thymocyte-depleted preparations of fetal thymic stromal cells by in situ hybridization as described previously.[20]

induce IL-2 gene expression in TcR⁻ but not TcR⁺ thymocytes in vitro. The authors also demonstrated that IL-1-dependent IL-2 producing TcR⁻ thymocytes appear before IL-1-independent IL-2-producing TcR⁺ thymocytes in the thymusesof radiation chimeras. This observation confirms the findings from our studies that the IL-2 gene locus is inducible in immature T cells[20] and quite possibly by IL-1. Likewise, there may be reciprocal signaling from the thymocytes that regulates the expression of genes such as those encoding MHC antigens on stromal cells.[28,29] IL-1 may also be able to induce the production of other cytokines, for example IL-6 by stromal cells which synergistically acts with IL-1 in stimulating thymocyte proliferation.[30] In response to IL-1, connective tissue fibroblasts have been shown to secrete high levels of IL-6,[31] suggesting that thymic reticular fibroblasts could respond to epithelial cell-derived IL-1 in a similar manner. Clearly, these studies represent only a preliminary attempt to determine the contribution thymic stromal cells make to cytokine production within the fetal thymus. More detailed studies of cytokine production by phenotypically and morphologically distinct populations of epithelial and other stromal cells need to be determined in order to obtain a clearer understanding of their role in thymic development.

The observation that day 12 fetal thymic rudiments stripped of their mesenchymal capsule fail to support T-cell development suggests that mesenchymal-derived fibroblasts play an important role in promoting T-cell development.[32,33] These findings have been confirmed by very recent in vitro thymic reconstitution studies in which the early stages of T-cell development (day 14 fetal precursors) have been shown to be dependent upon fibroblast products.[34]

In summary, the analyses of cytokine production within the fetal thymus have shown that it is characterized by: 1) their transient production, which for the majority of cytokines studied to date is defined by a peak of production by thymocytes[2] and stromal cells (Fig. 2) at around day 15 of gestation in the mouse; 2) the limited and selective production of cytokines; 3) the different frequencies of cells expressing different cytokine mRNA or protein and 4) a striking parallel in the expression of cytokine receptors by thymocytes during T-cell ontogeny.

Up until day 15 of fetal thymic development the vast majority of thymocytes have yet to express CD4, CD8 or the TcR/CD3 receptor complex. In addition, the initiation of CD3/TcR expression by thymocytes in the fetal[20,35-39] and adult[40] thymus is strikingly coordinate with the downregulation of IL-2 receptor (IL-2R) expression. Consequently, it is possible that the cytokines (in particular IL-2) produced within the thymus at this time play a role in initiating or promoting the activation and expression of the genes that encode the TcR/CD3 complex (Nikolic-Zugic, personal communication), thereby regulating the progression of T cell development. Alternatively, they may be utilized as autocrine or paracrine growth factors to promote the expansion and growth of developing T cells and/or stromal cell populations.

CYTOKINE UTILIZATION WITHIN THE FETAL THYMUS

The implication that the cytokines produced within the thymus can be productively utilized requires an indication that appropriate receptors for these molecules are expressed by developing T cells within the thymus. Although expression of several cytokine receptor complexes by T-cell precursors in the developing thymus have been analyzed to date, the IL-2R and the IL-2/IL-2R signaling pathway has been the most extensively studied.

THE IL-2 RECEPTOR

It is now widely accepted that the majority of thymocytes in the fetal thymus express receptors for IL-2 in a developmentally-regulated manner;[36-39] maximal numbers of IL-2R⁺ cells being apparent at day 15 of gestation. However, the functional significance of these receptors has been an area of considerable controversy. Experiments in which IL-2R⁺ fetal thymocytes have been shown to be unable to proliferate in response to exogenous IL-2[36-38] and the demonstration that these receptors are of only low affinity and are unable to internalize bound IL-2[41,42] all argue for these receptors being nonfunctional. On the other hand, studies demonstrating that day 15 and day 16 mouse fetal thymocytes express both high and low affinity IL-2R[43] and that IL-2 induced proliferation of IL-2R[+] mouse and human fetal thymocytes[44-49] argue that the IL-2/IL-2R signaling pathway is operational in IL-2R[+] fetal thymocytes. These apparently conflicting studies may be reconciled by a requirement for an intact thymic microenvironment for fetal thymocytes to respond to IL-2.[43,50,51] Indeed, it has been shown that intact fetal thymic lobes cultured in IL-2 exhibit an in vitro proliferative response to IL-2 at a concentration (20-40pM) corresponding to the equilibrium dissociation constant (kD of between 7 and 29pM) of high affinity IL-2Rs.[43] The requirement of an intact thymic environment may reflect the need for intercellular interactions between T-cell precursors and stromal cells. For example, such interactions may be required for the induction or upregulation of the β and/or γ-chain components of the IL-2R by fetal thymocytes, allowing the formation of IL-2Rαβ and/or IL-2Rαβγ receptors which have approximately 10- or 100-fold greater affinity, respectively, for IL-2 than receptors composed of the single α chain.[52] More direct evidence for the requirement of developing T-cell precursor populations to express functional IL-2Rs that are composed of β and/or γ chains has recently been obtained.

Structure-function studies of the IL-2R have demonstrated that the β-chain plays a critical role in transducing the IL-2-induced mitotic signal(s) in hematopoietic cell lines,[53-55] implying that the utilization of the IL-2 produced within the fetal thymus may be restricted to IL-2Rβ[+] precursor cells. In one study,[56] IL-2Rβ expression in the fetal thymus has been shown to be restricted to a subset of IL-2Rα[-], γδ-TcR[+] thymocytes that are the thymic precursors of the skin, Thy.1[+] dendritic epidermal cells. The requirement for IL-2 for the development of these γδ T cells was demonstrated by the ability of an

anti-IL-2Rβ specific antibody to block their generation in the developing thymuses of embryos in utero or in fetal thymic organ culture (FTOC).

A central role for the γ chain and the IL-2/IL-2R signaling pathway in T-cell development has recently been demonstrated from the studies of human X-linked severe combined immunodeficiency (XSCID).[57] In this study the IL-2Rγ chain gene was mapped to the same region of the X chromosome as the SCID locus and, in all of the XSCID patients examined, mutations in the IL-2Rγ chain were identified. These findings imply that the production of a nonfunctional IL-2Rγ chain by T-cell precursor populations prevents their development resulting in an absence or dramatic reduction in the number of peripheral T cells characteristic of the SCID phenotype. Identification and isolation of an equivalent IL-2Rγ[+] T-cell precursor population in the mouse thymus should define its role in lineage development of intrathymic stem cell(s) and the role that the IL-2/IL-2R signaling pathway plays in promoting or regulating their development.

OTHER CYTOKINE RECEPTORS

Considering the limited availability of antibodies specific for cytokine receptors other than IL-2, experimental approaches other than immunochemical ones must be adopted in order to determine their profile of expression by developing T cells. Our laboratory has employed three different but complementary approaches to the analysis of IL-1, IL-2, IL-4 and TNF receptor expression by fetal thymocytes. Hybridization in situ using cytokine receptor specific probes and a reverse transcriptase-PCR (RT-PCR) assay have been used to visualize and determine the kinetics of cells expressing cytokine receptor-encoding genes in the fetal thymus, respectively. In addition, we have used a cytokine-receptor-ligand binding assay to identify and enumerate populations of developing T cells that express cell surface receptors for a variety of cytokines. This assay utilizes saturating amounts of a biotinylated-recombinant cytokine (IL-1α, IL-2, IL-4 and TNF-α) and a secondary gold-conjugated

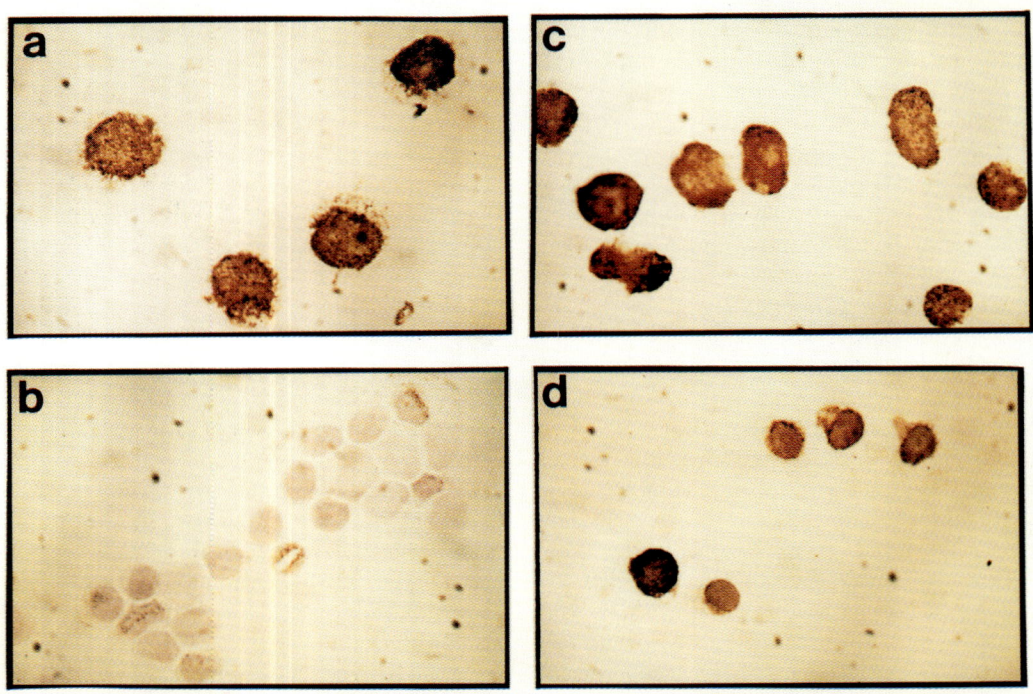

Fig. 3. Constitutive cytokine receptor expression by day 14 fetal thymocytes. Cell surface expression of IL-1 (a), IL-4 (c) and IL-2 (d) receptors were detected using a cytokine-ligand binding assay in which cytocentrifuge preparations of cells were incubated consecutively with biotinylated-recombinant cytokines, a monoclonal anti-biotin antibody conjugated to gold particles and a silver enhancement reagent to visualize receptor positive cells. Pre-incubation with excess native IL-1 virtually eliminates subsequent reactivity of biotinylated IL-1 with day 14 fetal thymocytes (b). Magnification x1600.

monoclonal anti-biotin antibody to visualize receptor-expressing cells. As can be seen in the photomicrograph of the results obtained from the analysis of cytokine receptor expression by day 14 fetal mouse thymocytes (Fig. 3), IL-1 (a), IL-2 (d) and IL-4 (c) receptors are expressed at high levels by the majority of these cells. The specificity of this assay is demonstrated by the capacity of native IL-1α to inhibit the binding of biotin-conjugated IL-1α (b). In presenting the results from a more comprehensive analysis of cytokine receptor expression throughout T-cell development (Table 2), it is apparent that the expression of receptors for all of the cytokines studied are developmentally regulated. Maximal numbers of IL-1, IL-2 and IL-4 receptor-positive thymocytes are evident between 13 and 15 of gestation, coincidental with the time in fetal thymic development at which the highest levels of IL-1, IL-2 and IL-4 were produced.

This coordinate production of many different cytokines by lymphoid and non-lymphoid cells of the fetal thymus may provide an explanation for the results obtained from several in vitro and in vivo experiments in which the influence of heterogenous cell populations on the development of T-cell precursors has been demonstrated.[2] In addition, these observations may also explain the general lack of responsiveness of in vitro cultured T-cell precursor populations to individual, exogenously supplied, cytokines.

Results from our own studies and those of several other groups investigating cytokine production and utilization in the fetal thymus are consistent with the hypothesis that several cytokines, particularly IL-1, IL-2 and IL-4, act in a coordinate manner to control the proliferation and differentiation of thymocytes in vivo. Clearly, there is now a need to develop experimental systems in which it is possible to selectively prevent the production of particular cytokines within the fetal thymus to more precisely define the role of these, and other, cytokines in T-cell development. It is important to acknowledge the contribution that the studies identifying the spatial and temporal production of cytokines and expression of cytokine receptors within the developing fetal thymus make to the design of functional studies. For example, as a result of these studies it is now possible to identify the stages of development and the target cell populations.

THE FUNCTION OF CYTOKINES IN FETAL THYMIC DEVELOPMENT

Historically, attempts at understanding the role(s) that cytokines play in T-cell development in the fetal thymus have relied upon the use of FTOC. FTOC supports

normal T-cell precursor proliferation and a program of T-cell development generating functionally competent T cells.[58] More recently, a variety of cytokine and cytokine receptor transgenic mice have been used to investigate the role cytokines play in T-cell development. Other approaches that have been used include the administration of anti-cytokine or anti-cytokine receptor antibodies to intact animals (reviewed in ref. 2).

FETAL THYMIC ORGAN CULTURE EXPERIMENTS

This system has been successfully used to demonstrate the developmental lineage of T-cell precursors and identify cytokines that are able to regulate proliferation and differentiation of thymocytes.[58] The addition of cytokine-specific antibodies and recombinant cytokines to cultured thymic lobes has demonstrated the direct involvement of several cytokines (IL-1, IL-4 and IL-7) in precursor proliferation and differentiation to functionally mature T cells (reviewed in ref. 2). For example the results from studies in which IL-4 or IL-7 were added to FTOC have

Table 2. Constitutive lymphokine receptor expression by populations of developing T cells

Cells (Source)	% Cells Expressing Lymphokine Receptors[#]			
	IL-1R	IL-2R	IL-4R	TNFR
Thymus (Embryo)				
13d	86 ± 3 (6)[*]	46 ± 3 (6)	81 ± 2 (9)	86 ± 4 (8)
14d	84 ± 2 (10)	87 ± 4 (6)	94 ± 5 (8)	82 ± 9 (9)
17d	64 ± 3 (8)	42 ± 5 (6)	49 ± 3 (5)	28 ± 5 (2)
18d	71 ± 6 (6)	23 ± 4 (4)	30 ± 4 (2)	17 ± 3 (6)
Thymus (Adult)				
CD4⁻, CD8⁻	63 ± 7 (3)	45 ± 5 (6)	62 ± 6 (6)	61 ± 4 (5)
Spleen (Adult)				
CD4⁺	3 ± 1 (1)	6 ± 2 (1)	31 ± 5 (3)	2 ± 1 (1)

Cytokine receptors were detected on surface of cells with biotinylated-recombinant lymphokines and a monoclonal anti-biotin/gold conjugated antibody. Receptor positive cells were visualized after development with a silver enhancement reagent.
[*] % Positive cells detected after pre-incubation of cells with excess native recombinant lymphokines.
[#] Values were obtained as the mean of the results from three independent experiments.

demonstrated that different cytokines are able to influence the development of T-cell precursors at different stages of their intrathymic development; the effects of IL-7 appear to be restricted to enhancing the growth of CD3$^-$4$^-$8$^-$ precursors[49] whereas IL-4 acts to regulate the development of more mature CD4$^+$8$^+$ thymocytes.[59] FTOC experiments investigating the role of IL-2 in T-cell development have, however, yielded apparently conflicting results. The addition of anti-IL-2 antibodies to FTOC has been shown to cause a 40% reduction in cell yield when compared to control cultures which appeared to be specific for IL-2R$^+$ subsets of CD3$^-$4$^-$8$^-$ fetal thymocytes, implying that IL-2 is required for their expansion.[43] However, contradictory results have been obtained from studies in which fetal thymic lobes have been cultured in the presence of exogenously added recombinant IL-2. Evidence for IL-2 being able to both promote[43,59] and abrogate[60,61] thymocyte proliferation and/or differentiation has been obtained. Similar conflicting results have been obtained from experiments in which anti-IL-2 receptor antibodies have been added to FTOC; the addition of antibodies specific for the α chain of the IL-2 receptor have been shown to either perturb[62] or have no effect[63] on T-cell precursor development. Although FTOC has not been as extensively used for the study of other cytokines in T-cell development as it has for IL-2, two different FTOC studies of IL-4 have also produced conflicting results. Whereas the addition of recombinant IL-4 to FTOC has been shown to impair the development of CD4$^+$8$^+$ fetal thymocytes,[59] the addition of neutralizing anti-IL-4 specific antibodies has been shown to have no obvious effects on the cellularity or thymocyte subsets in day 14 fetal thymic lobes after 12 days of culture.[64]

The contrasting results from the addition of antibodies and cytokines to FTOC may be related to differences in the accessibility of target cell populations within the thymus to each type of reagent; smaller cytokine molecules may be more effectively distributed throughout the thymus than much larger antibody molecules. In addition, slight variations in culture conditions may also contribute to conflicting FTOC results. For example, whether or not the lobes are cultured at an air-liquid interface or submerged in culture[48,49] and variations in the oxygen content of the media, the exact gestational age of the embryos from which thymuses are used and the timing of the addition of cytokines or antibodies to FTOC[65] can influence the outcome of these experiments. In addition, certain cytokines may be able to act as both positive and negative influences on T-cell precursors proliferation and/or differentiation. For example, whereas the addition of recombinant IL-7 to fetal thymuses in organ culture has been shown to preferentially enhance the proliferation of thymocytes SCA-1$^+$, CD3$^-$, 4$^-$ and 8$^-$. It also prevented this population from giving rise to CD4$^+$8$^+$ and αβ-TcR$^+$ thymocytes.[66] It is also possible that cytokines may act to promote or abrogate the expansion or differentiation of precursor cell populations at different stages of their development. In support of this concept preliminary results from our own studies using an IL-2-transgenic mouse, in which IL-2 producing cells in the fetal thymus can be selectively eliminated (see below), suggest that at different times in fetal thymic development IL-2 may act to promote and inhibit the proliferation and differentiation of T-cell precursor populations.

CYTOKINE/CYTOKINE RECEPTOR TRANSGENIC MICE

Until very recently the application of transgenic mice to the study of cytokines in T-cell development has used animals in which cytokines are constitutively produced or in which functional or nonfunctional cytokine receptors are expressed by cells in the thymus. Results from IL-2 receptor transgenic mice have provided evidence for the direct involvement of the IL-2/IL-2R signaling pathway in regulating the differentiation of T-cell precursor populations. The constitutive expression of the gene encoding the human IL-2Rα chain in the thymus of transgenic mice has been shown to allow thymocytes to respond to IL-2 in the absence of any other co-mitogen. This result implies that the additional chains (β and/or γ) required for expression of a functional IL-2R are normally constitutively expressed by subsets of thymocytes.[67] The generation of transgenic mice in which thymocytes express a non-functional hybrid IL-2R consisting of a human α-chain and a murine β-chain has been shown to result in a block in the development of CD4⁻8⁻ thymocytes,[68] consistent with the requirement for an intact and functional IL-2/ IL-2R signaling pathway in the development of T-cell precursor populations. Similarly, studies from mice that constitutively produce high levels of IL-4 in which the development and/or expansion of CD4⁺8⁺ cells was perturbed have been used as evidence for the stage-specific involvement of different cytokines in the intrathymic development of T cells.[69,70] The analysis of T-cell development in an IL-7-transgenic mouse has revealed a more subtle effect of constitutive cytokine production in the thymus.[71] Although there was no obvious difference in the distribution of the different thymocyte subsets as defined by CD4 and CD8 expression in these animals when compared to thymocytes from normal mice, a two to three-fold increase in total number of thymocytes was seen in the transgenic animals. From these results the authors have suggested that IL-7 may serve to promote the proliferation of T-cell precursors at several stages of their intrathymic development. However, due to the nonphysiological nature of all of these transgenic model systems the results they generate are difficult to interpret.

One of the most direct ways to study the role of any soluble factor in T-cell development would be to produce an animal defective in its expression of the gene that it encodes. Using homologous recombination in embryonic stem cells mice deficient in IL-2, IL-4, IL-10, IFN-γ and TGF-β have to date been generated and it is surely only a question of time before "knockout mice" for all of the other known cytokines are generated. In view of the large body of literature that has provided both indirect and direct evidence for the involvement of IL-2 and IL-4 in T-cell development it was disappointing to discover that the elimination of the expression of either the IL-2[72] or IL-4[73] gene

had no obvious effects on the generation of T cells in adult mice. In contrast to wild type mice, it would appear that in these "knockout mice" the IL-2 and IL-4 genes and the proteins they encode can be functionally replaced. This conclusion is supported by the observations made from the analyses of cytokine production and utilization within the fetal thymus: that cytokines appear to act together in a coordinated manner to regulate thymocyte proliferation and differentiation.[2] The elimination of one, therefore, may be masked or compensated for by qualitative or quantitative changes in the production of other cytokines. This is also not surprising considering the fact that all of these mice have successfully "adapted" and survived, albeit in the relatively protected environment of specific-pathogen free animal facilities, to adult life in the absence of these cytokines. Of course, another obvious, although less appealing, interpretation of the results from these "knockout mice" is that the IL-2 and IL-4 produced within the developing thymus is biologically inert and has no role in T-cell development. The results from the effects on T-cell development in mice deficient of both IL-2 and IL-4 may provide an indication of just how redundant the thymus is in its production and use of cytokines for regulating T-cell development.

Perhaps a better approach to investigating the role cytokines such as IL-2 and IL-4 might play in T-cell development would be to generate cytokine transgenic animals in which cytokine producing cells can be inducibly, specifically and selectively eliminated in vivo. In this system it may be possible to both minimize the effects of any compensatory mechanism(s) as well as identify qualitative and quantitative changes in the production of other cytokines within the fetal thymus made as a consequence of ablating IL-2 or IL-4 production. Such an experimental system would also be useful for studying not only the effects of cytokine deficiencies on T-cell development but also for identifying cooperative cytokine networks that might operate in the thymus during T-cell ontogeny in vivo. Such mice have recently been generated and we have begun to use them in our laboratory for investigating the role of IL-2 and IL-4 in T-cell development.

One conclusion that can be made from the functional studies of cytokines in T-cell development, including those using transgenic animals, is that perturbation of cytokine receptor expression and/or function appears to have a more profound effect on T-cell development than the blocking or raising the level of production of the corresponding cytokines. For example, defects in IL-2Rγ as seen in human XSCID result in a more dramatic loss of T cells than ablation of IL-2 production in the IL-2-knockout mice. One interesting possibility is that the IL-2Rγ chain may be shared by other cytokine receptors[57] which may enable cytokines other than IL-2 if present at sufficiently high enough concentrations and in the absence of IL-2 to interact with and deliver a mitotic signal via this chain of the IL-2R. Such a system would be analogous to the IL-3, IL-5 and GM-CSF receptors which share a common β-chain facilitating cross-talk among these cytokines at the receptor level.[74] Thus, the ability of cytokines other than IL-2 to signal through the IL-2R may provide the molecular basis for at least one compensatory mechanism that is operational in cytokine (IL-2)-deficient animals. Whether or not growth factor receptor chains are differentially expressed and participate in the reorganization of signaling pathways during T-cell development in the thymuses of wild type animals remains to be determined.

UNANSWERED QUESTIONS AND FUTURE DIRECTIONS

From the studies described here it is apparent that there are multiple and complex systems within the thymus that operate to regulate T-cell development. One of these systems may consist of a network of cytokines that act in a concerted and coordinate manner to initiate, promote or regulate the passage of developing T-cells through several stages of their intrathymic development.

Despite the many studies that have been carried out to investigate cytokines in T-cell development, we have still failed to answer several very important and fundamental questions. For example, we do not know with certainty the identity of the developing T cells within the fetal thymus that produce or respond to the cytokines detected in the fetal thymus. In addition, we do not know if all of the cytokines that can be or are produced within the thymus have in fact been identified. Even less is known about the nature of cytokine production and utilization by thymic stromal cells. Until these questions can be addressed, it will not be possible to design experiments to identify the molecules that mediate interactions between thymocytes and stromal cells resulting in cytokine production within the thymus and determine their function in T-cell development. Two important and recently developed model systems offer the promise of being able to answer some or all of these questions in the near future. The first advancement made is the development of a thymic reaggregation procedure which allows the effects of selectively removing different populations of lymphoid and non-lymphoid thymic cells on T-cell development to be studied in the in vitro-accessible FTOC system. Second, a novel cytokine transgenic mouse has been developed in which cytokine (IL-2 or IL-4)-producing cells can be inducibly and selectively eliminated. Thus, using this model system it should now be possible to identify the populations of IL-2 and IL-4-producing cells within the fetal thymus throughout T-cell ontogeny.

THYMIC REAGGREGATION CULTURES

In this system dispersed fetal thymic lobes are reaggregated using defined thymocyte and stromal cell populations under organ culture conditions that provide optimal support for T-cell development in vitro.[34,75] This procedure provides a means for determining the role of phenotypically distinct stromal cell populations on T cells at different stages of their intrathymic development. This model system has already been used to demonstrate that in the absence of a source of mesenchymal cells (fibroblasts) the thymus is unable to support the development of αβ TcR$^+$ T cells expressing CD4 and CD8 from day 14 fetal (CD4-,

CD8- and >97% αβ TcR-) thymocytes.[34] Interestingly 3T3 fibroblasts were able to substitute for fetal mesenchymal cells in supporting the maturation of 14-day precursors suggesting that thymic fibroblasts may influence T-cell development by contact-mediated mechanisms and by the production of soluble factors (cytokines?). In dispersing the lymphoid and stromal cell populations of the fetal thymus in this system cytokine-producing or -responding stromal cell populations are made more accessible to antibodies specific for cytokine or cytokine receptors enabling the role that the products of these cell types play in regulating specific developmental stages of T-cell ontogeny to be studied.

An Inducible Cytokine-Ablation Transgenic Mouse

Transgenic mice in which a toxic phenotype can be selectively induced in cells producing IL-2[76] and IL-4[77] have been produced. These mice were generated by injecting a suicide or toxic vector which was constructed by fusing the promoter sequences of the IL-2 or IL-4 gene to the coding sequence of the herpes simplex virus 1 thymidine kinase (HSV-TK) gene[78] into fertilized mouse eggs. When expressed, the viral TK enzyme is able to convert the exogenously supplied nucleoside analog ganciclovir (9[1,3-dihydroxy-2-propoxy (methyl)]guanine) to toxic intermediates which disrupt DNA replication and cause the death of any cytokine producing cell that coordinately expresses the HSV-TK gene product. The major advantage of this two-stage system is that neither component alone (TK or gancyclovir) is harmful yet together they yield a highly toxic phenotype. This achieves an important level of control over the potency and timing of cell death that is not possible with the conventional knockout system or that of other toxic transgenic mouse systems in which the diptheria toxin gene under the control of a specific promoter induces cell death.[79,80] This system not only allows the identification of cells producing IL-2 and IL-4 but also identifies those populations of developing T cells that do not produce but require these

cytokines for their growth or differentiation.

To date these animals have been incorporated into FTOC studies designed to identify at what stages in T-cell development IL-2 is produced and its cellular source in the fetal thymus. Using this system we have tentatively identified at least three different stages in T-cell development at which IL-2-producing cells are generated (Tannishtha, Flavell and Carding, unpublished observations). The first time period, identified from experiments in which stem cells from the TK-IL-2 transgenic mice were used to reconstitute deoxygauncsine-treated thymic lobes of nontransgenic fetal mice, occurs shortly after stem cells colonize the thymus. Subsequent to this stage of development IL-2-producing cells are also apparent among CD3-4-8- thymocytes. This is not surprising considering the large number of IL-2 mRNA+ cells that are also detected at this stage of development.[20,21,43] Finally, we have also demonstrated the production and subsequent ablation of IL-2-producing CD4+8- thymocytes in FTOC using fetal thymuses isolated from day 15-16 transgene-positive embryos. We are currently attempting to isolate and more extensively characterize the population(s) of cells, that may represent only a minor subset of developing T cells, that produce IL-2 at these different stages of T-cell ontogeny. More importantly, this inducible cytokine ablation system will allow us to design experiments, for example using the thymic reaggregation technique, to define the source of the inductive signals for IL-2 production by T-cell precursors and determine if IL-2 is required for their subsequent expansion and/or development.

In summary, these technical developments should enable us to more clearly understand the nature of the cellular mechanisms that operate to regulate normal T-cell development and the role(s) that cytokines play in them.

References

1. von Boehmer H. Developmental biology of T cells in T cell receptor transgenic mice. Ann Rev Immunol 1990; 8:531-549.
2. Carding SR, Hayday AC, Bottomly K. The

role of cytokines in T cell development: Immunol Today 1991; 12:239-245.

3. Jordan RK, Robinson JH, Waggot E. A qualitative and quantitative study of macrophages in the developing mouse thymus. J Anat 1979; 129:871-880.

4. Sminia T, van Arselt AA, van de Ende MB et al. Rat thymus macrophages: an immuno-histochemical study on fetal, neonatal and adult thymus. Thymus 1968; 8:141-150.

5. Boyd JD. Development of the thyroid and parathyroid glands and the thymus. Ann R Coll Surg Eng 1950; 7:445-459.

6. Le Douarin NM, Dieterlen-Lievre F, Oliver PD. Ontogeny of primary lymphoid organs and lymphoid stem cells. Am J Anat 1984; 170:261-299.

7. Owen JJT, Ritter MA. Tissue interaction in the development of the thymus lympho-cytes. J Exp Med 1969; 129:431-442.

8. Stutman O. Intrathymic and extrathymic T cell maturation. Transplant Rev 1978; 42:138-149.

9. Kindler V, Thorens B, Vassalli P. In vivo effects of murine recombinant interleukin 3 on early hematopoietic progenitors. Eur J Immunol 1987; 17:1511-1514.

10. Metcalf D. Hematopoietic growth factors and marrow transplantation: An overview. Transplant Proc 1989; 21: 2932-2933.

11. Heimfeld S, Weissman IL. Characterization of several classes of mouse hematopoietic progenitor cells. Curr Top Microbiol Immunol 1992; 177:95-105.

12. Moore MAS, Owen JJT. Experimental studies on the development of the thymus. J Exp Med. 1967; 126:715-725.

13. Jotereau FV, Houssaint E, Le Douarin NM. Lymphoid stem cell homing to the early thymic primordium of the avian embryo. Eur J Immunol 1980;10:620-627.

14. Fontaine-Perus JC, Calman FM, Kaplan C et al. Seeding of the 10-day mouse embryo thymic rudiment by lymphocyte precursors in vitro. J Immunol 1981; 126:2310-2316.

15. Jenkinson EJ, Franchi LL, Kingston R et al. Effects of deoxyguanosine on lympho-poiesis in the developing thymus rudiment in vitro; application in the production of chimeric thymus rudiments. Eur J Immunol. 1982; 12:583-587.

16. Pyke KW, Bach JF. The in vitro migration of murine fetal liver cells to thymic rudiments. Eur J Immunol 1979; 9: 317-323.

17. Champion S, Imhof BA, Savagner P et al. The embryonic thymus produces chemo-tactic peptides invovled in the homing of hematopoietic precursors. Cell 1986; 44:781-790.

18. Dunon D, Kaufman J, Salomonsen J et al. T cell precursor migration towards β_2-microglobulin is involved in thymus colonization of chicken embryos. EMBO J 1990; 9:3315-3322.

19. Picker LJ, Butcher EC. Physiological and molecular mechanisms of lymphocyte hom-ing. Ann Rev Immunol 1992; 10:561-591.

20. Carding SR, Jenkinson EJ, Kingston R et al. Developmental control of lymphokine gene expression in fetal thymocytes during T cell ontogeny. Proc Natl Acad Sci USA 1989; 86:3342-3347.

21. Yang-Snyder JA, Rothenberg EV. Devel-opmental and anatomical patterns of Il2-gene expression in vivo in the murine thymus. Dev Immunol 1993; 3:85-103.

22. Lampert IA, Ritter MA. The origin of the diverse epithelial cells of the thymus: Is there a common stem cell? In: Thymus Update. Vol. 1. New York: Harwood, 1990:5-25.

23. Brekelmans P, van Ewijk W. Phenotypic characterization of murine thymic micro-environments. Seminars Immunol 1990; 2:13-24.

24. Dardenne M, Bach J-F. Functional biology of thymic hormones. In: Thymus Update. Vol 1. New York: Harwood, 1990:101-133.

25. Haynes BF. Human thymic epithelium and T cell development: Current issues and fu-ture directions. Thymus 1990; 16:143-157.

26. Kyewski B. Seeding of thymic micro-environments defined by distinct thymocyte-stromal cell interactions is developmentally controlled. J Exp Med 1987; 166:520-538.

27. Rothenberg EV, Diamond RA, Pepper KA et al. IL-2 gene inducibility in T cells before T cell receptor expression. Changes in signalling pathways and gene expression requirements during intrathymic matur-ation. J Immunol 1990; 144:1614-1624.

28. Berrih S, Arenzana-Selsoedos F, Cohen S et al. Interferon-γ modulates class II antigen

expression on cultured human thymic epithelial cells. J Immunol 1986; 135: 1165-1171.

29. Kosaka H, Ogata M, Hikita I et al. Model for clonal elimination in the thymus. Proc Natl Acad Sci USA 1989; 86:3773-3777.

30. Helle M, Boeije L, Aarden LA. IL-6 is an intermediate in IL-1-induced thymocyte proliferation. J Immunol 1988; 142:4335-4338

31 Van Damme J, Cayphas S, Openakker G et al. Interleukin 1 and poly (rI) and ploy (rC) induce production of a hybridoma growth factor by human fibroblasts. Eur J Immunol 1987; 17:1-7.

32. Auerbach R. Morphogenetic interactions in the development of the mouse thymus gland. Dev Biol 1960; 2:271-284.

33. Auerbach R. Experimental analysis of the origin of cell type in the development of the mouse thymus. Dev Biol. 1961; 3:336-354.

34. Anderson G, Jenkinson EJ, Moore NC et al. MHC class II-positive epithelium and mesenchyme cells are both required for T cell development in the thymus. Nature 1993; 362:70-73.

35. Takacs L, Osawa H, Diamantstein T. Detection and localization by the monoclonal anti-interleukin 2 receptor antibody AMT-13 of IL-2 receptor-bearing cells in the developing thymus of the mouse embryo and in the thymus of cortisone-treated mice. Eur J Immunol. 1984; 14:1152-1156.

36. Raulet DH. Expression and function of interleukin-2 receptors on immature thymocytes. Nature 1985; 314:101-103.

37. Habu S, Okumuru K, Diamantstein T et al. Expression of interleukin 2 receptors on murine fetal thymocytes. Eur J Immunol 1985; 15:456-460.

38. von Boehmer H, Crisanti A, Kiesilow P et al. Absence of growth by most receptor-expressing fetal thymocytes in the presence of interleukin-2. Nature 1985; 314:539-540.

39. Penit C, Vasseur F. Cell proliferation and differentiation in the fetal and early postnatal mouse thymus. J Immunol 1989; 142:3369-3377.

40. Petrie HT, Pearse M, Scollay R et al. Development of immature thymocytes: Initiation of CD3, CD4 and CD8 acquisition parallels down-regulation of the interleukin

2 receptor alpha chain. Eur J Immunol 1990; 20:2813-2815.

41. Ceredig R, Lowenthal JW, Nabholz M et al. Expression of interleukin-2 receptors as a differentiation marker on intrathymic stem cells. Nature 1985; 314:98-100.

42. Lowenthal JW, Howe RC, Ceredig R et al. Functional status of interleukin 2 receptors expressed by immature (Lyt-2⁻/L3T4⁻) thymocytes. J Immunol 1986; 137:2579-2584.

43. Zuniga-Pflucker JC, Smith KA, Tentori L et al. Are the IL-2 receptors expressed in the murine fetal thymus functional? Dev Immunol. 1990; 1:59-66.

44. Hardt C, Diamantstein T, Wagner H. Developmentally controlled expression of IL-2 receptors and of sensitivity to IL-2 in a subset of embryonic thymocytes. J Immunol 1985; 134:3891-3894.

45. Hardt C, Fleischer S, Steinmetz M et al. Detection of rearranged T cell receptor β-chain gene and induction of cytolytic function in interleukin 2-responsive day 14-15 murine fetal thymocytes. Eur J Immunol 1986; 16:1087-1092.

46. Toribio ML, DeLaHera A, Marcos MAR et al. Activation of the interleukin 2 pathway precedes CD3-T cell receptor expression in thymic development. Differential growth requirements of early and mature intrathymic subpopulations. Eur J. Immunol 1989; 19:9-15.

47. Toribio ML, Gutierrez-Ramos JC, Pezzi L et al. Interleukin-2-dependent autocrine proliferation in T-cell development. Nature 1989; 342:82-85.

48. Ceredig R, Medveczky J, Skulimowski A. Mouse fetal thymus lobes cultured in IL-2 generate CD3⁺, TcR-γδ-expressing CD4⁻/CD8⁺ and CD4⁻/CD8⁻ cells. J Immunol 1989; 142:3353-3360.

49. Watson JD, Morrisey PJ, Namen AE et al. Effect of IL-7 on the growth of fetal thymocytes in culture. J Immunol 1989; 143:1215-1222.

50. Papiernik M, Penit C, Rouby SE. Control of prothymocyte proliferation by thymic accessory cells. Eur J Immunol 1987; 17:1303-1310.

51. Denning SM, Kurtzberg J, Le PT et al. Human thymic epithelial cells directly

induce activation of autologous immature thymocytes. Proc Natl Acad Sci USA. 1988; 85:3125-3129.

52. Minami Y, Kono T, Miyazaki T et al. The IL-2 receptor complex: Its structure, function and target genes. Ann Rev Immunol 1993; 11:245-267.

53. Tsudo M, Goldman CK, Bongiovani KF et al. The p75 peptide is the receptor for interleukin 2 expressed on large granular lymphocytes and is responsible for interleukin 2 activation of these cells. Proc Natl Acad Sci USA 1987; 84: 5394-5397.

54. Siegel JP, Sharon M, Smith PL et al. The IL-2 receptor βchain (p70): Role in mediating signals for LAK, NK and proliferative activities. Science 1987; 238:75-78.

55. Hatakeyama M, Mori H, Doi T et al. A restricted cytoplasmic region of IL-2 receptor β chain is essential for growth signal transduction but not for ligand binding and internalization. Cell 1989; 59:837-845.

56. Tanaka T, Takeuchi Y, Shiohara T et al. In utero treatment with monoclonal antibody to IL-2 receptor β-chain completely abrogates development of Thy.1+ dendritic epidermal cells. Int Immunol 1992; 4:487-491.

57. Noguchi M, Yi H, Rosenblatt HM, Modi WS et al. Interleukin 2 receptor γ-chain mutation results in X-linked severe combined immunodeficiency in humans. Cell 1993; 73:147-157.

58. Jenkinson EJ, Owen JJT. T-cell differentiation in thymus organ cultures. Sem Immunol 1990; 2:51-58.

59. Plum J, De Smedt M, Leclercq G et al. Inhibitory effects of murine recombinant IL-4 on thymocyte development in fetal thymus organ cultures. J Immunol 1990; 145:1066-1073.

60. Skinner M, Le Gros G, Marbrook J et al. Development of fetal thymocytes in organ cultures: effect of IL-2. J Exp. Med 1987; 165:1481-1493.

61. Waanders GA, Godfrey DI, Boyd RL. Modulation of T cell differentiation in murine fetal thymus organ cultures. Thymus 1989; 13:73-82.

62. Jenkinson EJ, Kingston, Owen JJT Importance of the IL-2 receptors in intrathymic

generation of cells expressing T cell receptors. Nature 1987; 329:160-162.

63. Plum J, deSmedt M. Differentiation of thymocytes in fetal organ culture: lack of evidence for the functional role of the interleukin-2 receptor expressed by prothymocytes. Eur J Immunol 1988; 18:795-799.

64. Plum J, De Smedt M, Tison B et al. Influence of antibodies neutralizing cytokines on murine fetal thymic organ culture. Thymus 1989; 13:83-93.

65. Kyewski B, Hunig T. Taking the thymus to pieces. Immunol Today. 1992; 13:288-290.

66. Plum J, De Smedt M, Leclercq G. Exogenous IL-7 promotes the growth of CD3⁻CD4⁻CD8⁻CD44+CD25+/⁻ precursor cells and blocks the differentiation pathway of TcR-αβ cells in fetal thymus organ culture. Int Immunol 1993; 150:2706-2716.

67. Nichi M, Ishida Y, Honjo T. Expression of functional interleukin-2 receptors in human light chain/Tac transgenic mice. Nature 1988; 331:267-269.

68. Gutierrez-Ramos JC, Martinez AC, Kohler G. Analysis of T cell subpopulations in human IL-2R-alpha transgenic mice: Expansion of Thy.1.2⁻ thymocytes and depletion of double-positive T cell precursors. Immunol Res 1990; 140:661-674.

69. Tepper RI, Levinson DA, Stanger BZ et al. IL-4 induces allergic-like inflammatory disease and alters T cell development in transgenic mice. Cell 1990; 62:457-467.

70. Lewis DD, Yu CC, Forbush KA et al. Interleukin 4 expressed in situ selectively alters thymocyte development. J Exp Med 1991; 173:89-100.

71. Samaridis J, Casorati G, Traunecker A et al. Development of lymphocytes in interleukin-7 transgenic mice. Eur J Immunol 1991; 21:453-460.

72. Schorle H, Holtschke T, Hunig T et al. Development and function of T cells in mice rendered interleukin-2 deficient by gene targeting. Nature 1991; 352:621-624.

73. Kuhn, R, Rajewsky K, Muller W. Generation and analysis of interleukin-4 deficient mice. Science 1991; 254:707-710.

74. Miyajima A, Kitamura T, Harada N et al. Cytokine receptors and signal transduction.

Ann Rev Immunol 1992; 10:295-331.

75. Jenkinson E, Anderson G, Owen JJT. Studies on T cell maturation on defined thymic stromal cell populations in vitro. J Exp Med 1992; 176:845-853.

76. Minasi L-A, Kamogawa Y, Carding SR et al. The selective ablation of interleukin 2-producing cells isolated from transgenic mice. J Exp Med 1993; 177:1451-1459.

77. Kamogawa Y, Minasi L-A, Carding SR et al. The relationship of IL-4 and IFN-γ producing T cells studied by lineage ablation of IL-4-producing cells. Cell 1993; 75:1220-1228.

78. Borelli E, Heyman R, Hsi M et al. Targeting of an inducible toxic phenotype in animal cells. Proc Natl Acad Sci USA 1988; 85:7572-7576.

79. Palmiter RD, Behringer RR, Quaife CJ et al. Cell lineage ablation in transgenic mice by cell-specific expression of a toxin gene. Cell 1987; 50:435-443

80. Breitman ML, Clapoff S, Rossant J et al. Genetic ablation: Targeted expression of a toxin gene causes microphthalmia in transgenic mice. Science 1987; 238:1563-1565.

81. De Luca D, Mizel SB. I-A-positive non-lymphoid cells and T cell development in murine fetal thymus organ cultures: Interleukin 1 circumvents the block in T cell differentiation induced by monoclonal anti-I-A antibodies. J Immunol 1986; 137:1435-1441.

82. Wiles M.V, Ruiz P, Imhof BA. Interleukin-7 expression during mouse thymus development. Eur J Immunol 1992; 22:1037-1042.

83. Deman J, Martin M-T, Delvenne P et al. Analysis by in situ hybridization of cells expressing mRNA for tumor-necrosis factor in the developing thymus of mice. Dev. Immunol. 1992; 2:103-109.

CYTOKINES
IN THE ADULT THYMUS

Albert Zlotnik

Gregory S. Kelner

In the past ten years increased attention has been focused on the possible role of cytokines in T-cell development. The goal of this chapter is to bring the field up to date on the importance and role of various cytokines during T-cell development. Recently, there have been several major developments that deserve special attention. Among these are the production of various cytokine-deficient mice by homologous recombination and the effects (or lack thereof) of these mutations on T-cell development in the thymus. This chapter is not intended to be a comprehensive review of the literature but rather to highlight what we consider the state of the art knowledge about the possible role of each cytokine during T-cell development in the adult mouse thymus.

As discussed in detail elsewhere in this book, T-cell development is a highly complex process that starts with pre-T-cell colonization of the thymic stromal component during fetal gestation. The interaction of pre-T cells with the stromal components of the thymus results in the proliferation and differentiation of these early pre-T cells, and it is likely that several cytokines mediate some of these processes. During early T-cell development two pivotal events include the irreversible commitment to the T-cell lineage and the rearrangement of the β and γ chain T-cell receptor (TcR) loci.[1] We have recently identified the stage of T-cell development (Fig. 1) where this rearrangement occurs within the adult murine thymus, as CD25$^+$ triple negative (TN)(CD3$^-$CD4$^-$CD8$^-$) thymocytes downregulate the expression of CD44 and *ckit*.[1] The latter molecule is the receptor for a cytokine, stem cell factor (SCF),[2] which is likely to play a pivotal role during T-cell development. Following these events, TN thymocytes become CD44$^-$25$^+$ and receive signal(s) that will induce the expression of CD4 and CD8 in these cells. These cells then downregulate CD25 to become CD44$^-$CD25$^-$"TN". The latter subset is known to undergo a process called "programmed differentiation" in vitro by which they spontaneously express CD4, CD8 and the

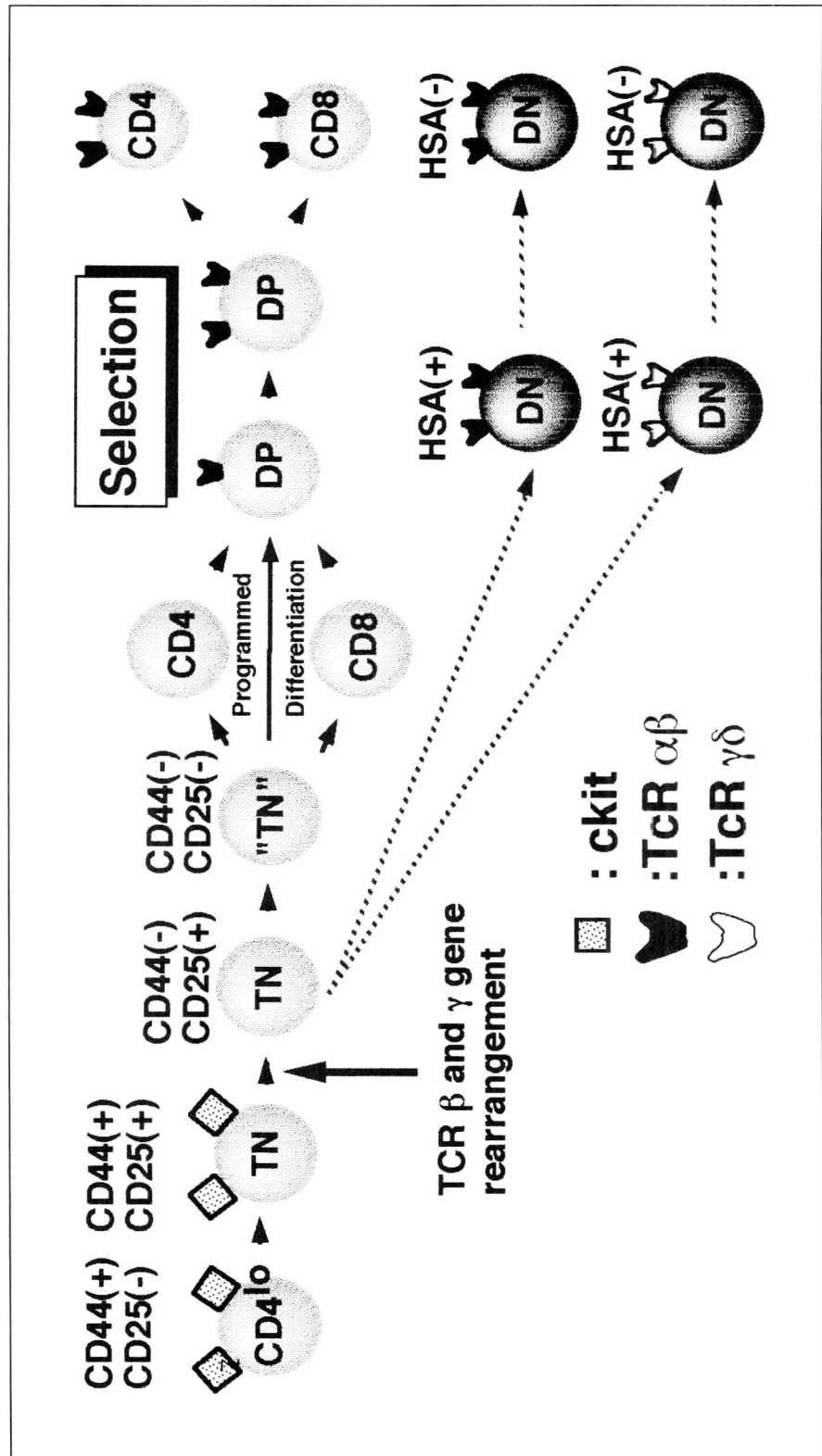

Fig. 1. Model of T-cell development in the mouse thymus. TN: triple negative CD4⁻CD8⁻CD3⁻ cells. DN: Double negative CD4⁻CD8⁻ cells. DP: Double positive CD4⁺CD8⁺ cells. Programmed differentiation refers to the acquisition of CD4 and CD8 markers by CD44⁻CD25⁻"TN" in vitro.

TcR αβ.[3,4] This phenomenon occurs because they are already actively transcribing mRNA for all of these molecules, as well as undergoing TcR α chain rearrangement. These cells are direct precursors of CD4+CD8+ thymocytes, and are, in fact, CD4loCD8lo although their expression of these cell surface molecules is very low making them appear phenotypically within the TN subset (hence the "TN" designation). These cells differentiate to become CD4+CD8+ and continue to upregulate the TcR and undergo positive and negative selection. Finally, the post-selection cells downregulate either CD4 or CD8 to become CD4+CD3+ or CD8+CD3+ thymocytes. The latter subsets are direct precursors of the cells that migrate to the periphery.

A summary of the cytokine production potential of various thymocyte subsets from the adult mouse thymus[1,5-8] is shown in Fig. 2 and the cytokine responsiveness of various subsets[1,5,8-16] is shown in Fig. 3.

CYTOKINES AND POSITIVE AND NEGATIVE SELECTION IN THE THYMUS

While the mechanisms of positive and negative selection have been the focus of attention in many laboratories for some time, the role that cytokines may play in these processes, if any, remains obscure. Specifically, we and others[5,6,8] have been unable to demonstrate detectable cytokine production by mouse CD4+CD8+ thymocytes, and these cells also fail to proliferate to any significant extent with a variety of cytokine combinations.[12,15] These observations are significant, since it has been possible to find cytokine production and/or combinations of cytokines that induce the proliferation of almost all other thymocyte subsets (including more mature and more immature subsets than CD4+CD8+). It could be argued that this failure to demonstrate immune function in CD4+CD8+ thymocytes is due to a high rate of apoptosis in these cells (due to positive and negative selection). However, we have recently observed that the direct precursors of CD4+CD8+ thymocytes (CD44-CD25-"TN"; see above) which are not likely to have been subjected yet to either positive or negative selection already show this inability

to produce cytokines.[5] This observation suggests that the lack of immune function is an event programmed in these cells prior to their differentiation to the CD4+CD8+ stage. Furthermore, we have recently observed that the early pre-T cells (that have not yet rearranged their TcR genes) are capable of producing high titers of IL-2, IFN-γ and TNF-α when activated with calcium ionophore, phorbol ester and IL-1 (Fig. 2).[1] As these cells progress down the TN differentiation pathway, they gradually lose their ability to produce cytokines until they reach the CD44-CD25-"TN" stage when the ability to produce cytokines is no longer detectable.[1] Taken together, these observations suggest that there is an active process to "shut down" immune functions in developing T cells prior to the CD4+CD8+ stage. These observations lead to a hypothesis we have proposed previously,[5,8] namely, that this lack of immune function reflects a "fail-safe" mechanism through which developing T cells that have not yet been selected as nonself reactive are rendered nonfunctional until selection is complete. Following selection, this hypothesis would predict that immune function is restored. The data in Figure 2 shows this prediction to be generally correct. However, some details do not necessarily fit this hypothesis. While CD4+CD3+ thymocytes have been shown to be active cytokine producers[5,8] there are two subsets within this population defined by expression of the heat-stable antigen (HSA). HSA+CD4+CD3+ cells are more immature than HSA-CD4+CD3+ thymocytes (the latter is essentially the phenotype of mature peripheral T cells). Only HSA-CD4+CD3+ cells produce cytokines in response to anti-CD3 stimulation[6] even though both HSA+ and HSA- subsets are likely to represent post-selection cells. Therefore, it appears that the restoration of cytokine production potential does not exactly correlate with successful positive and negative selection, but rather, it reappears later as the cells are about to exit the thymus.

These observations suggest that cytokines play little or no role during positive or negative selection. On the other hand, there are some predictions for the possible role of

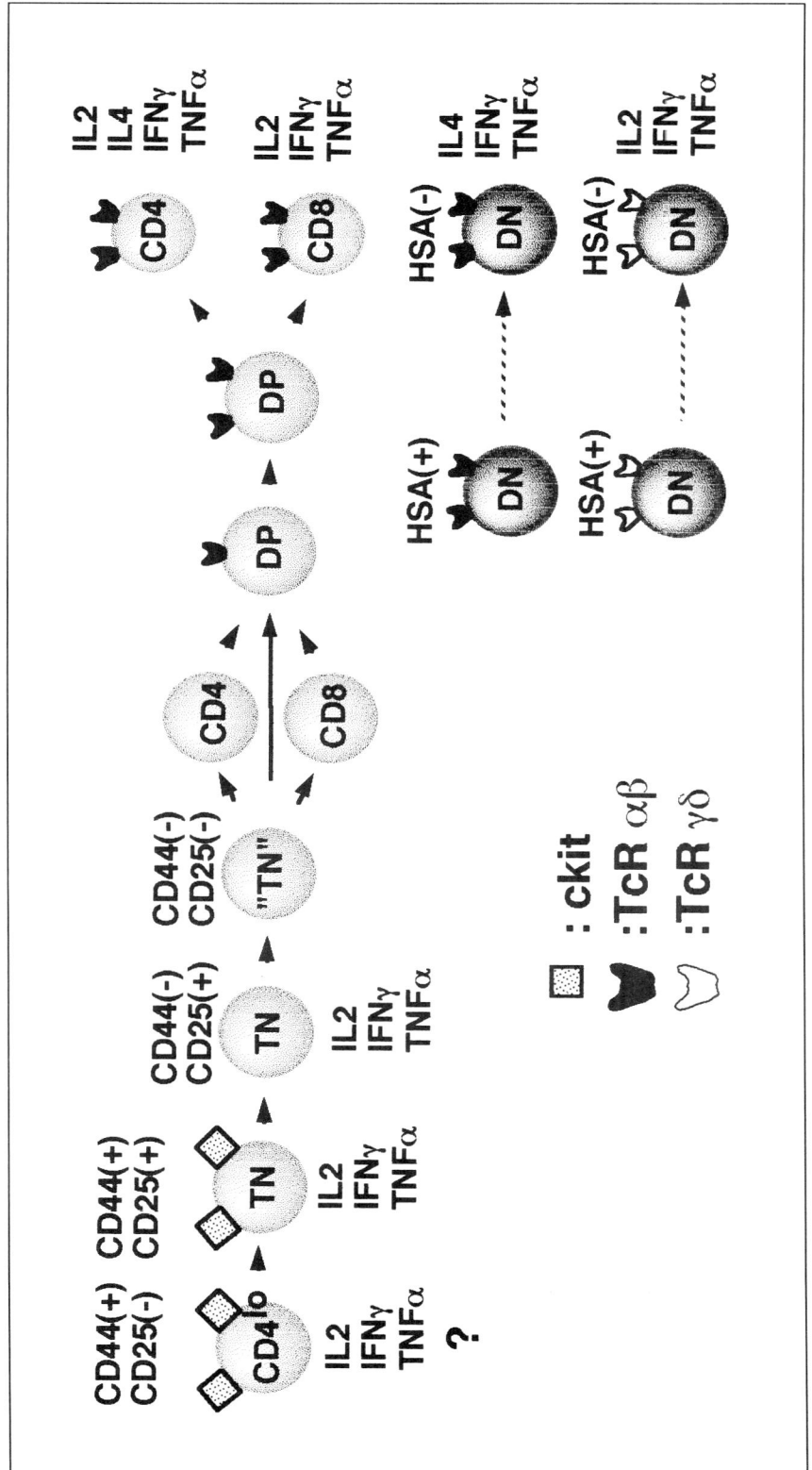

Fig. 2. Cytokine production potential of various thymocyte subsets during T-cell development. These studies refer only to the production capacity of four cytokines: TNF-α, IL-2, IL-4 and IFN-γ. The question mark indicates that the cytokine production potential of this subset was studied when these cells were contaminated with a CD44⁺CD25⁻ ckit⁻TN subset, probably belonging to the αβTcR+CD4-CD8-thymocyte lineage.[1]

cytokines during the CD4+CD8+ stage. One of these is that there must be a growth or maintenance factor for CD4+CD8+ thymocytes. This factor should be produced by either TN thymocytes, stromal cells or CD4+CD8+ thymocytes. We have not found such a CD4+CD8+ growth or maintenance factor, but this does not mean it does not exist. In fact, many of these CD4+CD8+ thymocytes (CD3[lo]) proliferate in the thymus.[17] If they require a signal to proliferate, it is likely that this signal involves an as yet unidentified cytokine. Alternatively, it is possible that CD4+CD8+ precursors may receive all the signals necessary to proliferate for up to three days and once these cells become CD4+CD8+ they may no longer require any additional proliferation stimuli. The latter hypothesis is supported by the fact that CD4+CD8+ thymocytes show significant viability for up to 2 days in vitro in regular culture media (A. Zlotnik and D.I. Godfrey, unpublished observation).

Finally, another potential role for cytokines may occur during selection, resulting in signals that initiate apoptosis. For example, IL-2 may induce apoptosis in certain thymocyte subsets.[18] And TNF-α has long been known to induce apoptosis in certain cell types. A new "cytokine" candidate that may also play a role in apoptosis is CD40 and its ligand, especially given the recent observation that CD40 is expressed by thymic epithelial cells,[19] an observation we have recently confirmed in the mouse thymus (A. Bean, M. Howard and A. Zlotnik, unpublished observation).

CYTOKINES PRODUCED BY STROMAL CELLS

Stromal cells are likely to be important sources of cytokines that may play critical roles in T-cell development. As discussed below, this prediction has already been shown to be correct in the case of IL-7 and SCF. A recent study has demonstrated that not only thymic epithelial cells are required, but fibroblastic cells and cells from the mesenchyme are necessary for successful T-cell development.[20] Thymic epithelial cells, and thymic macrophages have been studied for

their cytokine-producing ability,[12,20] which include IL-6, IL-7 and GM-CSF. In addition, we have observed IL-12 mRNA expression in thymic epithelial cells (J. Kennedy, G. Kelner and A. Zlotnik, unpublished observation).

ROLE OF CYTOKINES IN T-CELL DEVELOPMENT

INTERLEUKIN-1

IL-1 is one of the "oldest" cytokines available and one of the first to be reported to have effects during T-cell development.[21] One of the most commonly used methods to investigate the possible role of cytokines in T-cell development is the fetal thymus organ culture (FTOC). In this technique, a fetal mouse thymic lobe is cultured in vitro on a filter paper that sits on top of a gel-sponge (Gelfoam, Upjohn Co., Kalamazoo MI). The cytokine to be studied can be added in a known concentration to the culture medium and its effects on T-cell development can be monitored as the FTOC allows T-cell development to proceed to the point when the pattern of CD4 and CD8 expression of the thymocytes in the lobe resembles that observed in vivo in a normal thymus. This is the technique initially used by DeLuca and colleagues,[21] and subsequently by many other groups, to investigate the effects of cytokines or anti-cytokine antibodies during T-cell development. In some of these initial experiments, they observed that anti-Ia antibodies significantly inhibited FTOC development, whereas addition of exogenous IL-1 reversed this inhibition. A possible explanation for this effect comes from observations by Rothenberg et al[22] who reported that immature TN thymocytes were able to produce large amounts of IL-2 when activated with calcium ionophore, phorbol ester (PMA) and IL-1. We subsequently showed that the cells producing IL-2 in this fashion were located within the CD25+TN subset[8] and more recently that most early subsets of TN thymocytes produce various cytokines including IFN-γ (see Fig. 2) when activated by calcium ionophore, PMA and IL1.[1] A likely function of IFN-γ is the induction of class I

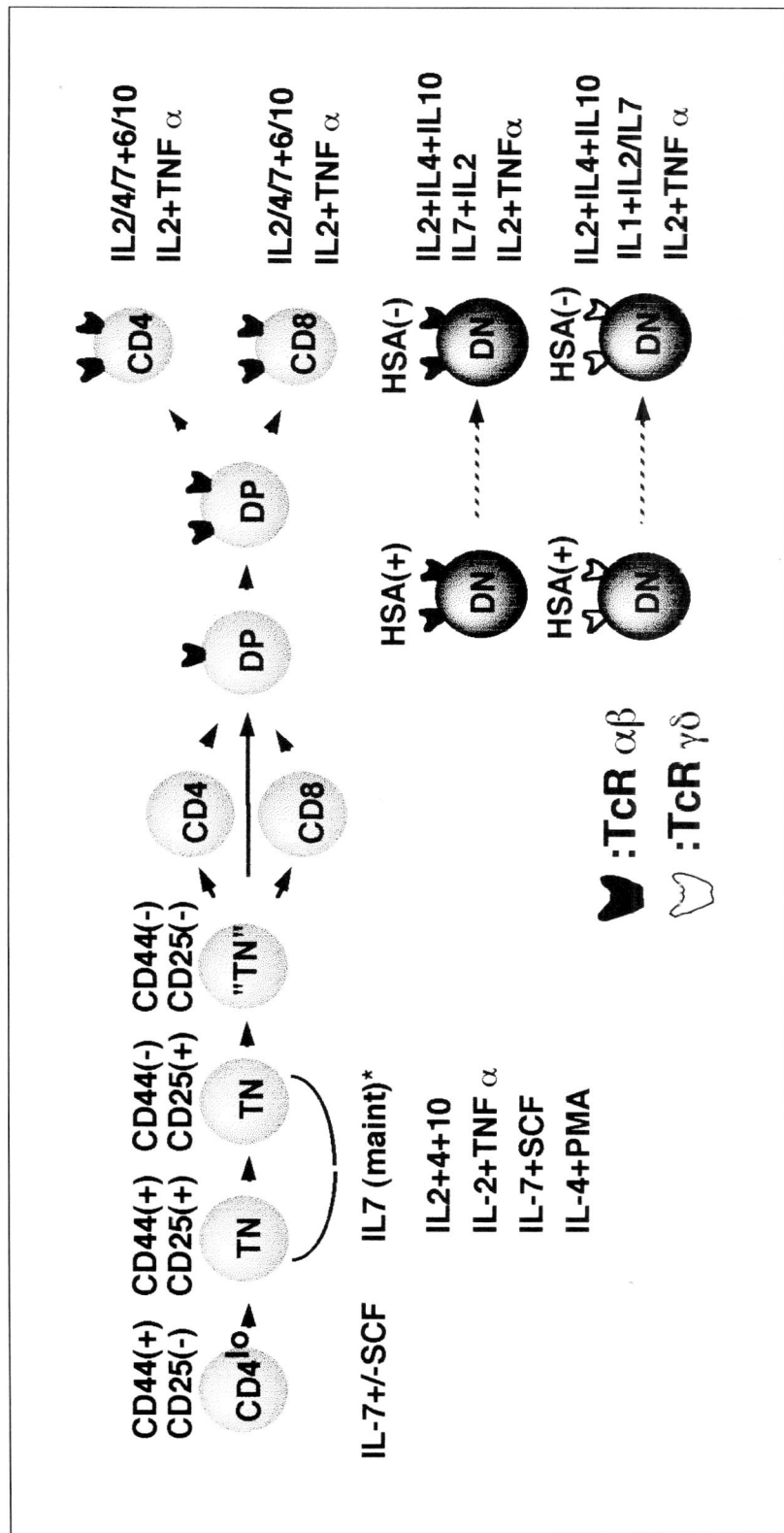

Fig. 3. *Proliferative ability of various thymocyte subsets to various cytokines or cytokine combinations. The (*) indicates that IL-7 plus SCF induce proliferation) only in the CD44+CD25+TN subset.¹ The target subset(s) (CD44+ or CD44+CD25+TN) of the other cytokine combinations (IL-2+IL-4+IL-10, IL-2+TNFa, IL-4+PMA) have not been defined yet.*

and class II MHC antigens in thymic stromal cells.[23] Thus, if IL-1 were neutralized in the early stages of TN development, it is possible that the production of IFN-γ may have been impaired. This in turn would lead to lower MHC antigen expression (which affects selection) and could explain the observations of DeLuca et al. We have recently reexamined this possible mechanism using IL-1 receptor antagonist (IL-1ra) to inhibit endogenous IL-1 in FTOC. We improved upon the earlier study by using a reconstituted FTOC system, where the thymic lobes are first depleted of lymphoid cells by culture in 2-deoxyguanosine. The lobe is then repopulated with defined purified precursor thymocytes (we used CD44⁻CD25⁺TN) (see Fig.1). In this system, the addition of IL-1ra led to a reduction in the number of cells recovered in the lobe (mostly in the CD4⁺CD8⁺) suggesting that IL-1 is necessary for the transition between TN and CD4⁺CD8⁺ thymocytes.

In addition, IL-1 has been implicated in the growth of γδTcR⁺CD4⁻CD8⁻ thymocytes.[16] In vitro, these cells grow well with IL-7, and their growth is costimulated with IL-1. However, there seems to be no data yet on the possible requirement for IL-1 for the development of these cells, although they probably arise from an IL-1 responsive CD25⁺TN precursor.[24]

INTERLEUKIN-2

IL-2 was also one of the first cytokines whose effects in T-cell development was investigated. Its perceived role was further supported by the fact that a subset of immature thymocytes expressed CD25, the α chain of the IL-2 receptor.[25] However, several studies have concluded that the expression of CD25 on these cells is probably not related to IL-2 responsiveness.[26] Nevertheless, these cells respond to IL-2 in combination with other cytokines (TNFa,[15] IL-4+IL-10[11]), and they are able to produce significant amounts of IL-2 in vitro, as discussed above. Recently, we have explored whether these cells make IL-2 in vivo, by probing by PCR for the presence of cytokine mRNA from freshly isolated, purified CD25⁺TN. We have found

positive signals for IL-2, IFN-γ and TNFa (G. Kelner and A. Zlotnik, unpublished observation). These data suggest that IL-2 is produced by these cells in vivo.

Schorle and colleagues have constructed an IL-2-deficient mouse by homologous recombination.[27] This mouse has been shown to have a phenotypically normal thymus, although it exhibits reduced immune responses and eventually dies from a syndrome resembling ulcerative colitis. While these observations suggest that IL-2 is not necessary for T-cell development, it is still possible that the changes caused by the absence of IL-2 reside in molecules or cell lineages that are still unknown. Thus, it is possible that the mature T cells present in these mice are not entirely normal, and that some of these abnormalities may be due to a lack of IL-2 during T-cell development.

INTERLEUKIN-4

IL-4 is a potent growth factor for various thymocyte subsets, especially in the presence of PMA.[28] However, we have been unable to detect its production by immature thymocytes in the adult thymus, although its production during fetal gestation in the mouse has been described by several groups.[29] As in the case of IL-2, an IL-4 deficient mouse has been constructed.[30] and its thymus appears phenotypically normal. In contrast to IL-2-deficient mice, these animals do not exhibit gross pathological conditions. It is therefore likely that IL-4 may not be necessary during T-cell development.

However, an interesting observation pertains to a novel subset of αβTcR⁺CD4⁻CD8⁻ T cells.[31] These cells are present in both the thymus and the periphery.[5] The expression of Vβ8.2 by many of these cells suggests that these cells undergo some kind of positive selection in the thymus.[24] possibly by an endogenous superantigen. We have observed that these cells produce large titers of IL-4 and IFN-γ in vitro.[5] In a related phenomenon, a subset of CD4+ thymocytes has also been shown to produce IL-4 upon activation in vitro. Both of these IL-4-producing cells (CD4⁺ or CD4⁻CD8⁻) exist in the spleen as well, and may participate in immune responses as sources of IL-4 that may drive TH0 cells to the TH2 (IL-4) producing phenotype.[6]

INTERLEUKIN-6

IL-6 is produced by a large variety of cells. In the thymus it is very likely that stromal cells produce large amounts of IL-6. We have observed that IL-6 is a thymocyte growth cofactor[6,12,15] and more specifically, its growth cofactor effect maps to CD4+CD3+ thymocytes.[10] An IL-6 deficient mouse has recently been produced at our Institute by R. Murray and S. Dalrymple, and its thymus is normal both in cell numbers and by extensive phenotypic analysis (D. Godfrey, A. Zlotnik , S. Dalrymple and R. Murray, unpublished observation). These results suggest that IL-6 is not required during T-cell development.

INTERLEUKIN-7

IL-7 was initially isolated and cloned on the basis of its pre-B cell activities.[32] It soon became clear that IL-7 had effects on both pre-T and T cells.[9] We observed that IL-7 induced proliferation of various thymocyte subsets and that thymic epithelial cells produced this cytokine.[12] IL-7 is a cytokine that is very likely to have important effects during early T-cell development. Another important observation concerns the effects of IL-7 on CD25+TN thymocytes. These cells can be cultured in IL-7 for several days, and then used to repopulate a lymphoid-cell depleted thymus successfully.[14] This is, to our knowledge, the first demonstration of the maintenance of a T-committed cell in vitro while maintaining its precursor potential intact. More recently, we have mapped the cells that survive under these conditions to the CD44+ subset of CD25+TN thymocytes. This observation is important since, as shown in Figure 1, these cells represent the last stage of T-cell development prior to TcR β and γ chain rearrangement.

Leclerq et al[33] have studied the effects of IL-7 in FTOC. Their results suggest that IL-7 may cause a delay in the maturation of pre-T cells. A similar conclusion has been reached by Rich et al[34] although Palacios et

al[45] observed larger cell numbers in all thymocyte subsets in another IL-7 transgenic mouse model. Taken together, these data suggest that IL-7 may be a critical factor in the development of TN thymocytes, by being responsible for the maintenance of their viability. It is likely that in conjunction with IL-7, SCF may be important in TN thymocyte development.

INTERLEUKIN-10

In 1989, we detected a novel cytokine that induced thymocyte proliferation in combination with IL-2 and IL-4.[13] This cytokine turned out to be the same as a new factor called cytokine synthesis inhibitory factor (CSIF)[36] and was eventually renamed IL-10.[37] IL-10 in combination with either IL-7 or IL-2 plus IL-4[11] induces proliferation in a variety of mature and immature thymocytes (essentially all subsets except CD4+CD8+ and their precursors; Figure 3). We performed a series of studies using IL-10 or anti-IL-10 in FTOC but were unable to demonstrate significant effects of this cytokine in these assays (I. MacNeil and A. Zlotnik, unpublished observations). Furthermore, an IL-10 deficient mouse has been produced by R. Kuhn, W. Mueller and K. Rajewsky and we have been able to analyze its thymus. Our phenotypic studies have failed to detect any abnormalities in the thymus of these mice (D.I. Godfrey and A. Zlotnik, unpublished observations). These results suggest that IL-10 is not required for normal T-cell development.

INTERLEUKIN-2

IL-12 is a novel cytokine[38] originally cloned from human B cells and called "cytotoxic T-cell maturation factor" that has also recently been cloned in the mouse.[39] We have recently observed that addition of IL-12 to FTOC results in altered T-cell development. It appears that IL-12 favors the development of CD3+ CD8+thymocytes, while having a negative impact on the transition between TN and CD4+CD8+ thymocytes. Interestingly, we have recently observed that IL-12 and SCF induce strong proliferation of CD44+CD25+ TN thymocytes. We are currently characterizing the cells that grow in these cultures.

Preliminary observations suggest that IL-12 mRNA is produced by thymic epithelial cells (J. Kennedy, D. Godfrey and A. Zlotnik, unpublished observation) and by freshly isolated CD44+CD25+TN thymocytes (G. Kelner and A. Zlotnik, unpublished observation). These results indicate that IL-12 is present during early T-cell development further suggesting that this cytokine plays an important role in T-cell development.

INTERFERON-γ

IFN-γ is an important cytokine that is likely to be involved in the expression of class I and class II MHC antigens by thymic stromal cells. The expression of these antigens is critical to successful positive and negative selection as both class I and class II MHC deficient mice have demonstrated.[40,41] Several reports have documented the ability of IFN-γ to induce class II MHC expression in thymic epithelial cells.[23] Furthermore, IFN-γ has been shown to be produced in the day 14 fetal thymus[29] and early pre-T cells in the thymus (CD44+CD25+TN) have the potential of producing IFN-γ (Fig. 2). While these observations strongly suggest that IFN-γ plays a role in the induction and maintenance of the expression of class II MHC antigens by the thymic stroma, a recent report documenting the production of an IFN-γ-deficient mouse indicates that this mouse has no apparent abnormalities in cell numbers or the distribution of CD4, CD8 and CD3 antigens in either the thymus or spleen.[42] While the latter observation implies that IFN-γ is not required during T-cell development, it is possible that there are other molecules capable of fulfilling the same function(s) that IFN-γ may have during T-cell development. The latter study did not document whether the expression of class I or class II MHC in the thymus of these animals was normal. Further experiments are also necessary to establish whether positive and negative selection are entirely unaffected by the IFN-γ deficiency during T-cell development.

STEM CELL FACTOR

SCF is a recently characterized cytokine that constitutes the defect of the Steel mouse.[2] While its name suggests that it acts on stem cells, formal proof of this contention is still lacking. Instead, it appears that this cytokine is a potent mast cell growth factor and also is capable of strongly synergizing the growth promoting activities of various other lineage-specific cytokines (GM-CSF, IL-2, G-CSF, etc.).[43,44] Insofar as T cells are concerned, very little information is available. However, a recent report[45] described the presence of c-kit (the receptor for SCF) on various thymocyte subsets, and our group has performed a more detailed analysis of the expression of this receptor.[46] c-kit is present on the most immature pre-T cells present in the thymus, and interestingly, its expression decreases at the exact point where T cells rearrange their TcR genes for the β and γ chain (Fig. 1). This observation suggests that SCF has effects on early progenitor cells that have not yet committed to the T-cell lineage. On CD44+CD25+TN thymocytes, SCF induces proliferation in combination with IL7 or IL-12 (D. Godfrey and A. Zlotnik, manuscript in preparation). We also observed that antibodies against c-kit exert a strong inhibitory influence on T-cell development in FTOC.[46] More recently, we have confirmed and extended these observations by demonstrating that the addition of anti-c-kit antibodies to FTOC depleted of lymphoid cells and repopulated with c-kit+CD44+CD25-TN thymocytes completely abrogates the ability of these cells to repopulate in FTOC.[46] This observation, to our knowledge, is the first demonstration of an absolute requirement for a cytokine during T-cell development, as well as mapping of the developmental step when this cytokine is required.

Galy and colleagues have documented the ability of thymic stromal cells to produce SCF.[47] This observation is not surprising since SCF was cloned from a stromal cell line[2] and further supports a role for SCF in pre-T-cell development. It remains to be defined what specific roles it may have during these events.

OTHER CYTOKINES

We have discussed the potential roles of various cytokines during T-cell development. There are other cytokines that may be important during T-cell development. These include TNF-α and TGF-β. We observed that the combination of these cytokines induces CD8 expression on CD25+TN cells maintained in culture in vitro with IL-7 (see above).[2,48,49] The cells generated in vitro with IL-7, TNF-α and TGF-β still have T-cell repopulation potential although some of them only expressed CD8α but not CD8β.[49] Based on these observations, we postulated that these cytokines were part of the normal signaling mechanisms that induce the expression of CD8 in TN thymocytes on their way to becoming CD4+CD8+ cells. We have since revised this opinion, given that the cells that survive in vitro under these conditions are mostly CD44+CD25+TN, not CD44⁻CD25+TN (the latter subset is normally the target of the signals that induce CD4 and CD8 for the transition from TN to CD4+CD8+ thymocytes, see Figure 1). It is nevertheless possible that these signals are part of this overall mechanism of differentiation, and that they also induce CD8 in the latter subset although this hypothesis at present is difficult to prove. We have not found conditions to maintain CD44⁻CD25+TN thymocytes alive in vitro while maintaining their repopulation potential.

Another cytokine with possible effects on T-cell development is IL-3. It has been implicated in the signals that induce commitment to the T-cell lineage in in vitro cultures based on embryonic stem cells.[50] It may have effects on the CD4ᴸᵒ earliest precursors (Fig. 1) but the difficulty of obtaining these cells in significant numbers makes these experiments technically difficult.

Other cytokines that can be demonstrated in the thymus include LIF, IFN-α, MCSF, IL-13, and GCSF. All of these are stromal cell products except IL-13. Very little information is available concerning possible effects of these cytokines in T-cell development, but they should be kept in mind in future experiments designed to investigate the signals that control T-cell differentiation.

CONCLUSION

We have reviewed the possible role that various cytokines may play in T-cell development. The amount of information that has become available on this topic has expanded significantly in the last few years, a trend motivated by the recognition of the important role that cytokines play in the control and development of the immune system. The future challenge should not focus as much on the individual role each cytokine plays, but rather, on studying specific steps along the developmental pathway that constitute important milestones for the developing T cell. These include: i) the commitment to the T-cell lineage of the immature lymphoid precursor that first enters the thymus; ii) the signals that induce rearrangement of the TcR β and γ chains, as well as the events that lead to the branching off of the γδ T-cell lineage from the main pathway; iii) the signals that induce CD4 and CD8 expression in the late TN thymocytes, and finally iv) possible roles of cytokines in positive and negative selection. The progress we have witnessed in the past few years suggests an optimistic view for the future resolution of these questions.

REFERENCES

1. Godfrey DI, Kennedy J, Zlotnik A. A developmental pathway involving four phenotypically and functionally distinct subsets of CD3-CD4-CD8- triple negative adult mouse thymocytes defined by CD44 and CD25 expression. J Immunol 1993; 150:4244-4252.

2. Zsebo KM, Wypych J, McNiece IK et al. Identification, purification, and biological characterization of hematopoietic stem cell factor from buffalo rat liver—conditioned medium. Cell 1990; 63:195-201.

3. Nakano N, Hardy RP, Kishimoto T. Identification of intrathymic T progenitor cells by expression of Thy-1, IL-2 receptor and CD3. Eur. J. Immunol 1987; 17:1567-1571.

4. Wilson A, Petrie HT, Scollay R et al. The acquisition of CD4 and CD8 during the differentiation of early thymocytes in short-term culture. Int. Immunol 1989; 1:605-612.

5. Zlotnik A, Godfrey DI, Fischer M et al. Cytokine production by mature and immature CD4-CD8- T cells. Alpha beta-T cell receptor+ CD4-CD8- T cells produce

IL-4. J Immunol 1992; 149:1211-5.

6. Bendelac A, Schwartz RH. CD4+ and CD8+ T cells acquire specific lymphokine secretion potentials during thymic maturation. Nature 1991; 353:68-71.

7. Hayakawa K, Lin BT, Hardy RR. Murine thymic CD4+ T cell subsets: a subset (Thy0) that secretes diverse cytokines and over-expresses the V beta 8 T cell receptor gene family. J Exp Med 1992; 176:269-74.

8. Fischer M, MacNeil I, Suda T et al. Cytokine production by mature and immature thymocytes. J Immunol 1991; 146:3452-6.

9. Conlon PJ, Morrissey PJ, Nordan RP et al. Murine thymocytes proliferate in direct response to interleukin-7. Blood 1989; 74:1368-1373.

10. Hodgkin PD, Cupp J, Zlotnik A et al. IL-2, IL-6, and IFN-gamma have distinct effects on the IL-4 plus PMA-induced proliferation of thymocyte subpopulations. Cell Immunol 1990; 126:57-68.

11. MacNeil I, Suda T, Moore KW et al. IL-10: a novel cytokine growth cofactor for mature and immature T cells. J. Immunol 1990; 145:4167-4173.

12. Murray R, Suda T, Wrighton N et al. IL-7 is a growth and maintenance factor for mature and immature thymocyte subsets. Int Immunol 1989; 1:526-31.

13. Suda T, O'Garra A, MacNeil I et al. Identification of a novel thymocyte growth-promoting factor derived from B cell lymphomas. Cell Immunol 1990; 129:228-40.

14. Suda T, Zlotnik A. IL-7 maintains the T cell precursor potential of CD3-CD4-CD8- thymocytes. J Immunol 1991; 146:3068-73.

15. Suda T, Murray R, Guidos C et al. Growth-promoting activity of IL-1 alpha, IL-6, and tumor necrosis factor-alpha in combination with IL-2, IL-4, or IL-7 on murine thymocytes. Differential effects on CD4/CD8 subsets and on CD3+/CD3- double-negative thymocytes. J Immunol 1990; 144:3039-45.

16. Lynch F, Shevach EM. Activation requirements of newborn thymic gamma delta T cells. J Immunol 1992; 149:2307-14.

17. Rothenberg EV. Death and transfiguration of cortical thymocytes: a reconsideration. Immunol Today 1990; 11:116-9.

18. Migliorati G, Nicoletti I, Pagliacci MC et al. Interleukin-2 induces apoptosis in mouse thymocytes. Cell Immunol 1993; 146:52-61.

19. Galy AH, Spits H. CD40 is functionally expressed on human thymic epithelial cells. J Immunol 1992; 149:775-82.

20. Anderson G, Jenkinson EJ, Moore NC et al. MHC class II-positive epithelium and mesenchyme cells are both required for T-cell development in the thymus. Nature 1993; 362:70-73.

21. DeLuca D, Mizel SB. I-A-positive nonlymphoid cells and T cell development in murine fetal thymus organ cultures: interleukin 1 circumvents the block in T cell differentiation induced by monoclonal anti-I-A antibodies. J Immunol 1986; 137:1435-41.

22. Rothenberg EV, Diamond RA, Pepper KA et al. IL-2 gene inducibility in T cells before T cell receptor expression. Changes in signaling pathways and gene expression requirements during intrathymic maturation. J Immunol 1990; 144:1614-24.

23. Ransom J, Fischer M, Mosmann T et al. Interferon-gamma is produced by activated immature mouse thymocytes and inhibits the interleukin 4-induced proliferation of immature thymocytes. J Immunol 1987; 139:4102-8.

24. Suda T, Zlotnik A. Origin, differentiation, and repertoire selection of CD3+CD4-CD8- thymocytes bearing either alpha beta or gamma delta T cell receptors. J Immunol 1993; 150:447-55.

25. Shimonkevitz RP, Husmann LA, Bevan MJ et al. Transient expression of IL-2 receptor precedes the differentiation of immature thymocytes. Nature 1987; 329:157-9.

26. Raulet DH. Expression and function of interleukin-2 receptors on immature thymocytes. Nature 1985; 314:101-3.

27. Schorle H, Holtschke T, Hunig T et al. Development and function of T cells in mice rendered interleukin-2 deficient by gene targeting. Nature 1991; 352:621-4.

28. Zlotnik A, Ransom J, Frank G et al. Interleukin 4 is a growth factor for activated thymocytes: Possible role in T cell ontogeny. Proc Natl Acad Sci USA 1987; 84:3856-3860.

29. Carding SR, Hayday AC, Bottomly K.

Cytokines in T-cell development. Immunol Today 1991; 12:239-45.

30. Kuhn R, Rajewsky K, Muller W. Generation and analysis of interleukin-4 deficient mice. Science 1991; 254:707-10.

31. Fowlkes BJ, Kruisbeek AM, Ton TH et al. A novel population of T-cell receptor alpha beta-bearing thymocytes which predominantly expresses a single V beta gene family. Nature 1987; 329:251-4.

32. Cosman D, Goodwin R, Lupton S et al. Molecular-cloning of interleukin-7—a novel cytokine involved in lymphopoiesis. Lymphokine Research 1988; 7:259.

33. Leclercq G, DeSmedt M, Plum J. Cytokine production and responsiveness of fetal T-cell receptor V gamma 3 thymocytes. Scand J Immunol 1992; 36:833-41.

34. Rich BE, Campos TJ, Tepper RI et al. Cutaneous lymphoproliferation and lymphomas in interleukin 7 transgenic mice. J Exp Med 1993; 177:305-16.

35. Samaridis J, Casorati G, Traunecker A et al. Development of lymphocytes in interleukin 7-transgenic mice. Eur J Immunol 1991; 21:453-60.

36. Fiorentino DF, Bond MW, Mosmann TR. Two types of mouse helper T cell. IV. Th2 clones secrete a factor that inhibits cytokine production by Th1 clones. J. Exp. Med 1989; 170:2081-2095.

37. Moore KW, Vieira P, Fiorentino DF et al. Homology of cytokine synthesis inhibitory factor (IL-10) to the Epstein Barr Virus gene BCRFI. Science 1990; 248:1230-1234.

38. Gately MK, Desai BB, Wolitzky AG et al. Regulation of human lymphocyte proliferation by a heterodimeric cytokine, IL-12 (cytotoxic lymphocyte maturation factor). J Immunol 1991; 147:874-82.

39. Schoenhaut DS, Chua AO, Wolitzky AG et al. Cloning and expression of murine IL-12. J Immunol 1992; 148:3433-40.

40. Zijlstra M, Bix M, Simister NE et al. Beta 2-microglobulin deficient mice lack CD4-8+ cytolytic T cells. Nature 1990; 344:742-6.

41. Grusby MJ, Johnson RS, Papaioannou VE et al. Depletion of CD4+ T cells in major histocompatibility complex class II-deficient

mice. Science 1991; 253:1417-20.

42. Dalton DK, Pitts-Meek S, Keshav S et al. Multiple defects of immune function in mice with disrupted interferon-γ genes. Science 1993; 259:1739-1745.

43. McNiece IK, Langley KE, Zsebo KM. Recombinant human stem cell factor synergises with GM-CSF, G-CSF, IL-3 and epo to stimulate human progenitor cells of the myeloid and erythroid lineages. Exp Hematol 1991; 19:226-31.

44. McNiece IK, Langley KE, Zsebo KM. The role of recombinant stem cell factor in early B cell development. Synergistic interaction with IL-7. J Immunol 1991; 146:3785-90.

45. Palacios R, Nishikawa S. Developmentally regulated cell surface expression and function of c-kit receptor during lymphocyte ontogeny in the embryo and adult mice. Development 1992; 115:1133-47.

46. Godfrey DI, Zlotnik A, Suda T. Phenotypic and functional characterization of c-kit expression during intrathymic T cell development. J Immunol 1992; 149:2281-5.

47. Galy AH, Spits H. IL-1, IL-4, and IFN-gamma differentially regulate cytokine production and cell surface molecule expression in cultured human thymic epithelial cells. J Immunol 1991; 147:3823-30.

48. Suda T, Zlotnik A. In vitro induction of CD8 expression on thymic pre-T cells. I. Transforming growth factor-beta and tumor necrosis factor-alpha induce CD8 expression on CD8- thymic subsets including the CD25+CD3-CD4-CD8- pre-T cell subset. J Immunol 1992; 148:1737-45.

49. Suda T, Zlotnik A. In vitro induction of CD8 expression on thymic pre-T cells. II. Characterization of CD3-CD4-CD8 alpha + cells generated in vitro by culturing CD25+CD3-CD4-CD8- thymocytes with T cell growth factor-beta and tumor necrosis factor-alpha. J Immunol 1992; 149:71-6.

50. Gutierrez RJ, Palacios R. In vitro differentiation of embryonic stem cells into lymphocyte precursors able to generate T and B lymphocytes in vivo. Proc Natl Acad Sci USA 1992; 89:9171-5.

===============CHAPTER 6===============

INTRATHYMIC DEVELOPMENT AND SELECTION OF TcRγδ CELLS

Faith B. Wells

Louis A. Matis

Two independent T-cell lineages can be distinguished by the type of T cell receptor (TcR) heterodimer expressed on the surface of the cell—αβ or γδ. We will discuss the development and selection of T cells bearing the γδTcR. γδ T cells have certain characteristics that are common to all T cells: the γ and δ subunits of the TcR are expressed on the cell surface in association with the CD3 complex; TcR receptor γδ preferentially recognizes cell bound antigen, although not necessarily presented by molecules of the major histocompatibility complex (MHC); and cells of the γδ lineage function like αβ T cells in that they perform cytolysis and produce cytokines following activation. Nevertheless, γδ T cells clearly constitute a distinct lineage from TcRαβ, a fact confirmed by recent genetic studies in knockout mice. Phenotypically, most γδ cells do not express the accessory molecules CD4 and CD8 on their surface (although some, particularly intraepithelial γδ lymphocytes, express CD8, and others become CD8⁺ following activation). A major area of investigation has centered on the developmental influences on the γδ lineage. We will discuss evidence for similarities as well as differences between γδ and αβ T-cell differentiation and will review recent data showing that at least some γδ T cells can undergo processes of negative and positive selection mechanistically similar to those that shape the TcR αβ repertoire.

STRUCTURE OF γδ RECEPTORS

As noted, the γδ TcR is similar in structure to the αβ TcR as well as to immunoglobulin (Ig) molecules, consisting of rearranged V, (D), and J elements encoding variable regions whose diversity is generated by combinatorial as well as junctional mechanisms (reviewed in ref. 1).

In mice, there are seven Vγ genes aligned in distinct groups situated upstream of four separate JC clusters. This is not the case in humans whose TcRγ locus is arranged similar to that of the TcRβ gene. The δ gene region is interesting in that it is located, both in mice and humans, in the midst of the TcRα locus. Thus, Vδ genes, interspersed among the Vα gene segments, are situated upstream of two Dδ, two Jδ, and one Cδ element, followed by the large Jα locus and the Cα gene. As a consequence, Vα-Jα rearrangements generally delete the entire TcRδ locus. There are now a number of examples in which the same V element has been expressed as part of either an αβ or γδ TcR, implying some degree of similarity in the potential specificities of the two receptor subtypes, but more often a unique Vδ element is found rearranged to the DJδ segments. The reason for this is not known but it is thought to relate to the fact that the Vδ genes are physically closer to the DJδ elements, facilitating rearrangement. The organization of the TcRδ locus often leads to productive Vδ-Dδ1-Dδ2-Jδ rearrangements, allowing for an unprecedented degree of junctional diversity in this receptor chain.

Thus, using mechanisms similar to those used in B cells and αβ T cells, γδ T cells generate a potentially large array of receptor specificities. It remains to be determined whether these specificities are selected during development in a fashion analogous to that of αβ T cells.

ORDERED APPEARANCE IN THE THYMUS AND TISSUE DISTRIBUTION OF γδ T CELLS

TcR γδ cells are the first antigen receptor bearing cells to appear in the fetal thymus and are present by day 14.[2,3] Until day 18, they remain the predominant T-cell subset in the thymus. Subsequently, αβ T-cell development accelerates such that γδ T cells ultimately comprise less than 5% of TcR-expressing thymocytes. In the mouse, programmed development of T cells expressing distinct γδ receptors begins early in fetal ontogeny (Table 1). Thymocytes expressing receptors with specific Vγ and Vδ elements and very limited junctional diversity appear in tightly programmed waves. Furthermore, these cells emigrate from the thymus and then predominate in distinct epithelial sites.[4,5] The existence of these waves of

Table 1. Ontogenic waves of γδ thymocyte development

Ontogenic appearance in thymus	γ variable region	δ chain association	Predominant junctional diversity	Peripheral location
Early fetal	Vγ3	Vδ1	none	skin (s-IELs)
Fetal	Vγ4	Vδ1	none	reproductive tract (r-IELs)
Late fetal, adult	Vγ2(Vγ1)	diverse	significant	spleen lymph node

Summary of programmed waves of γδ receptor development. Development of intestinal and lung γδ cells (i-IELs and RPLs) is complex and likely involves extrathymic as well as thymic pathways of development. For references, see text.

receptor development was initially found by examining rearrangement of γ and δ genes in fetal thymus. It was shown that Vγ3 and Vγ4 rearrangements predominated in early γδ T-cell development.[6,7] In addition, Vδ1 rearrangement was frequently seen in this same population.[8-10] Evaluation of the surface expression of thymic γδ receptors confirmed this pattern of development. Thus, Vγ3/Vδ1 bearing cells appear earliest in ontogeny, followed by cells expressing Vγ4/Vδ1.[11,12] Interestingly, an early fetal microenvironment appears to be absolutely required for the maturation of these cells. Thus, Vγ3/Vδ1 thymocyte development can only be reconstituted by fetal progenitor cells maturing in a fetal thymic environment. For example, precursors for these cells do not appear to exist in adult bone marrow, and fetal stem cells do not reconstitute the Vγ3/Vδ1 population in adult thymuses.[13]

Interestingly, the early developmental waves of TcRγδ cells seen in the thymus correspond to the Thy-1[+] cells found in distinct intraepithelial sites (IELs), such as skin (s-IEL), intestine (i-IEL) and reproductive organs (r-IEL), where, as noted, they may predominate.[4,5] For example, s-IELs express almost exclusively the Vγ3/Vδ1 receptors found in their thymic precursors.[14] Even more striking is the fact that s-IELs do not only utilize the same V region genes, but in fact possess identical receptors. Sequence analysis has shown that junctional and joining regions are the same for all s-IELs tested.[15,16] The same is true for r-IELs, which primarily express identical receptors consisting of the subunits Vγ4/Vδ1.[17] Thus, the earliest Vγ3/Vδ1 bearing thymocytes migrate to cutaneous epithelium and the second wave of Vγ4/Vδ1 thymocytes are the precursors of r-IELs. i-IELs are somewhat different from the other IELs. There is more heterogeneity in the T-cell receptors found in the intestinal epithelium, including the presence of significant numbers of αβ T cells. Nevertheless, most of the γδ cells in this organ express Vγ5 in conjunction with a variety of δ subunits.[16,18-20] Both s-IELs and r-IELs are absolutely dependent upon thymic development. In contrast, there are much data to indicate that many TcRγδ[+] i-IELs develop extrathymically.[21,22]

Cells with receptors present in these early waves disappear from the thymus in later stages of ontogeny, and a more diverse population of thymic γδ cells emerges expressing a greater diversity of surface receptors comprised of Vγ2, Vγ1.1, and Vγ1.2 elements in association with a number of different Vδ chains.[7,10,23-25] In contrast to their early fetal counterparts, all of these more "mature" γδ TcRs also display considerable junctional diversity. In the periphery, these receptor types seen in the late fetal and adult thymus such as Vγ2 and Vγ1.1 are primarily found in lymphoid organs such as lymph nodes and spleen.[24-26] These receptors display much more heterogeneity even than i-IELs, with considerable junctional diversity.

THYMIC DEVELOPMENT OF THE INVARIANT γδ T-CELL RECEPTORS

A fundamental feature of αβ T-cell development is that of TcR driven intrathymic selection: negative selection to eliminate potentially deleterious autoreactive T cells and positive selection to ensure a self-MHC restricted peripheral T-cell repertoire. In sum, the fate of an emerging αβ thymocyte is dictated by the specificity of its receptor.[27,28] A major aspect of the study of γδ T-cell development has been to determine whether similar principles apply.

With regard to the invariant receptors found on murine s-IELs, for example, it has been asked whether the homogeneous receptor usage is the result of intrathymic selection by a self antigen or rather represents a genetically programmed event independent of receptor driven signaling. Early studies to determine the basis for the homogeneity of these receptors were contradictory. Evaluation of junctional sequences of rearranged genes of early fetal thymocytes by the polymerase chain reaction (PCR) revealed essentially no diversity of in frame rearrangements of the genes studied.[29] In contrast, there was limited but significant junctional diversity of the out of frame rearrangements. Thus, because among the cells with productive rearrangements only those with the canonical (invariant) sequence were found, the authors of this study interpreted these results as supporting the theory that the invariant receptor was selected. However, other similar studies revealed the same striking lack of diversity of out of frame as well as the in frame rearrangements of these early fetal thymocytes.[4,8] This contradictory evidence was felt to support a genetically programmed development of the invariant receptors since the identical junctional sequences were present regardless of whether the rearrangement was productive or not.

Another study utilized fetal thymic organ culture (FTOC) to attempt to answer the question of selection vs. genetic programming.[30] FTOCs were treated with antibody to the γδ receptor and the junctional sequences of emerging T cells were analyzed by PCR. Untreated cultures had the same lack of junctional diversity as seen in fetal thymuses. However, data from anti-γδ treated cultures revealed a high (up to 38%) percentage of in-frame noncanonical junctional sequences. This evidence was cited in support of selection as the basis for the predominance of invariant receptors in these cells.

Further evidence for selection of invariant γδ receptors was provided by a previously undescribed invariant chain found in the lung. In general, γδ cells in the lung, termed resident pulmonary lymphocytes (RPL), are similar to i-IELs. A number of V regions are utilized in both the γ and δ chains, and there is significant diversity at the joining regions due to addition of nucleotides in the N regions. This pattern is similar to what is seen in γδ thymocytes found in adult mice. Nevertheless, several Vδ elements have been found to predominate, particularly Vδ5, Vδ6 and Vδ7.[31] Sequence analysis of receptors containing these Vδ subunits also revealed the interesting finding that many of the Vδ5 sequences analyzed contained identical rearrangements. These rearrangements were very similar in pattern to the invariant receptors seen in early fetal thymuses in that the rearranged genes retained their germline structure and there were no added nucleotides in the N regions. These RPLs were first discovered in BALB/c mice and thus the conserved receptor was called the BID (BALB/c invariant delta).

In an effort to determine the reason for the predominance of BID among Vδ5 receptors in BALB/c RPLs, the authors analyzed several other strains of mice for the presence of the invariant delta. C57BL/6 mice had no detectable sequences similar to the BID. However, C57BL/6 x BALB/c F1 mice contained a significant number of BID sequences. This finding was very similar to the pattern of expression that would be observed in positively selected αβ receptors. However, it was further determined that the selecting element could not be a classical MHC molecule because BID sequences were also found in BALB.B mice which express the H-2[b] haplotype on a BALB/c background. The authors concluded from this evidence that the BID chain is selected, but not by classical MHC molecules. Moreover, evidence from experiments with athymic and bone marrow transplanted mice indicated that the selection of this BID receptor was extrathymic.

New evidence has shed some light on this controversy. Two recent studies using genetically altered mice have clearly shown that the fetal thymic-dependent expression of invariant γδ receptors is determined at least in part by genetic programming. In one study, transgenic mice were constructed expressing mutated Vγ2, Vγ3 and Vγ4 gene constructs that could not produce surface receptor.[32] This was accomplished by introducing frameshift mutations which led to premature termination codons in the Vγ genes. However, these genes could still rearrange normally with the machinery provided in vivo by the fetal thymus. Sequence analysis of cloned PCR products from fetal and newborn thymocytes revealed that 82% of the in-frame sequences analyzed were the canonical sequence of the Vγ3 invariant chain. Preliminary analysis of Vγ4 revealed that two out of three of the sequences examined represented the invariant receptor. Finally, as had been previously reported, there was more, although still limited, diversity among the out-of-frame rearrangements found. The authors attributed this finding to the addition of P (palindromic) nucleotides that occurs prior to recombination.[29] The fact that the invariant sequences predominate in cells where no selection can occur due to lack of expression of a surface receptor strongly supports the theory that the invariant chains develop in the manner in which they do because of existing cellular machinery affecting the recombination process.

A second recent study confirms this notion. Utilizing gene knockout technology to disrupt the C region of the δ gene, mice were generated that did not express any $\gamma\delta$ receptors.[33] In this case, analysis by PCR of junctional sequences generated by V(D)J rearrangements revealed essentially no diversity of the in-frame canonical sequences of the invariant receptors. There was some diversity of out-of-frame sequences consistent with what had been described before. Again, since these mice could not express surface receptor, these findings cannot be attributed to ligand driven selection of the predominant receptor.

Several cellular mechanisms appear to be responsible for the striking lack of diversity of the early fetal thymocytes and the s-IELs and r-IELs. The preferential usage of specific V regions in the earliest rearrangements may be due to the fact that these V regions are in closest physical proximity to the J regions in both the γ and δ genomes.[34] Secondly, the absence of N region nucleotides in early fetal rearrangements appears to relate to reduced levels in fetal thymus of terminal deoxynucleotidyl transferase, the enzyme responsible for N nucleotide addition.[35] Thirdly, exonuclease activity which would trim nucleotides from unrearranged DNA "ends" is limited in the early fetal thymus.[29] Finally, and as the two recent studies strongly support, the specific rearrangement is directed by the germline sequence of the receptor itself. It has been reported that rearrangements tend to occur at sites of two base pair repeats.[32,36] These direct repeats can be germline or created by additions of P nucleotides. It has been proposed that P nucleotide addition plays a very important role in $\gamma\delta$ rearrangement in particular.[29] Thus, since the exact rearrangement seems to be targeted by the genomic sequences and the cellular

machinery used to modify the rearrangements is not present yet in early fetal thymuses, the result is the highly conserved receptors seen in the initial waves of $\gamma\delta$ cells of the thymus. It is important to note, however, that although the evidence strongly supports a programmed development of the invariant receptors, it cannot be ruled out that selection also occurs after the programmed appearance of these receptors. This is supported by the recent demonstration that Vγ3 bearing fetal thymocytes mature from a TcR^{lo} HSA^{hi} immature phenotype to a TcR^{hi} HSA^{lo} mature phenotype, and that this phenotypic maturation is inhibitable by cyclosporin A,[37] features characteristic of positive selection in $\alpha\beta$ T-cell development and "adult-type" $\gamma\delta$ receptors.

THYMIC SELECTION OF "ADULT-TYPE" $\gamma\delta$ RECEPTORS

Murine $\gamma\delta$ T cells that appear in the late fetal and adult thymus express a distinct set of receptors from those that have undergone the early waves of thymic maturation; moreover, following thymic egress they migrate primarily to peripheral blood and lymphoid tissue.[23-25] Their function in immune responses, like that of the intraepithelial $\gamma\delta$ subsets, remains ill-defined, although they have been shown to expand at sites of infection with various microbes, particularly mycobacteria.[38,39] Several reports have demonstrated a specificity for proteins of the heat shock family.[40] The consensus from a considerable body of data is that while there clearly are $\gamma\delta$ T cells with MHC specificity, the $\gamma\delta$ TcR repertoire does not exhibit the same fundamental MHC-directed specificity as that of TcR $\alpha\beta$.[41] Receptors on $\gamma\delta$ T cells that develop in the late fetal and adult murine thymus display greater diversity than the earlier maturing invariant receptors. These receptors utilize several V regions with a predominance of Vγ2 and two Vγ1 homologues. A variety of Vδ elements are also expressed, including several that belong to well characterized Vα families, although a few, such as Vδ5, predominate. Both γ and δ chains in these receptors display extensive junctional diversity.

We have previously characterized several γδ TcR with either class I or class II MHC specificity.[41] Employing one of these receptors in a transgenic mouse model, we have generated evidence for intrathymic selection of γδ TcR bearing T cells, and have also been able to characterize surface phenotypic changes that accompany intrathymic γδ development. The receptor studied was derived from a BALB/c (H-2^d) nu/nu mouse and was shown to recognize a class I MHC antigen mapping within the TL locus of H-2^b as well as several other murine haplotypes. This receptor consisted of a Vγ2/Jγ1/Cγ1 chain and a Vα11/Dδ1/Dδ2/Jδ1/Cδ chain. As noted above, this receptor included a γ chain characteristic of peripheral lymphoid γδ T cells and a δ chain expressing a Vδ element derived from a well characterized Vα family.[42] Genomic constructs of both of the receptor chains were isolated and used to construct TcRγδ transgenic mice.

In the H-2^d background, the thymuses of transgenic mice contained a significant number of cells expressing the transgenic receptor. These cells were CD4 and CD8 negative, and proliferated strongly in vitro to antigen presenting cells (APCs) from H-2^b mice.[43] The double negative phenotype of the transgenic bearing γδ cells recapitulated the findings from αβ transgenic mice that TcR receptor type dictates the surface phenotype of developing thymocytes. These cells also migrated to peripheral lymphoid tissues where significant numbers of transgene-bearing cells were found in the spleen and lymph nodes.

These mice were initially employed to address whether γδ T cells would be subject to intrathymic negative selection.[43] To this end transgenic mice were bred to H-2^b mice expressing the alloantigen recognized by the transgenic TcR. In contrast to H-2^d transgenic mice, in tg+ H-2^b mice, there were very few transgene bearing cells and those that were present had markedly lower levels of receptor on their surface. In addition, these cells did not migrate to peripheral lymphoid organs and thus very few were found in lymph nodes and spleen. Moreover, the residual CD4$^-$CD8$^-$ tg$^+$ thymocytes in these

mice did not proliferate in response to H-2^b antigen. When removed from thymuses and cultured in vitro, unlike thymocytes from H-2^d mice, the tg$^+$ H-2^b thymocytes died within 24 hours. These results demonstrated that a γδ receptor bearing thymocyte developing in an environment expressing the ligand recognized by the receptor would be negatively selected in a fashion analogous to that governing deletion of self-reactive αβ T cells. Similar results were reported by others with a distinct transgenic TcRγδ also specific for a Tl molecule.[44] In this case similar numbers of transgene-bearing cells were found in H-2^d and H-2^b transgenic thymuses, but the transgene bearing thymocytes from H-2^b mice were larger and had much lower levels of surface receptor than those from H-2^d mice, and were unable to proliferate to H-2^b antigen stimulation. There was a much lower number of transgenic cells in the spleen of H-2^b mice compared to H-2^d mice as well. These authors interpreted their study to mean that the γδ receptor bearing cells were rendered anergic in the thymus of H-2^b mice due to exposure to self-antigen during development. Whether the transgene bearing cells were deleted or inactivated, these studies show that γδ T cells exposed to self-antigen during development do not mature into functioning cells, and thus are negatively selected in a manner analagous to αβ T cells.

Studies in the same transgenic model systems have shown that γδ receptors can be positively selected as well. To study the importance of MHC class I molecules in T-cell development, mice with no MHC class I surface expression (classical and nonclassical) were created by disrupting the β$_2$-microglobulin (β$_2$M) gene by homologous recombination.[45,46] MHC class I molecules and peptide must combine with β$_2$M to be transported to the cell surface and serve effectively as antigen presenting molecules. Thus without β$_2$M, virtually no functional surface expression of MHC class I can occur. Nonclassical class I MHC molecules are also expressed on the cell surface in association with β$_2$M. Nonclassical class I molecules, encoded in the Qa and Tl regions of the MHC, are similar in structure to classical class I MHC molecules of the K, D and L regions. Both classical and nonclassical class I MHC molecules combine with β_2M to form the antigen presenting molecule. It is as yet not firmly established whether all nonclassical class I MHC surface molecules have peptides in their putative binding pockets. Nonclassical class I molecules also differ from classical MHC in tissue distribution and polymorphism. Classical class I MHC is found on most somatic cells in the body at varying levels whereas nonclassical class I has very limited tissue expression with each specific gene product having a unique pattern of tissue expression. In addition, classical class I molecules are extremely polymorphic, leading to a large number of potential antigenic peptide-presenting molecule combinations, whereas nonclassical class I MHC molecules have very limited polymorphism.[47] Nevertheless, the requirement for β_2M coexpression with Tl molecules provided a model for testing the requirement for positive selection in $\gamma\delta$ development.

The initial experiments in β_2M knockout mice revealed an almost complete absence of class I MHC expression and correspondingly an absence of CD8$^+$ single positive T cells, demonstrating the necessity for class I MHC molecule recognition during CD8$^+$ $\alpha\beta$ T-cell maturation.[45,46] To examine the requirement for TcR-mediated selection in $\gamma\delta$ differentiation, the $\gamma\delta$ transgenic mice[43] were bred to the β_2M knockout mice to generate tg$^+\beta_2$M$^-$ offspring. Since the $\gamma\delta$ tg was alloreactive for a nonclassical class I MHC molecule, by analogy to $\alpha\beta$ development it was reasoned that the self selecting element for such a receptor would also be a homologous nonclassical class I MHC molecule. If so, in the absence of β_2M, the cells expressing the $\gamma\delta$ transgene would not be exposed to their selecting ligand during development.

The results, duplicated in two independent TcR$\gamma\delta$ tg models, provided compelling evidence for TcR-mediated positive selection in $\gamma\delta$ development. They showed that although the thymuses of β_2M$^-$tg$^+$ mice had comparable numbers of tg$^+$ cells with similar levels of surface receptor as β_2M$^+$tg$^+$ mice, they were functionally and phenotypically immature.[48,49] Thus, the tg$^+\beta_2$M$^-$ thymocytes, in

contrast to their β_2M$^+$ counterparts, failed to proliferate to alloantigen and did not emerge from the thymus to populate peripheral lymphoid tissue. Moreover, detailed surface phenotype analysis revealed striking differences between β_2M$^+$ and β_2M$^-$ thymocytes consistent with a maturational arrest in the latter population. For example, the tg$^+\beta_2$M$^+$ thymocytes consisted of both immature and mature heat stable antigen (HSA) hi and lo populations, whereas the tg$^+\beta_2$M$^-$ thymocytes were exclusively HSA hi.[50] Independently it was shown that HSA^{hi} $\gamma\delta$ thymocytes cannot proliferate to receptor-mediated stimulation whereas HSA^{lo} $\gamma\delta$ thymocytes can, a correlation of phenotype with function also found in the $\alpha\beta$ lineage (A. Dent and S. Hedrick, personal communication). These data demonstrate that, similar to CD8$^+$ class I MHC-restricted $\alpha\beta$ T cells, a class I MHC-specific $\gamma\delta$ thymocyte also requires self class I MHC surface expression to mature in the thymus.

The TcR-mediated signals that occur during positive selection remain to be definitively determined, but several studies have provided evidence to suggest that $\alpha\beta$ T cells undergoing positive selection demonstrate phenotypic characteristics of activated T cells. Thus, thymocytes thought to be in the process of differentiation have been found to transiently express interleukin-2 receptor (IL-2R), CD44 (Pgp-1) and CD69, all markers of activated T cells.[51,52] Similar results were obtained for tg$^+$ $\gamma\delta$ thymocytes in the positively selecting (β_2M$^+$) environment, in that subsets of tg$^+$ cells in control β_2M$^+$ mice have significant levels of surface IL-2R and CD44. This cell population also has a significant number of Mel-14^{lo} cells.[50] This phenotype—IL-2R$^+$, CD44$^+$, Mel-14^{lo}—is indicative of activated cells.[53-55] However, no tg$^+$ cells that developed in β_2M$^-$ mice were found that expressed this activated phenotype (Fig. 1).[50] Again this suggested that $\gamma\delta$ T cells can undergo a form of intrathymic selection similar to $\alpha\beta$ T cells following a receptor-ligand interaction resulting in the transient activation of the selected cell.

This notion is also supported by evidence that cyclosporin A (CsA) inhibits thymic maturation of $\gamma\delta$ T cells. CsA is a potent immunosuppressant that blocks activation of T cells by inhibiting a critical signaling pathway from the TcR to the nucleus. It has recently been shown that this effect is due to binding and inhibition of the phosphatase calcineurin by the CsA/cyclophilin complex. This blockade of signals from the TcR has been shown to prevent positive selection of αβ T cells, supporting the idea that selection requires TcR-ligand interaction with the resulting signal transmission.[56,57] This has now been shown to be true for γδ T cells as well. Bone marrow stem cells from the above described γδ tg[+] mice were injected into lethally irradiated BALB/c mice. These mice were then treated either with CsA (20 mg/kg) or olive oil as a control. After 21 days, thymuses from each group of mice were evaluated for the development of tg[+] cells. Thymocytes from the control group revealed a significant number of tg[+] cells with normal levels of surface T-cell receptor and a large percentage of mature HSA[-] cells. Mice treated with CsA had a significant number tg[+] cells with normal TcR levels, but virtually all these cells were HSA[+], a sign of immaturity. In addition, peripheral migration of tg[+] thymocytes from CsA treated γδ tg[+] bone marrow reconstituted mice was significantly impaired.[50] In short, the phenotype of tg[+] cells from mice treated with CsA was identical to that seen in β_2M^- mice. Moreover, as mentioned above, parallel observations have now been made with regard to the development of γδ thymocytes expressing the invariant Vγ3/Vδ1 receptors that are the precursors of dendritic epidermal lymphoid cells. These cells were also shown to undergo a CsA-inhibitable conversion from HSA[hi] to HSA[lo] phenotype required for maturation.[37]

Other recent functional studies have established further parallels between γδ and αβ thymic development. For example, a recent report indicates that function of the lck kinase, shown in lck knockout mice to be critical for αβ thymocyte differentiation, is also required during γδ development. Mice with no functional lck due to disruption of the lck gene by homologous recombination were mated to the γδ tg mice and the effect

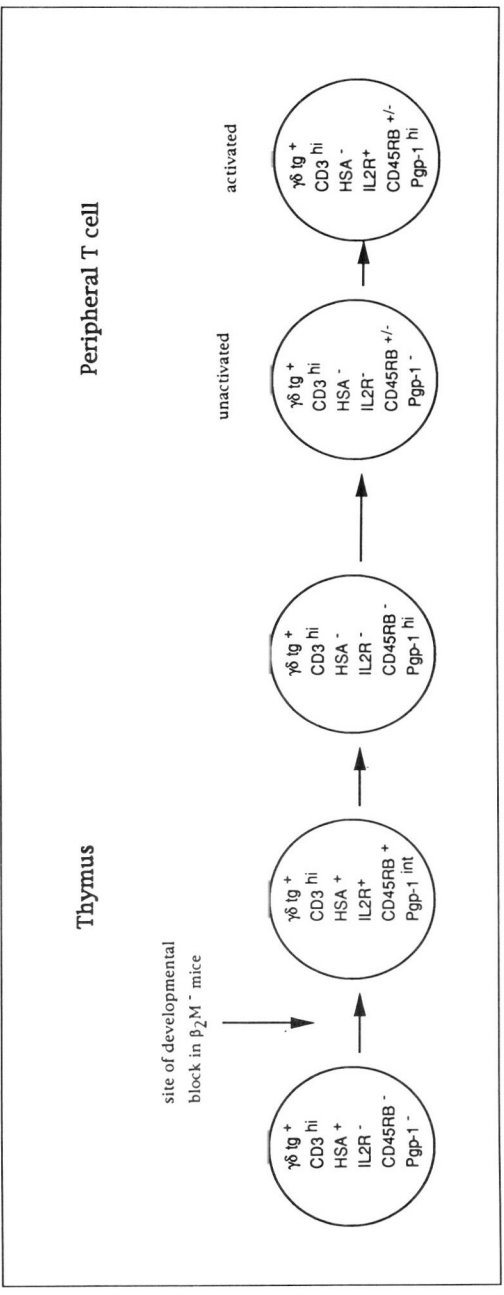

Fig. 1. Schematic representation of phenotypic changes that occur during development of a transgenic γδ TcR consisting of Vγ2/Vα11 variable chains. Tg-bearing cells that develop in the β_2M^- environment are not exposed to their selecting ligand during maturation and thus do not progress through these developmental stages.

on γδ T-cell development was evaluated.[58] Tg+ cells from lck knockout mice were present in normal numbers in the thymus and had normal levels of surface receptor. However, tg+ cells in lck knockout mice were immature as indicated by the fact that they were essentially all HSA+, did not proliferate in response to antigen and failed to exit the thymus and populate the periphery. This is contrasted with tg+ cells from mice with functional lck which developed normally. These results are of special interest because they imply that lck is required for TcRγδ signaling in general. Given that lck functions in αβ T cells through direct association with the CD4 or CD8 molecules, it will be of interest to determine how this kinase couples to CD4⁻CD8⁻ TcRγδ signaling. Regardless, the transgenic results indicate that a signaling pathway involving lck is important in both αβ and γδ maturation.

It has been shown that most γδ T cells develop normally in β_2M^- mice.[59] This is consistent with the fact that the TcR γδ repertoire is not fundamentally MHC specific as is αβ, and that many or most γδ T cells may not recognize MHC at all. In this light it will be important to determine whether, in a generic sense, TcRγδ selection occurs not to direct receptor repertoire specificity but because T-cell maturation in general involves TcR-mediated signals. If so, it will be of interest to identify the alternative self ligands involved in γδ selection.

SUMMARY

We have shown that, like αβ T cells, at least some γδ thymocytes undergo selection dictated by intrathymic receptor-ligand interactions. The mechanism of negative selection, as for αβ cells, remains to be determined, but appears to involve a form of programmed cell death. The molecular basis of the TcR/ligand interaction determining positive selection is also unclear but seems to require signaling via the pathway leading from the TcR to the nucleus which is blocked by CsA and involves phosphorylation of critical substrates by lck. This signaling causes a transient activation during development that results in differentiation.

At least in the mouse, γδ development involves a level of additional complexity characterized by the existence of programmed waves of development, beginning early in ontogeny, of subsets of thymocytes bearing specific receptors and destined to migrate to predetermined epithelial sites. These receptors that appear in uniform waves in the early fetal thymus appear to be programmed by genomic sequence and cellular machinery to develop as they do. It is currently not known if a selection step is necessary to allow further maturation of these cells after their programmed appearance in the thymus, although recent evidence suggests that this may be the case. This is followed by the intrathymic differentiation of γδ cells that populate the lymphoid organs. It has been demonstrated directly that at least subsets of these latter populations with MHC specificity undergo receptor mediated signaling during intrathymic development and selection, analogous to those observed within the αβ lineage. Also, it may be that γδ T cells, to a more significant degree than the αβ lineage, may develop extrathymically. Whether or not such extrathymically derived γδ T cells undergo any form of receptor-driven selection is currently under investigation. Finally, the antigen specific repertoire and the unique role in immune system function of TcRγδ T-cell subsets remains to be elucidated.

REFERENCES

1. Raulet DH. The structure, function and molecular genetics of the γ/δ T cell receptor. Ann Rev Immunol 1989; 7:175-207.
2. Bluestone JA, Pardoll D, Sharrow SO et al. Characterization of murine thymocytes with CD3-associated T cell receptor structures. Nature 1987; 326:82-84.
3. Pardoll D, Fowlkes BJ, Bluestone JA et al. Differential expression of two distinct T cell receptors during thymocyte development. Nature 1987; 326:79-81.
4. Allison JP, Havran WL. The immunobiology of T cells with invariant γδ antigen receptors. Ann Rev Immunol 1991; 9:679-705.
5. Raulet DH, Spencer DM, Hsiang Y-H et al. Control of γδ T-cell development. Immunological Reviews 1991; 120:185-204.

6. Garman RD, Doherty PJ, Raulet DH. Diversity, rearrangement, and expression of murine T cell γ genes. Cell 1986; 45:733-42.

7. Heilig JS, Tonegawa S. Diversity of murine γ genes and expression in fetal and adult T lymphocytes. Nature 1986; 322:836-40.

8. Chien YH, Iwashima M, Kaplan K et al. T cell receptor δ gene rearrangements in early thymocytes. Nature 1987; 330:722-27.

9. Elliot JF, Rock EP, Patten PA et al. The adult T cell receptor δ-chain is diverse and distinct from that of fetal thymocytes. Nature 1988; 331:627-31.

10. Korman A, Marusic-Galesic S, Spencer D et al. Predominant variable gene usage by γ/δ T cell receptor-bearing cells in the adult thymus. J Exp Med 1988; 168:1021-40.

11. Havran WL, Allison JA. Developmentally ordered appearance of thymocytes expressing different T cell antigen receptors. Nature 1988; 335:443-45.

12. Ito K, Bonneville M, Takagaki Y et al. Different γδ receptors are expressed on thymocytes at different stages of development. Proc Natl Acad Sci USA 1989; 86:631-635.

13. Ikuta K, Kina T, MacNeil I et al. A developmental switch in thymic lymphocyte maturation potential occurs at the level of hematopoetic stem cells. Cell 1990; 62:863-74.

14. Havran WL, Grell SC, Duwe G et al. Limited diversity of TcR γ chain expression of murine Thy-1⁺ dendritic epidermal cells revealed by Vγ3-specific monoclonal antibody. Proc Natl Acad Sci USA 1989; 86:4185-89.

15. Asarnow DM, Kuziel WA, Bonyhadi M et al. Limited diversity of γδ antigen receptor genes of Thy-1⁺ dendritic epidermal cells. Cell 1988; 55:837-47.

16. Asarnow DM, Goodman T, LeFrancois L et al. Distinct antigen repertoires of two classes of murine epithelium-associated T cells. Nature 1989; 341:60-62.

17. Itohara S, Farr AG, Lafaille JJ et al. Homing of a γ/δ thymocyte subset with homogenous T-cell receptors to mucosal epithelia. Nature 1990; 343:754-57.

18. Bonneville M, Janeway CA Jr, Ito K et al. Intestinal intraepithelial lymphocytes are a distinct set of γδ T cells. Nature 1988; 336:479-81.

19. Takagaki Y, DeCloux A, Bonneville M et al. Diversity of γ/δ T-cell receptors on murine intestinal intraepithelial lymphocytes. Nature 1989; 339:712-14.

20. Kyes S, Carew E, Carding SR et al. Diversity in T-cell receptor γ gene usage in intestinal epithelium. Proc Natl Acad Sci USA 1989; 86:5527-31.

21. Lefrancois L, LeCorre R, Mayo J et al. Extrathymic selection of TcR γδ⁺ T cells by class II major histocompatibility complex molecules. Cell 1990; 63:333-340.

22. Lefrancois L. Extrathymic differentiation of intraepithelial lymphocytes: generation of a separate and unequal repertoire? Immunol Today 1991; 12:436-438.

23. Takagaki Y, Nakanishi N, Ishida I et al. T cell receptor-γ and -δ genes preferentaially utilized by adult thymocytes for surface expression. J Immunol 1989; 142:2112-21.

24. Itohara S, Nakanishi N, Kanagawa O et al. Monoclonal antibodies specific to native murine T cell receptor γ/δ: Analysis of γ/δ cells during thymic ontogeny and in peripheral lymphoid organs. Proc Natl Acad Sci USA 1989; 86:5094-98.

25. Houlden BA, Cron RQ, Coligan JE et al. Systemic development of distinct T cell receptor-γδ T cell subsets during fetal ontogeny. J Immunol 1989; 141:3753-59.

26. Cron RQ, Koning F, Maloy WL et al. Peripheral murine CD3⁺, CD4⁻, CD8⁻ T lymphocytes express novel T cell receptor γδ structures. J Immunol 1988; 141:1074-82.

27. von Boehmer H, Kisielow P. Self-nonself discrimination by T cells. Science 1990; 248:1369-75.

28. Blackman M, Kappler J, Marrack P. The role of the T cell receptor in positive and negative selection of developing T cells. Science 1990; 248:1335-40.

29. Lafaille JJ, Cecloux A, Bonneville M et al. Junctional sequences of T cell receptor γδ genes: implications for γδ T cell lineages and for a novel intermediate of V-(D)-J joining. Cell 1989; 59:859-70.

30. Itohara S, Tonegawa S. Selection of γδ T cells with canonical T cell antigen receptors in fetal thymus. Proc Natl Acad Sci USA

1990; 87:7938-38.

31. Sim G-K, Augustin A. Dominantly inherited expression of BID, an invariant undiversified T cell receptor δ chain. Cell 1990; 61:397-405.

32. Asarnow DM, Cado D, Raulet DH. Selection is not required to produce invariant T-cell receptor γ-gene junctional sequences. Nature 1993; 362:158-160.

33. Itohara S, Mombaerts P, Lafaille JJ et al. T cell receptor δ gene mutant mice: independent generation of αβ T cells and programmed rearrangements of γδ TcR genes. Cell 1993; 72:337-348.

34. Goldman JP, Spencer DM, Raulet DH. Ordered rearrangement of variable region genes of T cell receptor γ locus correlated with transcription of unrearranged genes. J Exp Med 1993; 177:729-739.

35. Rothenberg E, Triglia D. Clonal proliferation unlinked to terminal deoxynucleotidyl transferase synthesis in thymocytes of young mice. J Immunol 1983; 130:1627-33.

36. Gu H, Forster I, Rajewsky K. Sequence homologies, N region insertion and JH gene utilization in VHDJH joining: implications for the joining mechanism and the ontogenetic timing of Ly 1 B cell and B-CLL progenitor generation. EMBO J 1990; 9:2133-2140.

37. Leclercq G, Plum J, Nandi D et al. Intrathymic differentiation of Vγ3 T cells. J Exp Med 1993; 178:309-315.

38. Janis EM, Kaufmann SHE, Schwartz RH et al. Activation of γδ T cells in the primary immune response to _Mycobacterium tuberculosis_. Science 1989; 244:713-716.

39. O'Brien RL, Happ MP, Dallas A et al. Stimulation of a major subset of lymphocytes expressing T cell receptor γδ by an antigen derived from _Mycobacterium tuberculosis_. Cell 1989; 57:667-674.

40. Born W, Hall L, Dallas A et al. Recognition of a peptide antigen by heat shock-reactive γδ T lymphocytes. Science 1990; 249:67-69.

41. Matis LA, Bluestone JA. Specificity of γδ receptor bearing T cells. Semin Immunol 1991; 3:75-80.

42. Bluestone JA, Cron RQ, Cotterman M et al. Structure and specificity of T cell receptor γ/δ on major histocompatibility complex antigen-specific CD3+, CD4-, CD8- T lymphocytes. J Exp Med 1988; 168:1899-1916.

43. Dent AL, Matis LA, Hooshmand F et al. Self-reactive gd T cells are eliminated in the thymus. Nature 1990; 343:714-19.

44. Bonneville M, Ishida I, Itohara S et al. Self-tolerance to transgenic γδ T cells by intrathymic inactivation. Nature 1990; 344:163-65.

45. Koller BH, Marrack P, Kappler J et al. Normal development of mice deficient in $\beta_2 M$, MHC class I proteins, and CD8+ T cells. Science 1990; 248:1227-31.

46. Zijlstra M, Bix M, Simister NE et al. β_2-microglobulin deficient mice lack CD4- CD8+ cytolytic T cells. Nature 1990; 344:742-6.

47. Flaherty L, Elliot E, Tine JA et al. Immunogenetics of the Q and TL regions of the mouse. Crit Rev Immunol 1990; 10:131-175.

48. Wells FB, Gahm S-J, Hedrick SM et al. Requirement for positive selection of γ/δ receptor-bearing T cells. Science 1991; 253:903-906.

49. Pereira P, Zijlstra M, McMaster J et al. Blockade of transgenic γ/δ cell development in β_2-microglobulin deficient mice. EMBO J 1992; 11:25-32.

50. Wells FB, Tatsumi Y, Bluestone JA et al. Phenotypic and functional analysis of positive selection in the γ/δ T cell lineage. J Exp Med 1993; 177:1061-70.

51. Bendelac A, Schwartz, RH. CD4+ and CD8+ T cells acquire specific lymphokine secretion potentials during thymic maturation. Nature 1991; 353:68-71.

52. Bendelac A, Matzinger P, Seder RA et al. Activation events during thymic selection. J Exp Med 1992; 175:731-40.

53. Budd RC, Cerottini J-C, Horvath C et al. Distinction of virgin and memory T lymphocytes. J Immunol 1987; 138:3120-29.

54. Jung TM, Gallatin WM, Weissman IL et al. Downregulation of homing receptors after T cell activation. J Immunol 1988; 141:4110-18.

55. Bradley LM, Duncan DD, Tonkonogy S et al. Characterization of antigen specific CD4+ effector T cells _in vivo_: immunization results in transient population of Mel-14-,

CD45RB⁻ helper cells that secrete interleukin-2 (IL-2), IL-3, IL-4 and interferon-γ. J Exp Med 1991; 174:547-59.

56. Gao E-K, Lo D, Cheney R et al. Abnormal differention of thymocytes in mice treated with cyclosporin A. Nature 1988; 336:176-79.

57. Jenkins MK, Schwartz RH, Pardoll DM. Effects of cyclosporine A on T cell development and clonal deletion. Science 1988; 241:1655-57.

58. Penninger J, Kishihara K, Molina T et al. Requirement for tyrosine kinase p56*lck* for thymic development of transgenic γδ T cells. Science 1993; 260:358-61.

59. Correa I, Bix M, Liao N-S et al. Most γδ T cells develop normally in β₂-microglobulin-deficient mice. Proc Natl Acad Sci USA 1992;89:653-660.

CHAPTER 7

POSITIVE INTRATHYMIC SELECTION OF TcRαβ THYMOCYTES

Janko Nikolić-Žugić

The central role of the thymus in T-cell development is evidenced by the obligatory requirement for thymic microenvironment in the conversion of multipotent precursors into immature thymocytes that express the TcR. But even more importantly, the thymus mediates selection of such thymocytes. The specificity of the TcR determines the fate of the thymocyte that bears it; the thymus permits the maturation of only those cells whose TcR can appropriately interact with the MHC molecules expressed by thymic cortical epithelium (positive selection). Cells whose TcR fail to do so will die in the thymus. In addition, negative selection eliminates all cells bearing TcRs reactive against self molecules. Such cells could potentially harm the organism by reacting against self and leading to autoimmunity. In short, the function of the thymus was perfectly summarized by von Boehmer et al in the title of their 1989 review article as: "The thymus selects the useful, ignores the useless and destroys the harmful."[1]

Separate chapters are devoted to discussing positive selection and deletional and nondeletional negative selection; with special attention on the debate on how the sum of these processes generates a broad, nonautoaggressive TcR repertoire.

DISCOVERIES OF MHC RESTRICTION AND POSITIVE SELECTION

The early 1970s were marked by one of the most important discoveries in immunology—that of major histocompatibility complex (MHC) encoded molecule restriction (reviewed in 2 and 3). This phenomenon was shown by several groups to apply to both classes of MHC encoded molecules, originally as a necessary requirement for T-B cooperation (class II restriction), and subsequently as a precondition for CTL-target interaction (class I restriction). It was characterized by the observation that T lymphocytes from a genetically inbred rodent of strain A, when confronted with foreign antigen presented on antigen-presenting cells (APC) of strain A or B, preferentially reacted with strain A antigen-presenting cells. T lymphocytes of strain

A were therefore "restricted" by strain A MHC molecules. A powerful theoretical speculation on the nature of antigen recognition by T cells, put forward by Zinkernagel and Doherty,[4] publicized these findings and placed them at the center of a debate in the following years. It quickly became clear that MHC restriction reflects a fundamental difference in the mechanism of antigen recognition between B and T cells. Namely, B cell receptors (surface immunoglobulins) recognize conformational (3-D) determinants on native antigens. By contrast, TcRs can recognize antigens only in a "processed," denatured form and in association with self MHC molecules. Neither the antigen nor the self MHC are recognized per se by T cells. The mechanism of restriction and its relationship to the process of intrathymic positive selection became apparent in the following years.

The late 1970s were marked by a number of experiments that established the concept of positive selection. These experiments took advantage of the radiation-induced bone marrow chimera system, where the hematopoietic system of an inbred animal of MHC haplotype A is ablated by total body irradiation in doses that do not substantially and/or irreversibly damage other tissues and organs. Such animals retain their radioresistant thymic epithelium, that continues to function in a relatively normal fashion. If such an irradiated mouse is then reconstituted by an injection of hematopoietic stem cells (in the form of bone marrow) of an allogeneic MHC haplotype, e.g., B, one can follow the

development of MHC B thymocytes in an MHC A thymus and investigate whether MHC restriction is dictated by the genotype of thymocytes or learned during development.

Using a complicated variation of this model—tetraparental [A + B → (A x B)F₁] chimeras—von Boehmer et al[5] demonstrated that mature T cells in such animals were restricted by both A and B MHC molecules. One explanation for these results was that in the F_1 host, parental cells must undergo some sort of adaptation that allows them to interact with the MHC molecules of the other parent. In 1977 Bevan published a landmark study[6] showing that in an (A x B)F₁ → P chimera, the genotype of the parental host dictated the MHC restriction of developing donor (F_1) cells. Namely, if (A x B)F₁ bone marrow cells mature in a type A host, an overwhelming majority of mature cytotoxic T lymphocytes (CTL) will be restricted by MHC A molecules (Table 1). The converse situation is found in an [(A x B) F₁→ B] chimera. In both cases the developing cells were genetically identical, and negative selection and antigenic stimulation were mediated by identical hematopoietic (donor) cells; it was concluded that the MHC restriction must be "learned" by a sort of "positive" selection during the development of donor T cells in a genetically disparate host. These results were in line with a proposal by von Boehmer and Sprent.[5] Similar studies were thereafter published by Zinkernagel's group.[7] Subsequently, both Fink and Bevan,[8] and Zinkernagel et al[9] showed thymus to be the

Table 1. Bevan's experiments that established positive selection

Thymocyte type	Thymus type	CTL activity against antigens presented by MHC molecules of type	
		A	B
(A x B) F₁	A	+++	—
(A x B) F₁	B	—	+++

F_1 → P chimeras were generated by lethal irradiation and bone marrow reconstitution. After 8-12 weeks, animals were immunized with minor histocompatibility antigens presented by (A x B)F₁ cells and the ability of spleen cells from immunized mice to generate a CTL response against minor histocompatibility antigens tested.[6] Similar results were reported by other groups.

learning site of MHC restriction (similar results were obtained by other groups[10,11]). Although numerous experiments attempted to challenge the concept of positive selection, a critical evaluation of experimental models and results strongly supported the original findings. (An excellent historical review of the controversial results obtained in the following years has been presented by Sprent and Webb.[2])

Positive selection is not absolute, but is still rather strict (reviewed in refs. 12 and 13). In the class I system radiation chimera, approximately 50-fold more CTL cells will be restricted to the intrathymically expressed MHC molecules. Class II molecules imprint less stringent selection, and approximately three- to five-fold more helper T lymphocytes (HTL) will be restricted by the MHC molecules present in the thymus of an F_1 chimera (possible reasons for this difference are discussed below). Importantly, even when the selected CTLs are restricted by molecules other than those expressed in the thymus, it can be demonstrated that some of these cells have learned their specificity on thymic (host) MHC.[14,15]

In the course of 15 years after the discovery of positive selection and 20 years after the discovery of MHC restriction, many critical features of these processes were elucidated. For example, we know now that MHC molecules physically bind short peptides derived from native antigens by cytosolic (class I) or endosomal/lysosomal (class II) processing (reviewed in ref. 3). We know the crystal structures of both class I[16,17] and class II[18] molecules, some of which have been determined with a single antigenic peptide bound to them.[19-21] It is clear that, in the course of antigen recognition, the TcR contacts the α-helices of class I and the peptide bound between them[22] (presumably, the same is true of class II). We know that an overwhelming majority of thymocytes die in the thymus,[23,24] and we know the outline of the molecular structure of the TcR.[25,26]

As early as in 1969, Jerne[27] postulated that lymphocyte receptors (at that time called "antibodies of lymphocytes" due to the fact that the division of lymphocytes into T and

B cells was not yet generally accepted[28]) bore some general affinity for MHC molecules. He also proposed that these receptors displayed on developing lymphocytes in any given animal were randomly specific for some of the MHC molecules of that species. This hypothesis proved to be essentially correct for the T-cell receptors. The rearrangement of the TcR genes is random with respect to the TcR specificity, and these molecules do have a general fold that "fits" the MHC.[29] Thymocytes have no way of knowing which particular MHC molecules await them in the thymus. During positive selection, the array of randomly displayed TcR specificities will be tested by the MHC molecules expressed on the stromal (epithelial) component of the thymus and only those that bind with an above-the-threshold affinity will be selected for further maturation. Therefore, in a haplotype A mouse, the thymus will select thymocytes bearing TcRs that bind MHC A molecules, because such a TcR will be able to recognize foreign antigens when presented by type A MHC molecules during an immune response. All other thymocytes (recognizing MHC molecules of types B, C, D, etc.) are completely useless to the type A animal, because they would never—under physiological circumstances—encounter antigen-presenting MHC molecules other than A during their lifetime. These thymocytes are therefore not allowed to mature into peripheral T cells. They die in the thymus due to a lack of positive selection, presumably by a form of programmed cell death.

A decade after the first description of positive selection, experiments with TcR transgenic mice[30-33] have unequivocally confirmed the tenets of this process at a single T-cell receptor level. To illustrate this, I shall use the model of anti-(H-Y +D^b) TcR Tg mice[30,34] (αH-Y in the text) as the first and well characterized TcR Tg model. Similar or essentially identical findings have been reported by other groups using other TcR transgenes restricted by either class I[31] or class II[32,33] MHC molecules. The production and characterization of α(H-Y) TcR Tg mice was performed at the Basel Institute of Immunology by von Boehmer, Steinmetz and colleagues. This group cloned TcR α and β genes from a

CD8⁺ CTL clone specific for the male minor histocompatibility antigen H-Y in the context of H-2Dᵇ class I molecules. When introduced into the germline of recipient mice by blastocyst injection, TcR transgenes heavily dominate the endogenous genes and create a nearly monoclonal mouse.[34] The β transgene blocks (allelically excludes) the rearrangement of endogenous β genes (the β transgene is expressed on > 95% thymocytes) while the α transgene dominates the endogenous α genes somewhat less efficiently, being expressed on about 70% thymocytes. In these mice, an efficient production of mature TcR tg⁺ T cells is possible only in the presence of selecting H-2Dᵇ molecules.[30,35] Essentially all mature TcR tg⁺ cells are of the CD8⁺ phenotype, in agreement with the phenotype of the CTL clone from which the genes were isolated and with the class I restriction of the TcR. These findings were also confirmed in a TcR tg scid mouse, where the contribution of endogenous TcR genes was excluded.[36] At this point, even the most diehard opponents of positive selection had to acknowledge the existence of this process.

The questions remaining were (and to some extent still are): Where, when and how does positive selection take place? These issues are still under intensive study, and the continuous flow of experimental evidence keeps these issues alive even when pieces of the puzzle appear to be solved. The divergent results on these issues is at least in part due to differences in the protocols used to generate radiation chimeras.[2]

CELL TYPE REQUIREMENTS FOR POSITIVE SELECTION

Which tissue mediates positive selection? An overwhelming body of experimental evidence demonstrates that thymocytes themselves cannot mediate positive selection of other thymocytes, and that other hematopoietic cells are also quite inefficient.[12,13,37] To date, thymic cortical epithelium is considered the best and physiologically the most important positively selecting tissue in the body (see Chapter 1), although recent evidence[38,39] has succeeded in reawakening the debate on this issue.

Results from F₁ → P chimeras quite clearly demonstrated that (donor) bone marrow elements cannot mediate positive selection (reviewed in ref. 2). Contrary results were obtained by Longo and Schwartz several years later (reviewed in refs. 40-42), but could not be reproduced by other investigators (reviewed in 2). A critical discovery by Lo and Sprent, that positive selection could be mediated by thymic lobes depleted of hematopoietic elements (including macrophages and dendritic cells) by deoxyguanosine treatment,[43]

Table 2. Positive selection of a tg TcR occurs only in the presence of the positively selecting MHC molecule

Thymocyte type	Thymus type	Positive selection (presence of tgTcR⁺CD8⁺ SP cells)
non-tg A	A	–
tg A	A	+++
tg A	B	–
Non-tg B	B	–
tg B	B	–
tg B	A	+++

This table illustrates findings obtained in several experimental models, most conclusively in bone marrow radiation chimeras using tg marrow and a panel of recombinant inbred mice as hosts.[35] A represents the positively selecting class I MHC molecule, whereas B is a neutral (nonselecting) molecule.

further suggested that the thymic epithelium must play a crucial role in this process. Genetic evidence also supports this view; targeted expression of MHC class II molecules on the thymic cortical epithelium leads to excellent positive selection by these molecules.[44,57] By contrast, if the same molecules are targeted to medullary epithelium, no positive selection is detectable. Therefore, it appears reasonable to conclude that thymic cortical epithelium is the tissue which normally mediates positive selection. Further support for this idea was recently lent by findings that isolated, cultured thymic epithelium can mediate positive selection when injected intrathymically.[45,46] Finally, in a re-aggregation system where selected elements of dissociated thymic lobes were allowed to reassociate, Jenkinson, Owen and co-workers[47,48] have elegantly shown that two types of cells are necessary and sufficient for the maturation (and presumably the positive selection) of DP cells into SP cells: thymic epithelium and fibroblasts.

What makes the thymic cortical epithelium capable of mediating positive selection, and are other cell types capable of doing so? The jury is still out on this issue. In a recent study, Muller and Kyewski[49] have demonstrated that positive selection can be mimicked using bispecific mAb that crosslink the TcR on thymocytes to a non-MHC antigen on the cortical epithelium. At face value, such a finding indicates that the TcR stimulation in the vicinity of the epithelial cell is sufficient for MHC-independent positive selection. Unfortunately, several idiosyncrasies are inherent in the experimental design and the results of that study. An obvious control, that of cross-linking of thymocytes to either medullary epithelium or a nonepithelial component, was lacking. Further, effect on positive selection was measured by quantifying the number and the percentage of SP thymocytes, but testing for antigen-specific responses or the repopulation of T-cell-deficient animals by such SP thymocytes in vivo was not done. Most importantly, the effect on positive selection was apparent only for the CD4[+] subset, a finding not explained at present. Therefore,

although this study suggests that cortical epithelium may be able to direct MHC-independent positive selection, the results are not conclusive.

Pawlowski et al[38] have recently shown that intrathymically injected fibroblasts can mediate the generation of functional, antigen-specific CD8[+] CTLs in β_2 -/- mice (findings confirmed in a class II model by Hugo et al[39]). These mice are deficient in the expression of MHC class I molecules and consequently have very few CD8[+] T cells, owing to a defect in positive selection. However, infection of such mice with a virus, as shown by Apasov and Sitkovsky,[50] can lead to accumulation of relatively high numbers of cytolytic CD8[+] cells. It is therefore possible that some selection occurs normally in these mice, either due to a leakiness in the "knock-out" or to the fact that some class I molecules, e.g., D^b, can fold in the absence of β_2-microglobulin and therefore, theoretically can mediate positive selection. In light of these possibilities and the results of Apasov and Sitkovsky,[50] it is difficult to interpret the data of Pawlowski et al.[38] An additional technical problem arises from the experimental design used by the latter authors. Namely, they injected very high numbers of fibroblasts per thymus (2×10^7) and waited only 10 days before observing wild-type levels of positive selection. In conventional bone marrow irradiation chimeras it is virtually impossible to obtain a functional immune response that reveals positive selection before six (and in the case of certain responses even 12) weeks after reconstitution.[2] Furthermore, a possibility that fibroblasts actually shed class I molecules that are then taken up by epithelial cells and thus serve as a source of class I molecules, has not been excluded. The data of Pawlowski could be alternatively explained if one considers that injected fibroblasts can stimulate and expand a small number of CD8[+] cells present in β_2-microglobulin -/- mice. The kinetics of the appearance of CD8[+] cells in these experiments would coincide quite well with the kinetics of proliferation. However, in other experiments Pawlowski et al have obtained evidence for positive selection by injecting fibroblasts into normal mice, and these results, although obtained using the same protocol described above, are not easily subject to the same criticism. Inasmuch as this topic is currently very much en vogue, I am sure that before long the issue will be clarified by additional experiments. Nevertheless, the physiological advantage of cortical epithelial cells over fibroblasts in mediating positive selection is considerable. Fibroblasts are clustered around thymic trabeculae and the blood vessels, and are therefore ill positioned to contact the majority of the developing thymocytes (Chapter 1 and references therein).

THE PHENOTYPIC STAGE AT WHICH POSITIVE SELECTION OCCURS

At which developmental stage are thymocytes positively selected? An answer to this question is impossible without a more precise biochemical definition of positive selection. It is quite likely that positive selection may consist of several signals mediated by cell-cell contacts (and, perhaps, soluble factors). If these signals are transmitted to a thymocyte over a long period of time or in different regions of the cortex [and even at the corticomedullary junction (see Chapter 2)] rather than as a "single hit", then it will be impossible to identify the "stage" of positive selection. This would also apply if positive selection occurs at several stages of development (a phenotypic "window" of positive selection). This situation is further complicated by findings that TcRα genes continue to rearrange during the DP stage.[51-54] As long as at least some cells can express TcRs of new specificities, there is a chance that these cells could be selected. But most of the older and even contemporary literature have assumed that positive selection is a "single-hit" event, and, with qualifiers, I shall discuss it as such.

Expression of the TcR (Chapter 3) is a prerequisite for positive selection, and therefore TcR- cells cannot be subject to this process. Significant TcR expression is evident on DP thymocytes, and these cells are the prime candidates for positive selection. However, the bona fide proof that positive selection occurs at a certain phenotypic stage

has so far been lacking. Such proof would be obtained by the transfer of one subset of thymocytes, e.g., from αH-Y TcR tg mice, from the selecting (D^b expressing) into a nonselecting (D^b negative) thymus. Normal maturation of this subset into functional CD8+TcRTg^{hi} cells would imply that such cells have been positively selected prior to being transferred into adoptive hosts. By contrast, a lack of maturation would imply that the subset has not been selected. Continuous rearrangement of the TcR α genes at the DP stage is terminated by positive selection, and this could be used as another indicator of selection. Alternatively, the expression of the transgenic α chain could be followed in such experiments. But the ultimate challenge is to come up with a quantitative (clonal) assay to test the stage at which positive selection occurs.

The best candidate for an early postselection intermediate is, at present, the TcR^{hi}DP subset. In αH-Y transgenic mice, these cells indeed have the characteristics of a postselection intermediate. They downregulate CD4 and become CD8+ in vitro, they express CD69 (an early activation marker) and show other features associated with thymocyte maturation.[55] An analogous subset in normal mice can also become CD8+ SP in vitro.[56] At face value, this result could be taken as evidence that CD8+ and CD4+ thymocytes get positively selected at different stages of development. However, when injected intrathymically, TcR^{hi}DP cells are perfectly capable of generating both lineages of SP cells.[56] Thus, although TcR^{hi}DP thymocytes are probably primed for further maturation, they most likely require additional signals from the thymus.

Some investigators have advocated that positive selection must be a late event, operating on SP cells. What is the evidence for such a model? In normal animals, increased levels of V$_\beta$6+ peripheral T cells can be observed if the expression of a class II I-E molecule is targeted to the thymic cortex.[57] When I-E is expressed in the medulla, no increase in V$_\beta$6+ cells can be detected. If subsets of thymocytes are analyzed for increased expression of V$_\beta$6, an increase is only detected in CD4$^+$ SP thymocytes, and not in DP cells. This evidence for the late onset of positive selection is indirect, in part because positive selection specific for V$_\beta$ fragments is poorly defined and may not be representative of normal, MHC:peptide-based positive selection, and in part because the function of these V$_\beta$6 cells has not been tested. More likely, and in accordance with the recent data from several groups,[58-60] it is possible that these results reflect the multi-hit nature of positive selection (as discussed above). Alternatively, it is possible that all signals have been received at the DP stage, but that additional time is needed for the change to become apparent. For example, one possibility is that positively selected V$_\beta$6$^+$ cells cannot be observed in increased numbers until cells bearing other V$_\beta$s are negatively selected, and that phenomenon is completed only at late developmental stages.

LIGAND(S) FOR POSITIVE SELECTION: MHC AND SELF PEPTIDES

Negative intrathymic selection, as discussed in the next chapter, involves the deletion or functional silencing of cells whose TcR are highly specific for self MHC and self peptides associated with them. What does the TcR then actually "see" during positive selection? This directly invites us to open the discussion on perhaps the most provocative question in thymology, (that will fully be discussed in Chapter 10): how do positive and negative selection operate to produce functional T cells? The T-cell ligand during an immune response consists of a complex of the antigenic peptide and the MHC (rev. in ref. 61). The idea was thus born that in the thymus T cells may be positively selected on self MHC alone ("empty MHC"), by loosely fitting with the MHC (TcR set A), and then negatively selected on complexes of self peptides and self MHC (TcR set B, a subset of A). This would explain how the first, broader set of TcR specificities gets purged of autoreactive cells without eliminating all positively selected cells.

Soon thereafter, it became clear that all immunologically relevant MHC molecules contain peptides. The first MHC molecule to be crystallized—a human class I molecule HLA-A2—was found to carry a non-MHC-derived extra electron density in its putative peptide-binding site.[16,17] The membrane-distal part of the molecule consisted of two α helices that rested on a set of β-pleated sheaths, forming a groove that contains an unexpected extra electron density. That groove was subsequently shown to be the peptide-binding site, and the density a mixture of peptides bound to MHC.[3] (The structure of MHC class II is similar, with some subtle differences.[18]) Subsequent biochemical experiments established that peptides are not only present in the groove of MHC molecules, but are in fact essential for the stable folding of the entire complex.[3] Cell lines defective for the expression of peptide-supplying transporters (TAPs) are unable to assemble stable MHC molecules and express them at the surface. The concept of "empty" MHC molecules therefore lost ground. However, it was still possible that peptides only play a stabilizing role during positive selection, and that only MHC molecules are recognized during positive selection.

To test whether peptides are recognized during positive selection, with Michael Bevan, I performed a series of experiments using bone marrow radiation chimeras.[62] We used the H-2K^b-restricted cytotoxic T-cell (CTL) response to ovalbumin (OVA) peptide 253-276 (OVA$_{253-276}$) and a set of naturally occurring mutants of the MHC class I K^b molecule (H-2K^{bm}) that differ from the wild type at residues located in the α$_1$ and α$_2$ domains (Table 3). We clearly demonstrated that positive selection of a CTL repertoire can be abrogated by amino acid substitutions at the bottom of the peptide-binding site (K^{bm8} mutation). These mutations are not likely to alter the configuration of the molecule, are inaccessible to the TcR and are strictly involved in peptide binding. The α helices of the mutant molecule are unchanged and the TcR contact area of the MHC should therefore be identical to that of the wild-type molecule. Thus, the effect on positive selection had to be mediated via the bound peptide(s), most likely originating from intracellularly derived self proteins. Our results therefore provided strong indirect evidence that self peptides, presented by class I molecules on thymic epithelial cells, are critically involved in positive selection of the T-cell repertoire. Studies in TcR transgenic (Tg) mice led to similar conclusions.[63-66]

Together, these experiments suggested that self peptides are specifically involved in positive selection. Subsequent experiments by Hogquist et al[67] demonstrated that exogenously added peptides that bind to and stabilize class I molecules can mediate positive selection, and that the efficacy of positive selection directly depends on the complexity of the peptides. By contrast, in a similar model, Ashton-Rickardt et al[68] demonstrated that even a single peptide can select a substantial number of $CD8^+CD4^-TcR^{hi}$ cells, and that peptide binding does not always correlate with selection, e.g., some peptides that bound very well were quite poor as selecting peptides. Both sets of experiments[67,68] were performed in a situation where MHC class I molecules are unstable and cannot positively select $CD8^+$ cells. Both obtained $CD8^+$ $CD4^+TcR^{hi}$ cells by adding peptides to fetal thymic organ cultures (FTOC), and in the latter case,[68] enormous amounts of peptides (0.5 mg/ml) had to be added to see an effect. Another critique is that neither of the above two studies demonstrated that obtained $CD8^+CD4^-TcR^{hi}$ cells are functional. The phenotype of these cells thus remains the only witness of positive selection. Together, although these experiments led to a wider acceptance of the role of peptides in positive

selection, they also left many questions open. Some of these questions are discussed below.

WHICH PEPTIDES?

Do all thymocytes require self peptides for positive selection? In answer to this question, it should be mentioned that whenever investigators searched for evidence of self peptide involvement, they found it. A widely accepted fact is that most MHC molecules cannot fold correctly and are biochemically unstable at the cell surface without a bound peptide. As these molecules by default carry self peptides, these peptides will be present at the time of positive selection. [Of course, if an organism is infected by a pathogen, all of the foreign peptides expressed in the host thymus at the time will also be treated as "self" peptides, until such an infection is cleared]. All the TcRs that have a "snug fit" for the MHC:self peptide complex will be critically dependent on the peptide. Whether there are other TcRs that can be selected by a loose interaction, and that are therefore less dependent on peptides, remains to be seen. But other MHC molecules may be relatively stable without a peptide, e.g, D^b and $L^{d\ 3}$, and it is critical to elucidate the requirements for positive selection in this case.

The length of peptides bound to class I (8-11 amino acids, but mostly 8 or 9) and class II molecules (14-25 amino acids, with large overhangs on one or both sides of the groove and a core of 6-10 residues making direct contacts with the groove) is strikingly different (reviewed in 69). Based on this observation, it is possible to speculate on the

---

Table 3. Self peptides play a role in intrathymic positive selection.

Thymocytes	Thymus	Mutation[1]	OVA-specific CTL
($K^b \times K^{bm8}$)	K^b	nil	+++
($K^b \times K^{bm8}$)	K^{bm8}	floor	–

Radiation-induced bone marrow chimeras were constructed and immunized as described.[62] Positive selection was judged by the ability of host MHC molecules to promote maturation of CTL specific for OVA + K^b. 1—refers to the part of the MHC molecule changed by the natural mutation in the MHC variant expressed by the host thymus.

differences in the mechanism of peptide recognition on these two types of molecules during positive selection. A more stringent positive selection by thymic class I molecules could result from the relatively fixed length (8-11 amino acids) of peptide ligands present in the thymus. More promiscuous selection by class II molecules could then be traced to a rather degenerate set of peptides that could conceivably look similar even when bound to different MHC alleles. To date, this argument remains purely speculative.

What is the tissue origin of positively selecting self peptides? In accordance with the processing pathways commonly used by class I and class II molecules, one would expect that both intracellular and extracellular proteins could provide the substrate to generate class I and class II positively selecting self peptides, respectively. It was hypothesized that the thymic cortex may express a unique set of self peptides used solely or mainly for positive selection.[70] According to this hypothesis, (discussed in greater detail in Chapter 10), negative selection would then occur on a set of ubiquitous peptides expressed on hematopoietic cells in the thymic medulla. This hypothesis explains the difference between positive and negative selection by postulating that the peptide ligand differs between the two. Unfortunately, there is little evidence to support this hypothesis. If the thymic cortex does express any tissue-specific peptides, these most likely originate from epithelium-specific proteins, and such peptides are quite efficiently used to tolerize the epithelium-reactive T cells.[71] As mentioned above, fibroblasts have been shown to induce positive selection,[38,39] arguing that positively selecting self peptides may be at least shared between the thymic epithelium and fibroblasts.

It is unclear whether some of the positively selecting self peptides may violate the prevalent processing pathways, and whether, for example, class I molecules in the thymus may use extracellularly processed peptides, that are not thymus-derived, but are present in extracellular fluids, to mediate positive selection. Perhaps more intriguingly, it is not known how many MHC:peptide complexes a thymocyte needs to be positively selected. A completely speculative, but rather attractive hypothesis has stemmed from the idea that the number of MHC:peptide complexes required for positive selection differs from that of negative selection and T-cell activation. This "determinant density" model is in fact a modification of the affinity model, and will be discussed in Chapter 10.

Another enigma is: what is the relationship between the positively selecting self peptide and the antigenic peptide? Some information has been obtained from the OVA/K^{bm} system. There is a striking correlation between the ability of four K^{bm} molecules to present the OVA peptide to CTLs and to select the OVA-plus-K^b—specific CTL repertoire.[62] This indicates that self peptides may somehow mimic foreign peptides during positive selection in the thymus. Comparison of the crystal structures of human[16,72] and murine[19,20] MHC class I molecules shows that the MHC polymorphism alters discrete subsites or pockets within the binding cleft while leaving the architecture of the molecule unperturbed. Different peptides have specific requirements for binding to individual pockets in the cleft.[72,73] According to the HLA-A model, the mutations in H-2K^{bm8} alter one of the antigen binding pockets of K^b, leaving the others unchanged. Indeed, a point mutant at residue 24 (predicted to form a part of the pocket B) abrogates presentation of OVA to polyclonal lines[74]. We showed that the alteration in K^{bm8} prevents it from presenting OVA peptides in a conformation recognized by CTLs.[62,75] In contrast to OVA, the vesicular stomatitis virus nucleocapsid peptide (VSV) binds to K^{bm8} and is presented by it to T cells. Thus, conformations of OVA and VSV peptides probably depend on different pockets in the K^b groove, the OVA-pocket being altered in K^{bm8}. K^{bm8} can also positively select a T-cell repertoire specific for VSV. The conformation of self peptides that positively select the repertoire for OVA and VSV therefore probably depends on the same pockets as OVA and VSV peptides, respectively, and this might form the structural basis for molecular mimicking. A case where a nonpresenting molecule can mediate positive selection of a class II-restricted transgenic TcR has been reported recently by Kaye et al[76] But the transgenic TcR heterodimer was engineered from α and β chains that do not naturally form a TcR.

Several studies have recently described the phenomenon of peptide antagonism, or partial agonism, for both class I[77] and class II[78,79] systems. Peptides differing from the antigenic peptide by a single amino acid residue, usually involved in a direct TcR contact, have been shown to act as classical competing antagonists—they inhibited T-cell activation despite the presence of sufficient quantities of stimulatory MHC:peptide complexes. Certain peptides acted at the same concentration as weak agonists, weakly sensitizing target cells for lysis, and as antagonists of peptides that strongly sensitize target cells for lysis. Partial agonists, on the other hand, were defined by the ability to induce some but not all biological responses. A single peptide can fall into more than one of these categories, and each cell clone appears to possess an exquisitely fine specificity not only for the antigen, but for the antagonists as well.[77] These attractive features of antagonism and/or partial agonism are immediately appealing to the aficionados of positive selection. If a peptide can elicit only part of the functional response in a notoriously fragile DP thymocyte, it may be able to transmit a survival signal to the cell without killing it (inducing apoptosis). I would not be surprised if the results from testing this hypothesis reach the public by the time this review is published.

The above scenario would be applicable if sequence homology were the sole relationship between positively selecting self peptides and the foreign peptides for which the selected TcR will be specific. However, it is also quite possible that some self peptides can positively select based on conformation, rather than sequence homology. It is currently difficult to design experiments in order to define those peptides, but our increasing knowledge of the MHC:peptide interactions should, in the future, permit a rational experimental design to fish out such

peptides. Another intriguing question is: how many TcR specificities can be selected on a single peptide:MHC complex. That is, how degenerate is positive selection? Designing unequivocal experiments to answer these questions remains a goal for years to come.

FUTURE DIRECTIONS

Intrathymic positive selection, although less mysterious than 15 years ago, still remains poorly chartered territory in molecular terms. Given the importance of this phenomenon for the generation of a diverse TcR repertoire, this field is bound to remain active and bring excitement to immunologists in the future. I expect that most attention will focus on physical contact of the TcR with the peptide:MHC complex, on sequence and origin of positively selecting self peptides, and on the biochemical signaling pathways that are initiated by positive selection.

SUMMARY

MHC restriction is imprinted on T cells in the thymus, by the process of positive selection. The TcR on a maturing thymocyte must contact MHC molecules expressed on the thymic cortical epithelium to ensure further maturation. A failure to do so results in death by neglect. The process of recognition involves a TcR and a complex of self peptide:self MHC. The precise stage at which thymocytes are selected, the nature of self peptides mediating the process and the mechanism of selection are still elusive at present.

REFERENCES

1. von Boehmer H, Teh HS, Kisielow P. The thymus selects the useful, neglects the useless and destroys the harmful. Immunol Today 1989; 10:57-61.
2. Sprent J, Webb SR. Function and specificity of T-cell subsets in the mouse. Adv Immunol 1987; 41:39.
3. Yewdell JW, Bennink JR. Cell biology of antigen processing and presentation to MHC class I molecule-restricted T lymphocytes. Adv Immunol 1992; 52:1.
4. Zinkernagel RM, Doherty PC. MHC-restricted cytotoxic T-cells: studies on the biological role of polymorphic major

transplantation antigens determining T-cell restriction-specificity, function, and responsiveness. Adv Immunol 1979; 27:51.

5. von Boehmer H, Sprent J, Nabholz M. Tolerance to histocompatibility antigens in tetraparental bone marrow chimeras. J Exp Med 1975; 141:322-334.

6. Bevan MJ. In a radiation chimera host H-2 antigens determine the immune responsiveness of donor cytotoxic cells. Nature 1977; 269:417-418.

7. Zinkernagel RM, Callahan GN, Althage A et al. On the thymus in the differentiation of "H-2 self-recognition" by T cells: evidence for dual recognition?. J Exp Med 1978; 147:882-896.

8. Fink PJ, Bevan MJ. H-2 antigens of the thymus determine lymphocyte specificity. J Exp Med 1978; 148:776.

9. Zinkernagel RM, Calahan GN, Klein J et al. Cytotoxic T cells learn specificity for self H-2 during differentiation in the thymus. Nature 1978; 271:251.

10. von Boehmer H, Haas W, Jerne NK. Major histocompatibility complex-linked immune-responsiveness is acquired by lymphocytes of low responder mice differentiating in thymus of high-responder mice. Proc Natl Acad Sci USA 1978; 75:2439-2443.

11. Kappler J, Marrack P. The role of H-2 linked genes in helper T-cell function. IV. Importance of T-cell genotype and host environment in I region and Ir gene expression. J Exp Med 1978; 128:1510.

12. Vukmanovic S, Bevan MJ, Hogquist KA. The specificity of positive selection: MHC and peptides. Immunol Rev 1993; 135. In press.

13. Hugo P, Kappler JW, Marrack PC. Positive selection of TcRαβ thymocytes: is cortical thymic epithelium an obligatory participant in the presentation of major histocompatibility complex protein? Immunol Rev 1993; 135, in press.

14. Bevan MJ, Hunig T. T cells respond preferentially to antigens that are similar to self H-2. Proc Natl Acad Sci USA 1981; 78:1843-1847.

15. Hunig TR, Bevan MJ. Antigen recognition by cloned cytotoxic T lymphocytes follows rules predicted by the altered-self hypothesis. J Exp Med 1982; 155:111.

16. Bjorkman PJ, Saper MA, Samraoui B et al. Structure of the human class I histocompatibility antigen, HLA-A2. Nature 1987; 329:506.

17. Bjorkman PJ, Saper MA, Samraoui B et al. The foreign antigen binding site and T-cell recognition regions of class I histocompatibility antigens. Nature 1987; 329:512.

18. Brown JH, Jardetzky TS, Gorga JC et al. Three-dimensional structure of the human class II histocompatibility antigen HLA-DR1. Nature 1993; 364:33-39.

19. Fremont DH, Matsumura M, Stura EA et al. Crystal structures of 2 viral peptides in complex with murine MHC class-I H-2K^b. Science 1992; 257:919.

20. Matsumura M, Fremont DH, Peterson PA et al. Emerging principles for the recognition of peptide antigens by MHC class-I molecules. Science 1992; 257:927.

21. Silver ML, Guo H-C, Strominger JL et al. Atomic structure of a human MHC molecule presenting an influenza virus peptide. Nature 1992; 360:367.

22. Ajitkumar P, Geier SS, Kesari KV et al. Evidence that multiple residues on both the α-helices of the Class I MHC molecule are simultaneously recognized by the T-cell receptor. Cell 1988; 54:47.

23. McPhee D, Pye J, Shortman K. The differentiation of T-lymphocytes. V. Evidence for intrathymic death of most thymocytes. Thymus 1979; 1:151.

24. Scollay R, Butcher E, Weissman I. Thymus migration: Quantitative studies on the rate of migration of cells from the thymus to the periphery in mice. Eur J Immunol 1980; 10:210.

25. Hedrick SM, Cohen DI, Nielsen EA et al. Isolation of c-DNA clones encoding T-cell specific membrane-associated proteins. Nature 1984; 308:149-153.

26. Yanagi Y, Yoshikai Y, Leggett K et al. A human T-cell-specific cDNA clone encodes a protein having extensive homology to immunoglobulin chains. Nature 1984; 308:145.

27. Jerne NK. The somatic generation of immune

recognition. Eur J Immunol 1970; 1:1-9.

28. Davies AJ. The tale of T cells. Immunol Today 1993; 14:137-140.

29. Chothia C, Boswell DR, Lesk AM. The outline structure of the T-cell α/β receptor. EMBO J 1988; 7:3745.

30. Teh H-S, Kisielow P, Scott B et al. Thymic major histocompatibility complex antigens and the αβ/T-cell receptor determine the CD4/CD8 phenotype of T cells. Nature 1988; 335:229.

31. Sha WC, Nelson CA, Newberry RA et al. Positive and negative selection of an antigen receptor on T cells in transgenic mice. Nature 1988; 336:73-76.

32. Kaye J, Hsu M-L, Sauron M-E et al. Selective development of CD4+ T cells in transgenic mice expressing a class II MHC-restricted antigen receptor. Nature 1989; 341:746.

33. Berg LJ, Pullen AM, Fazekas de St Groth B et al. Antigen/MHC-specific T cells are preferentially exported from the thymus in the presence of their MHC ligand. Cell 1989; 58:1035.

34. Bluthmann H, Kisielow P, Uematsu Y et al. T-cell-specific deletion of T-cell receptor transgenes allows functional rearrangement of endogenous α- and β-genes. Nature 1988; 334:156-159.

35. Kisielow P, Teh H-S, Bluthmann H et al. Positive selection of antigen-specific T cells in thymus by restriting MHC molecules. Nature 1988; 335:730.

36. Scott B, Bluthmann H, Teh H-S et al. The generation of mature T cells requires interaction of the αβ T-cell receptor with major histocompatibility antigens. Nature 1989; 338:591-593.

37. Bix M, Raulet D. Inefficient positive selection of T cells directed by haematopoietic cells. Nature 1992; 359:330.

38. Pawlowski T, Elliott JD, Jaenisch R et al. Positive selection of T lymphocytes on firboblasts. Nature 1993; 364:642.

39. Hugo P, Kappler JW, McCormack J et al. Fibroblasts can mediate thymocyte positive selection in vivo. Proc Natl Acad Sci USA 1993.

40. Longo DL, Schwartz RH. T-cell specificity for H-2 and Ir gene phenotype correlates with the phenotype of thymic antigen-presenting cells. Nature 1980; 287:44.

41. Longo DL, Davis ML. Early appearance of donor-type antigen presenting cells in the thymuses of 1,200 rad radiation-induced bone marrow chimeras correlates with self recognition of donor I region gene products. J Immunol 1983; 130:2525.

42. Longo DL, Kruisbeek AM, Davis ML et al. Bone marrow-derived thymic antigen presenting cells determine self-recognition of Ia resticted T lymphocytes. Proc Natl Acad Sci USA 1985; 82:5900.

43. Lo D, Sprent J. Identity of cells that imprint H-2-restricted T-cell specificity in the thymus. Nature 1986; 318:672-675.

44. Widera G, Burkly LC, Pinkert CA et al. Transgenic mice selectively lacking MHC class II (I-E) antigen expression on B cells: an in vivo approach to investigate Ia gene function. Cell 1987; 51:175.

45. Vukmanovic S, Grandea AG, Faas SJ et al. Positive selection of T-lymphocytes induced by intrathymic injection of a thymic epithelial cell line. Nature 1992; 359:729.

46. Hugo P, Kappler JW, Godfrey DI et al. A cell line which can induce thymocyte positive selection. Nature 1992; 360:679.

47. Jenkinson EJ, Anderson G, Owen JJT. Studies on T-cell maturation on defined thymic stromal cell populations in vitro. J Exp Med 1992; 176:845.

48. Anderson G, Jenkinson EJ, Moore NC et al. MHC class II-positive epithelium and mesenchyme cells are both required for T-cell development in the thymus. Nature 1993; 362:70.

49. Muller K-P, Kyewski BA. T-cell receptor targeting to thymic cortical epithelial cells in vivo induces survival, activation and differentiation of immature thymocytes. Eur J Immunol 1993; 23:1661-1670.

50. Apasov S, Sitkovsky M. Highly lytic CD8+, αβ T-cell receptor cytotoxic T cells with major histocompatibility complex (MHC) class I antigen-directed cytotoxicity in $β_2$-microglobulin, MHC class I-deficient mice. Proc Natl Acad Sci USA 1993; 90:2837.

51. Turka LA, Schatz DG, Oettinger MA et al. Thymocyte expression of RAG-1 and RAG-2: Termination by T-cell receptor

cross-linking. Science 1991; 253:778-781.

52. Petrie HT, Livak F, Schatz DG et al. Multiple rearrangements in T-cell receptor α chain genes maximize the production of useful thymocytes. J Exp Med 1993; 178:615-622.

53. Borgulya P, Kishi H, Uematsu Y et al. Exclusion and inclusion of α and β T-cell receptor alleles. Cell 1992; 69:529-537.

54. Brandle D, Muller C, Rulicke T et al. Engagement of the T-cell receptor during positive selection in the thymus down-regulates RAG-1 expression. Proc Natl Acad Sci USA 1992; 89:9529-9533.

55. Swat W, Dessing M, Baron A et al. Phenotypic changes accompanying positive selection of CD4+CD8+ thymocytes. Eur J Immunol 1992; 22:2367.

56. Petrie HT, Strasser A, Harris AW et al. CD4+8- and CD4-8+ mature thymocytes require different post-selection processing for final development. J Immunol 1993; 151:1273-1279.

57. Benoist C, Mathis D. Positive selection of the T-cell repertoire: where and when does it occur? Cell 1989; 58:1027.

58. Chan SH, Cosgrove D, Waltzinger C et al. Another view of the selective model of thymocyte selection. Cell 1993; 73:225.

59. Davis CB, Killeen N, Crooks MEC et al. Evidence for a stochastic mechanism in the differentiation of mature subsets of T lymphocytes. Cell 1993; 73:237.

60. van Meerwijk JPM, Germain RN. Development of mature CD8+4-thymocytes: Selection rather than instruction? Science 1993; 261:911-915.

61. Townsend A, Bodmer H. Antigen recognition by class I-restricted T lymphocytes. Ann Rev Immunol 1989; 7:601-624.

62. Nikolic-Zugic J, Bevan MJ. Role of self-peptides in positively selecting the T-cell repertoire. Nature 1990; 344:65.

63. Berg LJ, Frank GD, Davis MM. The effects of MHC gene dosage and allelic variation on T-cell receptor selection. Cell 1990; 60:1043.

64. Sha WC, Nelson CA, Newberry RD et al. Positive selection of transgenic receptor-bearing thymocytes by Kb mutations that involve peptide binding. Proc Natl Acad Sci USA 1990; 87:6186.

65. Jacobs J, von Boehmer H, Melief CJM et al. Mutations in the major histocompatibility complex class I antigen-presenting groove affect both negative and positive selection of T cells. Eur J Immunol 1990; 20:2333.

66. Bhayani HR, Hedrick SM. The role of polymorphic amino acids of the MHC molecule in the selection of the T-cell repertoire. J Immunol 1991; 146: 1093.

67. Hogquist KA, Gavin MA, Bevan MJ. Positive selection of CD8+ T cells induced by major histocompatibility complex binding peptides in fetal thymic organ culture. J Exp Med 1993; 177:1469-1473.

68. Ashton-Rickardt PG, Van Kaer L, Schumacher TNM et al. Peptide contributes to the specificity of positive selection of CD8+ T cells in the thymys. Cell 1993; 73:1041-1049.

69. Rammensee H-G, Falk K, Rotzschke O. MHC molecules as peptide receptors. Curr Opinion Immunol 1993; 5:35-44.

70. Marrack P, Kappler J. The T-cell receptor. Science 1987; 238:1073.

71. Bonomo A, Matzinger P. Thymus epithelium induces tissue-specific tolerance. J Exp Med 1993; 177:1153-1164.

72. Garrett TPJ, Saper MS, Bjorkman PJ et al. Specificity pockets for the side chains of peptide antigens in HLA-Aw68. Nature 1989; 342:692-696.

73. Falk K, Rotzschke O, Stevanovic S et al. Allele-specific motifs revealed by sequencing of self-peptides eluted from MHC molecules. Nature 1991; 351:290-296.

74. Pullen JF, Hunt HD, Pease LR. Peptide interactions with the Kb antigen recognition site. J Immunol 1991; 146:2145-2151.

75. Nikolic-Zugic J, Carbone FR. The effect of mutations in the MHC class I peptide binding groove on the cytotoxic T lymphocyte recognition of the Kb-restricted ovalbumin determinant. Eur J Immunol 1990; 20:2431.

76. Kaye J, Vasquez NJ, Hedrick SM. Involvement of the same region of the T-cell antigen receptor in thymic selection and foreign peptide recognition. J Immunol 1992; 148:3342.

77. Jameson SC, Carbone FR, Bevan MJ. Clone-specific T-cell receptor antagonists of major

histocompatibility complex class I-restricted cytotoxic T cells. J Exp Med 1993; 177:1541-1550.

78. Evavold BD, Allen PM. Separation of IL-4 production from Th cell proliferation by an altered T-cell receptor ligand. Science 1991; 252:1308.

79. De Magistris MT, Alexander J, Coggeshall M et al. Antigen analog-major histocompatibility complexes act as antagonists of the T-cell receptor. Cell 1992; 68:625.

CHAPTER 8

CLONAL DELETION IN INTRATHYMIC NEGATIVE SELECTION

Janko Nikolić-Žugić

T cells are in charge of defending an organism against foreign invaders. However, in the course of their normal function, T cells follow an old physicians' principle: *primum non nocere* (first, do no harm). In order to do no harm to normal, uninfected tissue, and focus their destructive action solely on infected of altered cells, T cells must be tolerant to self. The idea that the thymus may be critical in inducing and maintaining tolerance to self was pioneered by Jerne[1] in the late sixties. Indeed, neonatal—but not adult—thymectomy results in systemic autoimmunity.[2] In principle, tolerance to self in the thymus can be achieved by two mutually nonexclusive mechanisms: by physical elimination of self-reactive T cells (tolerance by clonal deletion) or by functional silencing of self-reactive cells (nondeletional tolerance or anergy) (reviewed in ref. 3). {Two other major mechanisms that could operate to prevent self-aggression, peripheral tolerance and suppression by regulatory T cells or veto cells, by definition act extrathymically, and will not be discussed here.} Direct evidence that both mechanisms indeed do operate in the organism came about with the advent of monoclonal antibodies against various TcR V_β segments and transgenic technology. Since the thymus remains the central organ that imparts deletional tolerance to strong, MHC-like self antigens, this mechanism will be discussed before nondeletional tolerance.

CLONAL DELETION IN THE THYMUS

In 1987 Kappler, Roehm and Marrack published a study which de facto demonstrated that clonal deletion was the dominant form of intrathymic negative selection.[4] Using an antibody directed against the $V_\beta 17^a$ segment of the TcR, they showed that in certain mouse strains bearing the class II molecule I-E, essentially all mature TcR^{hi} $V_\beta 17^a$-bearing T cells were deleted in the thymus (Table 1). By contrast, the majority of immature TcR^{lo} cells bearing this V_β segment were not deleted. Based on the intensity of TcR expression, the authors correctly postulated that, in the case of this particular antigen, deletion occurs at the post-DP developmental stage.

Table 1. MMTV-mediated tolerance by clonal deletion.

Mouse strain	I-E	% of total $V_\beta 17a^+$ thymocytes	
		$V_\beta 17a^{lo}$ cells	$V_\beta 17a^{hi}$ cells
SJL	–	56.1	43.9
SWR	–	76.3	24.7
C57BR	+	96.6	3.4
(AKR x SWR)F$_1$	+	94.7	5.3

Thymocytes of indicated strains were analyzed for the expression of $V_\beta 17a$ by flow cytometry, and the percentage of high and low expressors determined using a program described in.[4] In a separate experiment, the authors have documented that most $V_\beta 17a^{hi}$ cells are SP and that $V_\beta 17a^{lo}$ cells are DP. Details are described in 4.

Soon thereafter, similar phenomenology was reported for the $V_\beta 6^5-$ and $V_\beta 8.1$-bearing[6] T cells, and later for other V_βs (reviewed in refs. 3 and 7). Several years later it became apparent that the deleting ligands in these experiments were actually the products of endogenous mouse mammary tumor viruses (MMTVs).[7] These antigens, along with certain bacterial and mycoplasma products, belong to a group of microbial products named "superantigens" (SAG) by Marrack and Kappler.[8] By contrast to conventional antigens that bind to the peptide-binding site of the MHC molecules, superantigens combine with class II molecules (preferentially I-E molecules and DR molecules in the mouse and the human, respectively) by binding to the sites away from the peptide-binding groove. Likewise, these antigens bind to the TcR at the site distinct from the one that contacts the peptide:MHC complex (namely to the $V\beta$ segment, although other parts of the molecule may also be involved).

Given the unorthodox (and at the time very mysterious) nature of SAGs, it was important to demonstrate clonal deletion in other systems. Indeed, in 1988 results documenting clonal deletion were obtained from TcR transgenic mice.[9,10] In the αH-Y TcR tg model, it was shown that the male-specific H-Y antigen deletes almost all thymocytes bearing the transgenic TcR, including the vast majority of DP cells (Table 2A); thus reducing the number of cells in such a thymus to one-hundredth of control values.[9] These results were confirmed in other transgenic models, most importantly in those where the peptide antigen was well defined.[11-13] For example, clonal deletion was elegantly demonstrated in TcR tg animals whose TcR was specific for the soluble foreign antigen ovalbumin (OVA) and the class II molecule I-A^d after in vivo injection of the OVA peptide[13] (Table 2B). Likewise, in the {pigeon cytochrome C (pCyt) + I-E^k}-specific TcR Tg mice, DP cells were deleted in vitro by the pCyt peptide on APCs expressing I-E^k.[14]

Important experiments carried out by Smith et al indicated that the main biochemical mechanism for clonal deletion is the apoptotic death induced by TcR stimulation.[15] In these and other studies, it was demonstrated that thymocytes undergo characteristic DNA fragmentation and suicide upon TcR ligation by TcR-specific mAb (mimicking the antigen) or upon the elevation of intracellular calcium.[15,16] Subsequent experiments directly demonstrated that in vivo interaction of the TcR with self peptide:MHC complex induces apoptosis in immature thymocytes.[13] (The importance of apoptosis in clonal deletion and the development of T cells is such that it will be addressed in Chapter 12.)

Clonal deletion has lent itself to stricter scrutiny than positive selection; we therefore know much more about the stage, molecular requirements and biochemical events in deletional negative selection.

THE SITE OF INTRATHYMIC DELETION

A vast body of evidence shows that the most effective tolerizing tissues are of hematopoietic origin. In particular, macrophages (MØ) and dendritic cells (DC) are exquisitely potent in tolerizing against graft rejection in vivo and the MLR (mixed lymphocyte reaction) in vitro.[17,18] Thymocytes themselves are also effective in tolerizing other thymocytes against the MHC molecules expressed on their surface.[19] It seems certain that intrathymic MØ and DC actually delete, rather than induce nondeletional tolerance of self-reactive cells. Genetic evidence also supports such compartmentalization of tasks in the thymus. When a deleting element is expressed in the thymic cortex, essentially no deletion is detectable in an MMTV system. However, deletion is readily observed if the same element is selectively targeted to the medullary section of the thymus, and more precisely, to MØ and DC.[20,21] At the face value, this would mean that the thymic cortex possesses little or no ability to delete thymocytes, and that the medullary hematopoietic elements are crucial for this process. Alternatively, cortical thymocytes

could be too immature to process/detect a deleting signal "correctly" administered by the cortical epithelium.[22] In line with these experiments, a series of experiments failed to demonstrate tolerization of thymocytes when thymic grafts were depleted of hematopoietic cells.[17,18] In other experiments, however, evidence of split tolerance was obtained: the thymic epithelium was capable of inducing tolerance to graft rejection in vivo and to class I determinants in vitro, but could not establish tolerance to class II determinants in vitro.[23,24]

From the literature[17, 18] and the above discussion, it is quite clear that the thymic epithelium is not necessary for the induction of tolerance, and that the most efficient deleting tissue is the hematopoietic one. Controversy surrounds the ability of the thymic epithelium to imprint tolerance, and, in particular, to delete thymocytes. In addition to several elegant studies by Sprent et al,[23,24] which strongly indicated that the epithelium can tolerize (and, in some cases, delete), a recent study of Bonomo and Matzinger[25] has offered data that may help reconcile some of the old controversies. In an ingenious set of experiments, these authors demonstrated that thymic epithelium very effectively renders thymocytes tolerant to all antigens that it

---

Table 2. Clonal deletion in TcR transgenic mice.

TcR specificity	Deleting antigen/MHC	# DP thymocytes (x 10^{-6})
Exp. model #1		
H-Y + D^b	-/ D^b	63.0
H-Y + D^b	H-Y / D^b	1.4
Exp. model #2		
$OVA_{323-339}$ + A^d	-/ A^d	158.4
$OVA_{323-339}$ + A^d	$OVA_{324-334}$ / A^d	192.5
$OVA_{323-339}$ + A^d	$OVA_{323-339}$ / A^d	7.8

The details of these experiments are provided in references 9 and 13 for Experimental models #1 and #2, respectively. In the first model, the deleting antigen is cell-bound and was introduced into the transgenic background by mating. In the second model, OVA peptides were injected for three consecutive days i.p. and thymocytes examined for the evidence of deletion thereafter.

expresses. These antigens include MHC class I antigens, MHC class II antigens, and tissue-specific antigens, some of which are shared between the thymic epithelium and other epithelia, e.g., the skin. By contrast, other tissue-specific antigens not expressed by thymic epithelium could readily be recognized and eliminated (both in vivo and in vitro) by epithelium-tolerized T cells. These results are entirely consistent with the older literature, where thymic lobes depleted of hematopoietic elements were used to test tolerance induction. The lack of tolerance, especially that directed to class II molecules, was in most cases detected upon in vitro stimulation with spleen cells, and these cells must express an array of peptides not expressed by the thymic epithelium.

Although I clearly favor the above explanation for the controversy surrounding the tolerogenic capacity of thymic epithelium, other mutually nonexclusive explanations for the "poor" tolerogenicity of thymic epithelium are also valid, e.g., the one postulating a lack of expression of adhesion/co-stimulatory molecules by cortical epithelium. Indeed, certain[26] (but not other[27-29]) adhesion/costimulatory molecules have been shown to play an active role in clonal deletion. Furthermore, by the time thymocytes reach the medullary region, most of them actually express higher levels of TcR than in the cortex, and may even activate different signaling pathways than cortical thymocytes. These changes may be necessary to confer the ability to be deleted to certain thymocytes. Finally, it is possible that the density of certain self-peptide determinants may be rather low in the cortex compared to the medulla (where, for example, the expression of MHC class I molecules appears higher than in the cortex, judged by tissue section staining[22]).

THE STAGE AT WHICH THYMOCYTES ARE DELETED

Again, this question can be answered more precisely than the similar issue in positive selection. As mentioned above, Kappler et al in their original description of clonal deletion were the first to demonstrate that thymocytes are deleted rather late, i.e., after

upregulation of the TcR[4]. This upregulation generally occurs after the DP stage of development, although a minor subset of DP cells also expresses high levels of TcR (see Chapter 3). The same results were obtained with other MMTV-mediated deletions. Controversy arose when it became apparent that in TcR tg mice bearing class I-restricted transgenes the deletion affects the majority of DP thymocytes.[9] It was originally postulated that the artificially high levels of TcR expression in TcR tg mice (five- to ten-fold higher than in normal animals) led to early deletion in the thymus. However, the elegant experiments of Ohashi et al[30] clearly demonstrated that in their TcR tg system the stage of clonal deletion varies with the site of antigen expression. This tg TcR had dual specificity for the LCMV peptide + D^b and for an MMTV product (based on its V_β segment). When the deleting antigen was the LCMV peptide, expressed throughout the cortex, deletion occurred at the DP stage. By contrast, the MMTV product induced deletion of thymocytes at a later stage, without affecting most of the DP cells. MMTV products are poorly or not at all expressed in thymic epithelial cells, but are expressed abundantly on the medullary APCs. Thus the expression of the deleting antigen by thymic APCs can determine the stage at which thymocytes are deleted.

Despite studies that proposed an orderly sequence of intrathymic selection[31,32]—positive selection would precede negative according to this view—a number of experiments have de facto shown that negative selection can occur independently of positive selection and at several stages of development.[18,33] Thus, there exists a developmental window during which a thymocyte can be deleted.[34] Such a window most probably begins with the TcR[lo] thymocytes, some of which are clearly deleted in TcR Tg mice. The other boundary of such window is less clear. Several lines of evidence indicate that the most mature, HSA⁻ SP thymocytes can no longer be deleted (induced to undergo apoptosis) as easily as the DP cells. SP cells are generally spared after the acute corticosteroid treatment that kills most DP thymocytes, and, unlike the majority of DP cells, express an anti-apoptotic protooncogene *bcl-2*.[35-37] The most mature thymocytes thus probably acquire a degree of resistance to deletion just before leaving the thymus (see Chapter 12). This resistance is not absolute: peripheral T cells can undergo antigen-specific deletion under the circumstances where massive doses of antigen are injected in vivo.[38,39] The difference really lies in the ease with which the cells can be induced to die: immature DP cells require only subtle stimulation, whereas mature T cells need excessive stimulation that rarely occurs in vivo. Therefore, the window for "easy" clonal deletion may exist from the moment the TcR is expressed at the surface of thymocytes to the very last stage of intrathymic development, just prior to emigration.

THE LIGAND AND THE MOLECULES INVOLVED IN INTRATHYMIC DELETION

There is little doubt that the ligand for clonal deletion consists of self peptides coupled to self MHC molecules. Indeed, when a foreign peptide is introduced into the thymus, T cells specific for it are deleted as if the peptide is a self component;[13] from the standpoint of developing T cells, it seems such—it is encountered at the time when self/foreign distinction is being learned, and foreign is defined as "not present".

From the thymocyte point of view, the TcR has a decisive role in clonal deletion—its specificity determines the fit for self antigens. Accessory CD4 and CD8 molecules[40,41,42] as well as the costimulatory LFA-1 molecule[26] and their respective ligands are known to participate in negative selection by modulating the avidity of the interaction between a thymocyte and the APC and/or by transducing signals that are crucial to cellular activation. Other molecules and molecular pairs may also play a role in these processes. But it appears that some accessory interactions are redundant and that clonal deletion can proceed even in the absence of such obligatory signaling mediators such as the protein-tyrosine kinases.[43] Teleologically, this would suggest that the importance of clonal deletion is such that a duplication of signaling mechanisms have evolved, each of which can singlehandedly ensure that autoaggressive thymocytes are eliminated.

Of the sum of peptides to which T cells must be tolerant, a number are expressed neither in the thymus nor in extracellular fluids that could transport them to the thymus. Thus, the thymus deals quite effectively with all peptides that are present. But there is a clear safeguard built in the system for other peptides/proteins. Thus, it has been experimentally shown that both deletional[39,38] and nondeletional[44] tolerance can operate in the periphery. In addition, active mechanisms of suppression by regulatory T cells could also play a role in the maintenance of tolerance. It is not known what is the relative importance of each of these mechanisms for the induction and maintenance of tolerance in vivo. Personally, my bias is that the thymus has a lion's share, perhaps taking care of more than 99% of physiologically available self products, as discussed by Sprent.[18,23] The argument is purely speculative and teleological: if peripheral tolerance operates on a daily basis, one has to explain how T cells decide when to be activated and mount an immune response, as opposed to being inactivated or deleted. Although one attractive possibility may be to provide a different context of a signal, e.g., by costimulation, for activation versus deletion or anergy, I believe that such a regulation via costimulation plays a more important role in sustaining and regulating the magnitude and duration of an immune response, rather than tolerance. Without the experimental back-up, this remains just one possible scenario.

SUMMARY

Physical elimination of autoaggressive cells is the main mechanism of tolerance induction in the thymus. It can occur at several stages of T-cell development, before or after positive selection. A special role in deletional tolerance belongs to bone marrow-derived APCs, although the epithelial component of the thymus can also delete.

Mechanisms of deletion are now being heavily investigated at molecular and biochemical levels. The main challenge in the field is to elucidate the biochemical difference between the signals that mediate positive and negative selection.

REFERENCES

1. Jerne NK. The somatic generation of immune recognition. Eur J Immunol 1970; I:1-9.
2. Smith H, Chen I-M, Kubo R et al. Neonatal thymectomy results in a repertoire enriched in T cells deleted in adult thymus. Science 1989; 245:749-752.
3. Nossal GJV. Immunologic tolerance: collaboration between antigen and lymphokines. Science 1989; 245:147-153.
4. Kappler JW, Roehm N, Marrack P. T-cell tolerance by clonal elimination in the thymus. Cell 1987; 49:273-281.
5. MacDonald HR, Schneider R, Lees RK et al. T-cell receptor V_β use predicts reactivity and tolerance to Mls^a-encoded antigens. Nature 1988;332:40.
6. Kappler JW, Staerz U, White J et al. Self-tolerance eliminates T cells specific for Mls-modified products of the major histocompatibility complex. Nature 1988; 332:35-40.
7. Janeway C. Mls: makes a little sense. Nature 1991; 349:459-461.
8. Marrack P, Kappler J. The T-cell receptor. Science 1987;238:1073.
9. Kisielow P, Bluthmann H, Staerz UD et al. Tolerance in T-cell receptor transgenic mice involves deletion of nonmature CD4$^+$CD8$^+$ thymocytes. Nature 1988; 333:742.
10. Sha WC, Nelson CA, Newberry RD et al. Positive and negative selection of an antigen receptor on T cells in transgenic mice. Nature 1988; 336:73-76.
11. Berg LJ, Fazekas de StGroth B, Pullen AM et al. Phenotypic differences between $\alpha\beta$ and β T-cell receptor transgenic mice undergoing negative selection. Nature 1989; 340:559.
12. Kaye J, Hsu M-L, Sauron M-E et al. Selective development of CD4$^+$ T cells in transgenic mice expressing a class II MHC-restricted antigen receptor. Nature 1989; 341:746.
13. Murphy KM, Heimberger AB, Loh DY. Induction by antigen of intrathymic apoptosis of CD4$^+$8$^-$ TcR^{lo} thymocytes in vivo. Science 1990; 250:1720.
14. Vasquez N, Kaye J, Hedrick SM. In vivo and in vitro clonal deletion of double-positive thymocytes. J Exp Med 1992; 175:1307.
15. Smith CA, Williams GT, Kingston E et al. Antibodies to CD3/T-cell receptor complex induce death by apoptosis in immature T cells in thymic cultures. Nature 1989; 337:181.
16. Shi Y, Bissonnette RP, Parfrey N et al. In vivo administration of monoclonal antibodies to the CD3 T-cell receptor complex induces cell death (apoptosis) in immature thymocytes. J Immunol 1991; 146:3340.
17. Sprent J, Webb SR. Function and specificity of T-cell subsets in the mouse. Adv Immunol 1987; 41:39.
18. Sprent J, Lo D, Gao E-K et al. T-cell selection in the thymus. Immunol Rev 1988; 101:172.
19. Shimonkevitz RP, Bevan MJ. Split tolerance induced by the intrathymic adoptive transfer of thymocyte stem cells. J Exp Med 1988; 168:143-156.
20. Widera G, Burkly LC, Pinkert CA et al. Transgenic mice selectively lacking MHC class II (I-E) antigen expression on B cells: an in vivo approach to investigate Ia gene function. Cell 1987; 51:175.
21. Benoist C, Mathis D. Positive selection of the T-cell repertoire: where and when does it occur? Cell 1989; 58:1027.
22. Boyd RL, Tucek CL, Godfrey DI et al. The thymic microenvironment. Immunol Today 1993; 14:445-459.
23. Gao E-K, Lo D, Sprent J. Strong T-cell tolerance in parent $\rightarrow$ F$_1$ bone marrow chimeras prepared with supralethal irradiation. J Exp Med 1993; 171:1101-1121.
24. Gao E-K, Kosaka H, Surh CD. T-cell contact with Ia antigens on nonhemopoietic cells in vivo can lead to immunity rather than tolerance. J Exp Med 1991; 174:435-446.
25. Bonomo A, Matzinger P. Thymus epithelium induces tissue-specific tolerance. J Exp Med 1993; 177:1153-1164.
26. Carlow DA, Oers NSCvan, Teh S-J et al.

Deletion of antigen-specific immature thymocytes by dendritic cells requires LFA-1/ICAM interactions. J Immunol 1992; 148:1595-1603.

27. Tan R, Teh S-J, Ledbetter JA et al. B7 costimulates proliferation of CD4⁻8⁺ T lymphocytes but is not required for the deletion of immature CD4⁺8⁺ thymocytes. J Immunol 1992; 149:3217-3226.

28. Page DM, Kane LP, Allison JP et al. Two signals are required for negative selection of CD4⁺CD8⁺ thymocytes. J Immunol 1993; 151:1868-1880.

29. Killeen N, Stuart SG, Littman DR. Development and function of T cells in mice with a disrupted CD2 gene. EMBO J 1992; 11:4329-4340.

30. Ohashi PS, Pircher H, Burkl K et al. Distinct sequence of negative or positive selection implied by thymocyte T-cell receptor densities. Nature 1990; 346:861-863.

31. Guidos CJ, Danska JS, Fathman CG et al. T-cell receptor-mediated negative selection of autoreactive T lymphocyte precursors occurs after commitment to the CD4 or CD8 lineages. J Exp Med 1990; 172:835.

32. Finkel TH, Cambier JC, Kubo RT et al. The thymus has two functionally distinct population of immature αβ T cells: one population is deleted by ligation of αβ TcR. Cell 1989; 58:1047.

33. Spain LM, Berg LJ. Developmental regulation of thymocyte susceptibility to deletion by "self"-peptide. J Exp Med 1992; 176:213-223.

34. Nikolic-Zugic J. Phenotypic and functional stages in thymocyte development. Immunol Today 1991; 12:65.

35. Gratiot-Deans J, Ding L, Turka LA et al. bcl-2 proto-oncogene expression during human T-cell development. J Immunol

1993; 151:83-91.

36. Veis DJ, Sentman CL, Bach EA et al. Expression of the Bcl-2 protein in murine and human thymocytes and in peripheral T lymphocytes. J Immunol 1993; 151: 2546-2554.

37. Andjelic S, Jain N, Nikolic-Zugic J. Immature thymocytes become sensitive to calcium-mediated apoptosis with the onset of CD8,CD4, and the T-cell receptor expression: A role for bcl-2. J Exp Med 1993; 178:1745-1751.

38. Rammensee H-G, Kroschewski R, Frangoulis B. Clonal anergy induced in mature Vβ6⁺ T lymphocytes on immunizing Mlsᵇ mice with Mlsᵃ expressing cells. Nature 1989; 339:541-544.

39. Webb S, Morris C, Sprent J. Extrathymic tolerance of mature T cells: Clonal elimination as a consequence of immunity. Cell 1990; 63:1249-1256.

40. Ramsdell F, Fowlkes BJ. Engagement of CD4 and CD8 accessory molecules is required for T-cell maturation. J Immunol 1989; 143:1467.

41. Robey EA, Fowlkes BJ, Gordon JW et al. Thymic selection in CD8 transgenic mice supports an instructive model for commitment to a CD4 or CD8 lineage. Cell 1991; 64:99.

42. Lee NA, Loh DY, Lacy E. CD8 surface levels alter the fate of α/β T-cell receptor-expressing thymocytes in transgenic mice. J Exp Med 1992; 175:1013.

43. Nakayama K-I, Loh DY. No requirement for p56Lck in the antigen-stimulated clonal deletion of thymocytes. Science 1992; 257:94-96.

44. Ramsdell F, Fowlkes BJ. Maintenance in vivo tolerance by persistence of antigen. Science 1992; 257:1130.

CHAPTER 9

Negative Intrathymic Selection by Nondeletional Mechanisms

Fred Ramsdell

Although clonal deletion is the best studied system for removing potentially autoreactive cells from the mature T-cell pool, an alternate mechanism of tolerance involves the inactivation of self-reactive T cells. Nondeletional tolerance has been observed in a number of transgenic and superantigen-induced systems. The major characteristic of this form of tolerance is that cells reactive to a particular antigen are not removed from the mature T-cell pool but persist in an inactive state. This is most commonly referred to as clonal anergy, although there are probably multiple biochemical states that have been grouped together under the heading of anergy. Functionally, anergy consists of an inability of cells to respond to a normal stimulatory encounter with antigen. Anergy has been described for both T cells and B cells. This section will focus on the state of nonresponsiveness that can be induced during T-cell development, and the implications that this has for both positive and negative selection of the T-cell repertoire.

Several groups have described the induction of nondeletional tolerance in a developmental situation. Studies have involved the grafting of tissue onto allogeneic hosts including frogs and birds,[1] generation of transgenic animals[2] and the irradiation and bone marrow reconstitution of mice.[3] These studies have suggested that the thymic epithelium has significant tolerance-inducing capabilities, but that the mechanism is distinct from clonal deletion.

Chimeric animals have been produced by grafting tissue onto early embryos or by using thymic rudiments prior to stem cell colonization as donor grafts.[1] Animals bearing such grafts would subsequently tolerate additional skin grafts of the donor (but not third party) type. Tolerance appears to be nondeletional, however, because cells from these animals would react to donor-type MHC molecules in vitro. The precise specificity of the cells could not be examined in these experiments, however.

Using transgenic mice and radiation bone marrow chimeras, it has been possible to follow the fate of specific antigen reactive cells. Transgenic mice in which the MHC class II antigen IE was specifically localized to the thymic epithelium have provided evidence for a nondeletional mechanism for tolerance.[2] Although some reduction in the number of T cells reactive to IE occurs in these transgenic mice, most cells are not deleted. When tested in vitro, the functional responses of the potentially IE reacive T cells are dramatically decreased.

In bone marrow chimera studies, mice that possess and present a particular superantigen are lethally irradiated and subsequently reconstituted with bone marrow from mice that lack the relevant superantigen. The superantigens used in these studies are proteins derived from retroviral (usually MMTV) open reading frames (ORFs) capable of binding and stimulating T cells bearing particular $V\beta$ proteins in their T-cell receptor (TcR).[4] The presentation of these ORFs to T cells requires the presence of class II MHC molecules but is not dependent upon antigen processing. When the bone marrow donors expressed MHC class II molecules (IE) capable of efficiently presenting MMTV proteins, those T cells reactive with these ORFs are deleted.[5, 6] In other studies, the bone marrow donors lack the MHC class II mol-

ecules necessary for appropriate presentation of the particular MMTV ORF proteins also known as viral superantigen (vSAG). Following bone marrow engraftment in these animals, donor T cells develop normally within the host thymus, except that T cells bearing specific $V\beta$ chains fail to be efficiently deleted by the vSAGs of the host animal. An example of such chimeras (along with control chimeras) and the resulting T-cell $V\beta$ repertoire can be seen in Table 1. These data indicate that in these bone marrow chimeric animals, clonal deletion of potentially autoreactive T cells is most efficient when the bone marrow donor expresses the necessary MHC molecules. Further, the data indicate that deletion may fail to occur when the MMTV ORF proteins are presented exclusively by thymic epithelial (TE) cells.

When the T cells from chimeras in which deletion failed to occur were examined for their responses to host-type vSAGs, they were markedly suppressed despite the fact that the mice possessed T cells with $V\beta$ chains known to normally react to the specific vSAGs.[5, 7] Upon further study, it was discovered that those T cells normally deleted in an intact animal were

---

Table 1. Deletion of potentially autoreactive T cells in bone marrow chimeric mice depends upon IE expression by donor cells.

Control Mice	Donor				% Positive	
	vSAG	IE			$V\beta6$	$V\beta17$
SJL	–	–			10.6	10.4
CBA/Ca	–	+			10.2	NA
AKR	+	+			0.3	NA
(BIO.SxAKR)	–/+	–/+			0.2	NA
(SJLxAKR)	–/+	–/+			0.5	2.1
Chimeric Mice	**Donor**		**Host**		**% Positive**	
	vSAG	IE	vSAG	IE	$V\beta6$	$V\beta17$
SJL → B10.S	–	–	–	–	10.3	10.3
SJL → B10.SxAKR	–	–	+	+	9.7	7.4
CBA/Ca → B10.SxAKR	–	+	+	+	0.5	NA

Mature thymocytes were analyzed for the percent of $V_\beta6^+$ and $V_\beta17^+$ cells in the absence or presence of specific vSAGs and MHC class II IE molecules.

rendered nonresponsive to direct stimulation through their T-cell receptor. This is seen in Table 2 in which chimeric animals which possess potentially self-reactive cells or control chimeras are stimulated with antibodies directed to T cells bearing particular TcRβ chains. As noted above, the relative number of cells that express these TcRβ chains is approximately the same in both of these chimeric animals. Thus, although they are present in relatively normal numbers, T cells reactive with host-type vSAGs are functionally nonresponsive to direct TcR stimulation, suggesting that tolerance can be mediated by a mechanism distinct from clonal deletion.

The precise mechanism by which this nondeletional form of tolerance occurs is not clear. One possibility is that this represents an in vivo corollary to the in vitro clonal anergy described for T-cell clones.[8] The data from T clones indicate that to achieve complete activation of a T cell, two distinct signals are required. One of these signals is provided by occupancy of the T-cell receptor; the other, or costimulatory signal, is provided through a distinct cell surface protein. The engagement of the costimulatory receptor(s) initiates an apparently separate biochemical pathway. The interaction of CD28 on the T cell with B7/BB1 on an antigen presenting cell seems to fulfill the criteria for this costimulatory interaction, although other molecules may also possess this ability.[9] The lack of a costimulatory interaction leads to an inability to transcribe the IL-2 gene and a decrease in the transcription of other lymphokine genes. The failure to produce IL-2 results in an inability to proliferate. It is this lack of proliferation which is critical for induction of anergy in T-cell clones.[10] Evidence to suggest that the nonresponsiveness seen in bone marrow chimeras results from this type of anergy comes from studies on thymic antigen presenting cells. Lorenz and Allen have shown that purified TE cells are deficient at stimulating T-cell clones in vitro and in fact induce clonal anergy.[11] These TE cells are MHC class II positive but are presumably deficient at providing costimulation. Presentation of MMTV ORFs by host-type TE cells could therefore

induce anergy in developing T cells.

It is also possible that the nonresponsiveness seen in bone marrow chimeras results from a form of receptor desensitization. This model again derives from work using T-cell clones in which it has been shown that once a T cell has been stimulated, it requires a period of rest before it can be restimulated by antigen. Thus, chronic stimulation of a T cell can lead to an inability to respond to subsequent activation. Whether the ultimate mechanism of this nonresponsiveness is related to the clonal anergy described above is not clear. The mechanism for initiating this state is clearly distinct however, since receptor desensitization can occur in the presence of continuous stimulation involving both TcR occupancy and the provision of a costimulatory signal. Using a transgenic model of tolerance, Blackman et al suggest that in vivo nonresponsiveness may result from such chronic stimulation.[12] In this system, MMTV reactive T cells in an MMTV-bearing host are refractory to stimulation by either antigen or antibodies to their T-cell receptor. Unlike the situation described for T-cell clones, the T cells from this animal are unable to initiate a normal rise in intracellular Ca^{++} following TcR ligation. This characteristic is more indicative of receptor desensitization than the type of anergy described for T clones. Since T cells in the bone marrow chimeras may be constantly exposed to antigen, they may in fact be constantly stimulated, although their ability to initiate a Ca^{++} rise following TcR cross-linking has not been evaluated.

One other characteristic of nondeletional mechanisms of tolerance appears to be the ability to reverse this state. Although anergy may eventually lead to cell death, there exists a period of time in which an anergic T cell may revert to a state of normal responsiveness. This has been demonstrated both for T-cell clones[10] and for the nonresponsive cells found in bone marrow chimeras.[13] In the latter case, T cells were removed from the antigen bearing hosts and transferred to new recipients that either did or did not express the relevant vSAGs. If the new hosts failed to express the vSAGs, the anergic T

Table 2. Potentially self-reactive T cells are nonresponsive to direct TcR stimulation.

	Stimulating Antibody[a]		
	Anti-TcRαβ	Anti-Vβ17	Anti-Vβ6
SJL → B10.S	16,928	2,844	4,688
SJL → B10.SxAKR	28,727	339	793

[a]Antibodies to the TcR$_{\alpha\beta}$ complex or to Vβ17 or Vβ6 T cells were immobilized on microtiter plates. T cells from the chimeras were added and their proliferative response measured 3 days later. Values represent counts per minute of ^{3}H-TdR incorporation.

cells returned to a state of normal responsiveness (Table 3). Thus, the anergic state in the bone marrow chimeras requires the persistence of antigen. This does not allow us to distinguish between the two potential mechanisms for inducing this state however, since both anergy and receptor desensitization may be reversible conditions.

The mechanism of tolerance is probably related to the nature of the cell inducing this state. Clonal deletion appears to be most efficiently mediated by bone marrow-derived cells such as dendritic cells. The results from a variety of chimeric studies suggest that radioresistant elements within the host are relatively poor at inducing clonal deletion, although other chimeric model systems have shown that the epithelium does possess this capability.[14] The most straightforward model then suggests that tolerance induced by the radioresistant thymic epithelium is nondeletional, whereas bone marrow-derived cells mediate deletional tolerance. This notion also fits with the concept that TE cells are unable to provide costimulatory signals to T-cell clones in vitro. Data from Speiser et al, however, challenge this interpretation and suggest that the nondeletional tolerance seen in chimeras is induced by bone marrow-derived cells.[15] In these experiments, the presence and functional status of potentially autoreactive cells was associated with the MHC haplotype of the bone marrow donor and appeared to be independent of the host. Clonal deletion, anergy and normal responsiveness were all observed, depending upon donor MHC class II molecules. This contrasted with the original chimeric studies in which anergy was observed when the ability to efficiently present the MMTV proteins was

Table 3. Maintenance of T-cell tolerance requires the persistence of antigen.

	Pre-transfer analysis		Post-transfer analysis	
BM Recipient	Anti-Vβ17	Anti-Vβ6	Anti-Vβ17	Anti-Vβ6
B10.S	23,400	18,365	12,045	8,337
(B10.SxAKR)	1,202	966	10,347	7,934

Following reconstitution with SJL bone marrow, T cells from the chimeric mice were tested for their ability to respond to stimulation through their TcR as in Table 2. T cells were also transferred to irradiated mice that lacked the relevant self antigens. After 14 days, the T cells were again analyzed for functional responses.

relegated to the thymic epithelium.[5] Speiser et al have thus suggested that the overall avidity of interaction between an developing T cell and an MMTV-bearing cell may determine whether deletion or anergy (non-responsiveness) occurs. Using transgenic model systems, data has been obtained to support the concept that the balance between positive and negative selection is related to the avidity of T cells for their ligands.[16]

Determining the nature of the cell responsible for tolerance induction (either deletional or nondeletional) has important implications for overall T-cell development and positive selection. If thymic epithelial cells, which are known to be capable of positive selection, are also involved in negative selection, this places additional constraints on the mechanism of positive selection. Clearly not all those cells that are positively selected are also negatively selected, and several major models have been proposed to deal with the dichotomy of positive versus negative selection.[3,17] The first suggests that TE cells are primarily responsible for positive selection and that whatever negative selection is induced by thymic epithelium only represents a fraction of the T cells that are positively selected. This could be accomplished by having one subset of epithelial cells mediate positive selection and a distinct subset mediate negative selection. The nature of the MHC-associated peptides may also vary greatly between these subsets of TE cells. The second major model to deal with positive versus negative selection suggests that the affinity of the interaction for these two selections is different. Thus, positive selection may occur at a lower affinity than negative selection and the affinity achieved will probably be influenced by the nature of the antigen presenting cell. In this case, TE cells may only delete clones with high affinity for self ligands. One final model to deal with the issue of selection is that there is a sequential, restricted order to selection such that positive selection must precede negative selection. Thus, a cell could only be induced into a deletion (or anergy) susceptible stage after first undergoing positive selection. At the moment, there exists evidence for each of these models,

and the ultimate model may incorporate components of all of them.

The need to tolerize T cells to epithelial antigens provides a rationale for the tolerizing ability of TE. Although most studies on selection have focused on superantigens because of their ease of study, the MHC molecules of thymic antigen presenting cells possess a variety of peptides. This may affect both positive and negative selection, as the peptides associated with TE cells are almost certainly different from those associated with thymic dendritic cells. If at least a portion of the peptides in TE cells are common to epithelial cells throughout the body, then the tolerance induced by TE cells would be cross-reactive for other epithelial tissues. One potential source for such peptides would be the cytokeratin family of proteins which are common to all epithelial tissues.

The importance of nondeletional tolerance to the animal is not clear. Whether there is an advantage to possessing T cells that can recognize, but not react to self antigens has not been examined. Cells in this anergic state have also been described for antigens isolated to peripheral mesenchymal tissues as well.[18] It has been suggested that anergic cells can serve to potentially dampen an autoimmune response by binding to self antigen and absorbing cytokines produced by self-reactive cells, but not mediating effector functions themselves.[19] In this respect they would serve as antigen-specific suppressor cells. The ability of nonresponsive cells to revert to a responsive state would seem to make this type of tolerance potentially dangerous to the host however. At present, the only data to suggest that such nonresponsive cells are generated by the thymus (or in the periphery) comes from bone marrow chimeras and transgenic animals and use superantigens or allogeneic MHC molecules as a model system. As with most of the studies on clonal deletion, this is due to the inability to study antigen-specific cells in normal mice because of their low frequency.

SUMMARY

Bone marrow chimeras and transgenic animals have suggested that the thymus is capable of generating a nondeletional form of tolerance. This is characterized by the presence of relatively normal numbers of T cells bearing potentially autoreactive receptors. These cells are functionally silent in vivo and are nonresponsive to direct TcR stimulation in vitro. Like T-cell clones, the nonresponsive state induced in vivo is reversible upon withdrawal of the relevant antigen. The mechanism by which such cells are generated is as yet unknown, although this has implications for both positive selection and clonal deletion. Finally, if they exist in normal animals, the role of such cells may be to control autoimmune reactions by acting to specifically suppress self-reactive cells. Conversely, the ability to reverse the nonresponsive state also makes such cells prime suspects for the initiation of autoimmune responses.

REFERENCES

1. Houssaint E, Flajnik M. The role of thymic epithelium in the acquisition of tolerance. Immunol Today 1990; 11:357-360.

2. Lo D, Burkly LC, Flavell RA et al. Tolerance to class II MHC in transgenic mice. Semin Immunol 1989; 1:147-153.

3. Ramsdell F, Fowlkes BJ. Clonal deletion versus clonal anergy: the role of the thymus in inducing self tolerance. Science 1990; 248:1342-1348.

4. Huber BT. Mls superantigens: how retroviruses influence the expressed T-cell receptor repertoire. Semin Immunol 1992; 4:313-318.

5. Ramsdell F, Lantz T, Fowlkes BJ. A nondeletional mechanism of thymic self tolerance. Science 1989; 246:1038-1041.

6. Speiser DE, Lees RK, Hengartner H et al. Positive and negative selection of T-cell receptor V-β domains controlled by distinct cell populations in the thymus. J Exp Med 1989; 170:2165-2170.

7. Roberts JL, Sharrow SO, Singer A. Clonal deletion and clonal anergy in the thymus induced by cellular elements with different radiation sensitivities. J Exp Med 1990; 171:935-940.

8. Mueller DL, Jenkins MK, Schwartz RH. Clonal expansion versus functional clonal inactivation: a costimulatory signaling pathway determines the outcome of T-cell antigen receptor occupancy. Annu Rev Immunol 1989; 7:445-480.

9. Schwartz RH. Costimulation of T lymphocytes: the role of CD28, CTLA-4, and B7/BB1 in interleukin-2 production and immunotherapy. Cell 1992; 71:1065-1068.

10. Beverly B, Kang SM, Lenardo MJ et al. Reversal of in vitro T-cell clonal anergy by IL-2 stimulation. Int Immunol 1992; 4:661-671.

11. Lorenz RG, Allen PM. Thymic cortical epithelial cells lack full capacity for antigen presentation. Nature (London) 1989; 340:557-559.

12. Blackman MA, Finkel TH, Kappler J et al. Altered antigen receptor signaling in anergic T cells from self-tolerant T-cell receptor β-chain transgenic mice. Proc Natl Acad Sci USA 1991; 88:6682-6686.

13. Ramsdell F, Fowlkes BJ. Maintenance of in vivo tolerance by persistence of antigen. Science 1992; 257:1130-1134.

14. Gao EK, Lo D, Sprent J. Strong T-cell tolerance in parent → F1 bone marrow chimeras prepared with supralethal irradiation. Evidence for clonal deletion and anergy. J Exp Med 1990; 171:1101-1121.

15. Speiser DE, Chvatchko Y, Zinkernagel RM et al. Distinct fates of self-specific T cells developing in irradiation bone marrow chimeras: clonal deletion, clonal anergy, or in vitro responsiveness to self-Mls-1[a] controlled by hemopoietic cells in the thymus. J Exp Med 1990; 172:1305-1314.

16. Lee NA, Loh DY, Lacy E. CD8 surface levels alter the fate of α/β T-cell receptor-expressing thymocytes in transgenic mice. J Exp Med 1992; 175:1013-1025.

17. Blackman M, Kappler J, Marrack P. The role of the T-cell receptor in positive and negative selection of developing T cells. Science 1990; 248:1335-1341.

18. Miller JF, Morahan G. Peripheral T-cell tolerance. Annu Rev Immunol 1992; 10:51-69.

19. Lo D, Burkly LC, Flavell RA et al. Tolerance in transgenic mice expressing class II major histocompatibility complex on pancreatic acinar cells. J Exp Med 1989; 170:87-104.

CHAPTER 10

A Relationship Between Positive and Negative Selection

Janko Nikolić-Žugić

What is the mechanism that ensures that at least certain positively selected cells do not undergo negative selection? How do cells know whether they are positively or negatively selected? These issues are central to our understanding of thymic selection, and are at the same time far from being solved. In fact, these issues are probably the most attractive queries remaining in thymology. The biological outcomes of positive and negative selection are diametrically opposite: the first process makes the cell differentiate further and live, whereas the second induces the cell to kill itself. Yet, as described in previous sections, it is believed that during both processes the TcR on an immature thymocyte recognizes a complex of a self peptide and a self MHC molecule on a thymic stromal APC. If this is so, one might expect that all thymocytes positively selected on a given self peptide:MHC complex would be negatively selected on the same self peptide:MHC complexes. Since we all have a good deal of functional T cells, this obviously does not happen.

At present, there is no adequate molecular explanation for the above controversy. In the next section, I shall discuss several models put forward to explain the relationship between positive and negative selection. There are three distinct underlying premises on which most of these models are based (Fig. 1). The first group of models is based on the premise that the decision as to whether a cell will be positively or negatively selected is determined at the level of the affinity/avidity of the T cell for the APC. The second set of models presupposes that the difference is achieved at the level of the ligand, i.e., that positive selection occurs on a set of peptide:MHC complexes different from that used for negative selection. Finally, the third set of models would have that thymocytes themselves can, under certain conditions, perceive a signal exclusively as positively or only as negatively selecting. This would depend on the maturational stage of the thymocyte or on the context of the signal, e.g., adequate costimulation, accessory interactions, etc. These premises are not mutually exclusive, and some models draw upon more than one of them.

Relationship between positive and negative selection

MODEL	Difference between positive and negative selection
I. Affinity	Affinity of the TCR
II. Special peptide	Different peptides bound to MHC
III. Signalling difference	A. Coupling of TCR to signalling pathways
	B. Co-stimulatory signals

Fig. 1. Characteristics of the main models explaining the relationship between positive and negative selection.

For the sake of debate, I would also like to emphasize that the term "autoaggressive" will be used to denote a functional property of cells that can mount a response to self antigens. By contrast, the term "autospecific" is applicable to mature T cells, autoaggressive or not, from the standpoint that since all T cells were positively selected on self peptide:self MHC, they must possess some specificity for self. Another terminological and semantic clarification needs to be made concerning the terms "affinity" and "avidity". In a strict sense, "affinity" applies to the contact between two molecules, e.g., an antigen and an antibody. Thus one can measure the affinity of this reaction by determining the K_d. Since both TcR and peptide:MHC are cell-bound structures, their contact is dependent on the sum of affinities of an X number of TcR and an Y number of peptide:MHC complexes, and a sum of affinities is termed "avidity". Therefore, whichever term is used for historical or other reasons,

the reader should be aware that in this biological system we are dealing with avidity.

THE AFFINITY (AVIDITY) MODEL

This model, proposed by Sprent and coworkers,[1,2] belongs to that group of models that postulates quantitative differences in determining whether a thymocyte will be positively or negatively selected. According to this model, TcRs expressed on immature thymocytes are judged according to the affinity they possess for self MHC molecules (and peptides associated with them). Some TcRs would have virtually no affinity towards self peptide:MHC complexes expressed on cortical epithelial cells (Fig. 2). The cells bearing such TcR would die owing to a lack of positive selection. At and above a certain threshold of low affinity towards self peptide:MHC (the positive selection threshold), thymocytes would be positively selected. Negative selection would then eliminate the cells whose TcRs have an affinity at or above a second, higher threshold (the negative selection threshold). According to the affinity model, the organism would thus possess functional T cells whose TcR have low affinity for self, and this affinity would fall into the area between the two thresholds—this area is also called "a window of affinities". Inasmuch as there exist solid experimental evidence that interactions in the thymus can be modulated by the density (number) of TcRs (and other molecules) expressed by a thymocyte, this model is more accurately called the avidity model.

The avidity model is the oldest model explaining the relationship between positive and negative selection, and is among the rare models that have not been disproved so far. This model views selection as a function of quantitative events: affinity/avidity would dictate whether a threshold for one or both selections will be crossed. It also postulates that positive selection would occur at a lower threshold (avidity) than negative selection, and it does not put constraints upon the

temporal succession of positive or negative selection (solid experimental evidence supports the idea that negative selection indeed can occur before, during or after positive selection).[3-5] The difficulties in directly testing this theory come from three directions. First, it is very difficult to obtain soluble reagents, in particular soluble TcR, that could be used to inhibit positive or negative selection.[6] Second, even when such reagents are successfully produced,[7,8] none of them could be used in functional studies of intrathymic selection, owing to extremely low affinity of the soluble reagents for the respective peptide:MHC complexes. Finally, the nature of positively selecting self peptides is not known, and it is therefore impossible to measure their affinity for TcR.

Direct and indirect measurements of the affinity of TcR: peptide/MHC interaction have estimated that the affinity of the contact is at the level of $K_d = 10^{-5}$ M,[7,8] and that value is on the border of detection by affinity-measuring assays. Furthermore,

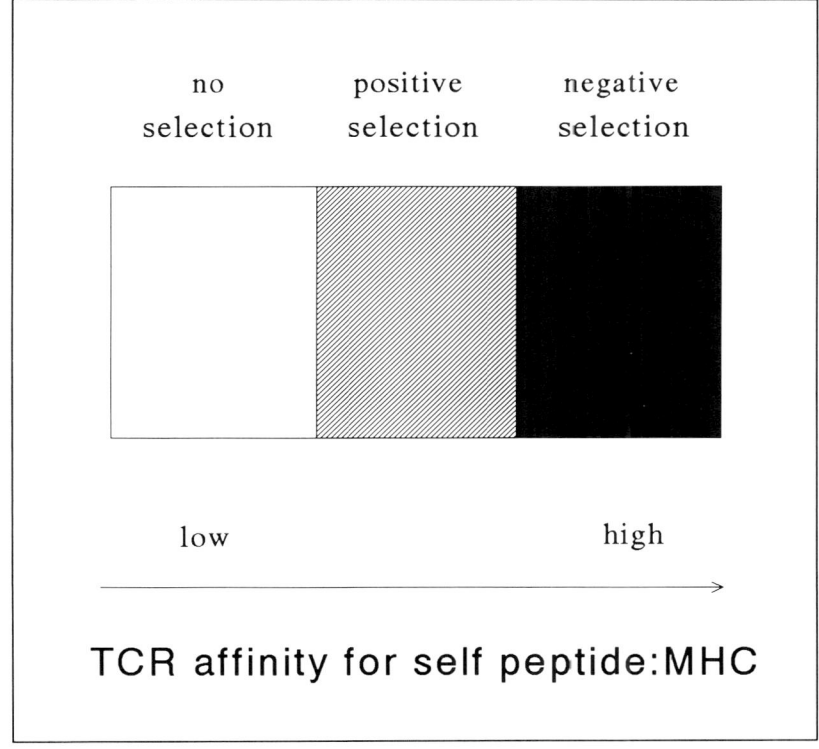

Fig. 2. The affinity/avidity model of intrathymic selection.

soluble TcRs could not inhibit activation of peripheral T cells by peptide:MHC. It is thus possible that additional structures could be involved in generating a stable contact between a thymocyte and a thymic epithelial cell, similar to the situation in peripheral T cells.[9,10] It is also possible that the affinity of a TcR monomer for the thymic APC could be augmented by membrane associations into multimers or by heterophilic interactions with other membrane or intracellular molecules.

What experimental evidence favors the avidity model? Certain TcRs were judged to be of low affinity because their interaction with peptide: MHC complexes can easily be inhibited with antibodies against accessory molecules, e.g., CD8. Thus, such TcRs depend on other molecules in order to form a meaningful interaction with antigen-carrying APC. One such TcR was used to make TcR transgenic mice (the αH-Y receptor). In the presence of the H-Y antigen, most cells bearing this TcR are eliminated by clonal deletion. However, some cells bearing the receptor survive, but only at the expense of down-regulating CD8.[11] Such cells are tolerant to self, i.e., they are unable to mount an αH-Y response. Since the downregulation of CD8 occurs in the thymus, the easiest explanation is that this mechanism decreases the avidity of a thymocyte for a deleting cell, permitting an otherwise autoaggressive cell to leave the thymus and become innocuous.*

In other experiments (summarized in Chapter 11), where accessory molecules were overexpressed in transgenic mice, the threshold of negative* selection was changed in a manner consistent with the avidity model. Namely, a positively selecting interaction was transformed into a negatively selecting one, presumably due to an increase in the avidity of thymocyte: APC contact.[12,13] Admittedly, such alterations could have been caused by

augmented signaling from overexpressed accessory molecules. As mentioned above, there is no direct evidence against the avidity model. A study by Kaye and Ellenberger[14] showed that positive selection-like events can be induced in a DP thymoma either by injecting it intrathymically in the absence of antigenic peptides, or by incubating it in vitro with fibroblasts expressing the restricting MHC molecules in the presence of the antigenic peptide. One may interpret these results as evidence against the avidity model, and in favor of the "special peptide" hypothesis (see below). But phenotypic signs of "positive selection" were temporary, and selected cells could neither be maintained nor shown to be functional. It is therefore possible that this thymoma actually reacted by delayed death, rather than by positive selection, to peptide:MHC stimulation.

A "DETERMINANT DENSITY" VARIANT OF THE AVIDITY MODEL

This model essentially draws upon the avidity model and uses a modification of the hypothesis put forward by Bevan[15] to explain alloreactivity. It differs from the avidity model by introducing another variable in the system—the relative density of peptide:MHC complexes available to selectable thymocytes. The relevance of this model has become apparent with the demonstration that positive, as well as negative selection, occurs on self peptide:MHC complexes (Chapter 7).

Self peptides are present at the surface of APCs—including thymic epithelial cells—at various densities, based on their ability to competitively occupy the available MHC molecules. This density presumably depends on the relative abundance of a given protein and the relative efficacy of its proteolytic processing and import into the endoplasmic reticulum, as well as on the affinity of the generated peptide for the restricting MHC allele. Some peptides will be abundantly present in association with MHC molecules and therefore clearly be of relevance to the immune system. Other peptides would be present at levels below the threshold level at which they provoke a biologically relevant

---

* Why some and not other cells use this alternative mechanism of tolerance induction is not clear. One possibility is that a specialized type of APC can induce downregulation of accessory molecules. A similar mechanism may operate in the periphery.

response (selection, deletion, anergy, activation, etc.).

Measurements of the number of peptide: MHC molecules required for activation of peripheral T cells (the activation threshold) have put an estimated number of such complexes between 180 and 500 (although this may be an overestimate).[16-18] I shall discuss the determinant density model using the example of the foreign antigen X that has to be present at densities of 300 or more peptides per APC to induce T-cell activation. The determinant density model postulates that positive and negative selection require different densities of self peptides to be present at the surface of thymic antigen-presenting cells (this term here includes various thymic epithelial cells, as well as thymic MØ, DC, B cells etc.). All peptides present at densities less than 10/APC would not provoke any response (negligible density), and TcRs specific for them would not be selected. Among peptides that can select TcRs specific for X, self peptides present at densities above 10 complexes/cell would mediate positive selection. By contrast, only abundantly present (more than 50/cell) self peptides would mediate negative selection. (Peptide density numbers mentioned above are completely speculative, and are used solely to illustrate the model.)

From the standpoint of peripheral activation, positively selecting self peptides that do not participate in negative selection could pose a problem. However, this model postulates that such peptides are ignored by peripheral T cells, since their density is insufficient to cause T-cell activation, i.e., is less than 300/cell. This model directly predicts that self-specific T cells exist in the organism and are perfectly compatible with health. Should the density of a positively selecting peptide increase above the activation level, these potentially pathogenic T cells may become autoaggressive. Indeed, a case of autospecificity compatible with health was demonstrated by Schild et al.[19] These authors showed that a peptide isolated from liver could sensitize target cells for in vitro lysis by naive (unprimed) CTLs of a syngeneic animal. But such peptide had to be used at a high concentration for in vitro sensitization and obviously provoked neither negative selection nor peripheral T-cell activation in vivo. These experiments are in full accord with the determinant density model. Their only drawback was that the nature of the liver peptide material was not defined by sequencing.

The determinant density model also predicts that thymocytes can be positively or negatively selected at various stages of development. However, unlike the avidity model, it stipulates that the decision on whether the T cell is positively or negatively selected (or not selected) would be made based on the receptor occupancy and not on the affinity of the receptor. In this model, a window of receptor occupancies (determinant densities) between low and intermediate would be characteristic of successfully selected thymocytes. An indirect argument in favor of the determinant density model comes from studies in TcR tg mice. If TcR avidity plays a decisive role, than an overexpression of the TcR by five- to ten-fold (common in most TcR tg mice)[20-23] would be expected to lead to negative selection owing to increased avidity. By contrast, TcR tg mice exhibited enhanced positive selection, most likely due to the fact that most thymocytes in a TcR tg animal bear a potentially selectable TcR.

To distinguish between the avidity and the determinant density models, one would need to clarify the relationship of the TcR affinity to T-cell activation, or more precisely to the biological response of the cell. At limited antigen concentrations, a high affinity receptor (and the T cell that bears it) will selectively be activated over a low affinity receptor, owing to superior binding. But even the high affinity receptors have to be cross-linked by the antigen to induce cell activation. Indeed, homo- and heterotypic receptor aggregation is a common first step in signaling in a variety of biological systems. Transient superunits, made of more than one receptor that interact in the process of signal transduction, have been suggested to operate in the immune and other systems.[24,25] The key question is: can a high affinity receptor trigger a biological response at a lower receptor occupancy per cell than a low affinity receptor? Or is it that once the receptor binds the ligand with strength over a certain threshold, it produces a signal regardless of the "extra" affinity it has for the ligand? At a single cell level, it is not clear how the TcR-generated signals evoke biological responses. If signals from the same TcR differ depending on the affinity of this TcR for the ligand, additive signals could be summed into a quantitatively increased response. Alternatively, it may be enough for a signal to reach a discrete threshold to provoke an all-or-none response. This question is valid for the activation of peripheral T cells as well as for selection in the thymus, and we unfortunately at present have no information that would help solve it.

Another related issue concerns the time-course of the selection events. It is known that sustained activation of mature T cells requires prolonged production of intracellular signaling messengers critical for the activation, such as PI turnover-generated calcium influx, etc.[24] If, as suggested by some studies, a prolonged contact of a T cell with an APC is necessary for such an intracellular response, one may draw a parallel with the selection processes. In this scenario, prolonged contact, predicted by the avidity model for high avidity interactions and by the determinant density model for cells specific for highly abundant peptides, would lead to negative selection. A short contact, produced by low avidity or low density interactions, would yield positive selection. Elucidating the relationship between the TcR affinity, receptor occupancy/determinant density, thresholds of the biological response[25] and the time of T cell: APC contact is essential for the complete understanding of thymic selection and T-cell activation. This formidable task is certain to keep immunologists busy in the future.

THE "UNIQUE PEPTIDE" MODEL

An alternative theory, put forward by Marrack and Kappler[26] and, in a modified version by Kourilsky and Claverie,[27] proposes that tissue-specific peptides are crucial for positive selection (Fig. 3). Positive selection, according to this hypothesis, occurs on a specialized set of peptides that are expressed solely by thymic epithelial cells. Since no other tissue in the body would express these peptides, there would be no need to delete positively selected cells specific for them. By contrast, other ubiquitously present peptides would be expressed on APCs in the medulla and would therefore induce clonal deletion of cells specific for them. A modification of this theory by Kourilsky and Claverie[27] proposes that "erroneous" peptides, originating from molecules that arose from aberrant transcription (chiefly due to frameshift and similar mutations) would be the driving force of positive selection. Inasmuch as the likelihood of repeating the exact mutation in a protein is rather small, most T cells selected on "erroneous" peptides would not be subject to negative selection.

What experimental evidence speaks about these hypotheses? Two predictions of the "unique peptide" model are that: 1) mature T cells should be reactive against cortical epithelium; and 2) cortical epithelium, but not other tissues, should be able to induce positive selection. The first prediction was tested by intrathymically injecting mature, peripheral T cells and following the fate of injected thymi. In the course of several weeks after injection, no macroscopic injury, decrease in size, weight or cellularity of injected thymuses was observed (J. Nikolic-Zugic, unpublished observation). Mature T cells are therefore not overly reactive against self thymic epithelium in vivo. Marrack et al[28] could, by contrast, demonstrate a weak level of reactivity of T-cell hybridomas against syngeneic thymic nurse cells, measured by IL-2 secretion. These results meant that either thymic cortex has no "special" peptides, or that a lack of or low reactivity is a consequence of poor stimulatory function of TEC. The latter was in fact demonstrated by Lorenz and Allen,[29] but these results did not directly address this hypothesis. In another study, Vukmanovíc et al (manuscript submitted) have shown that a positively selecting TEC line cannot stimulate CTL responses. The second, and critical

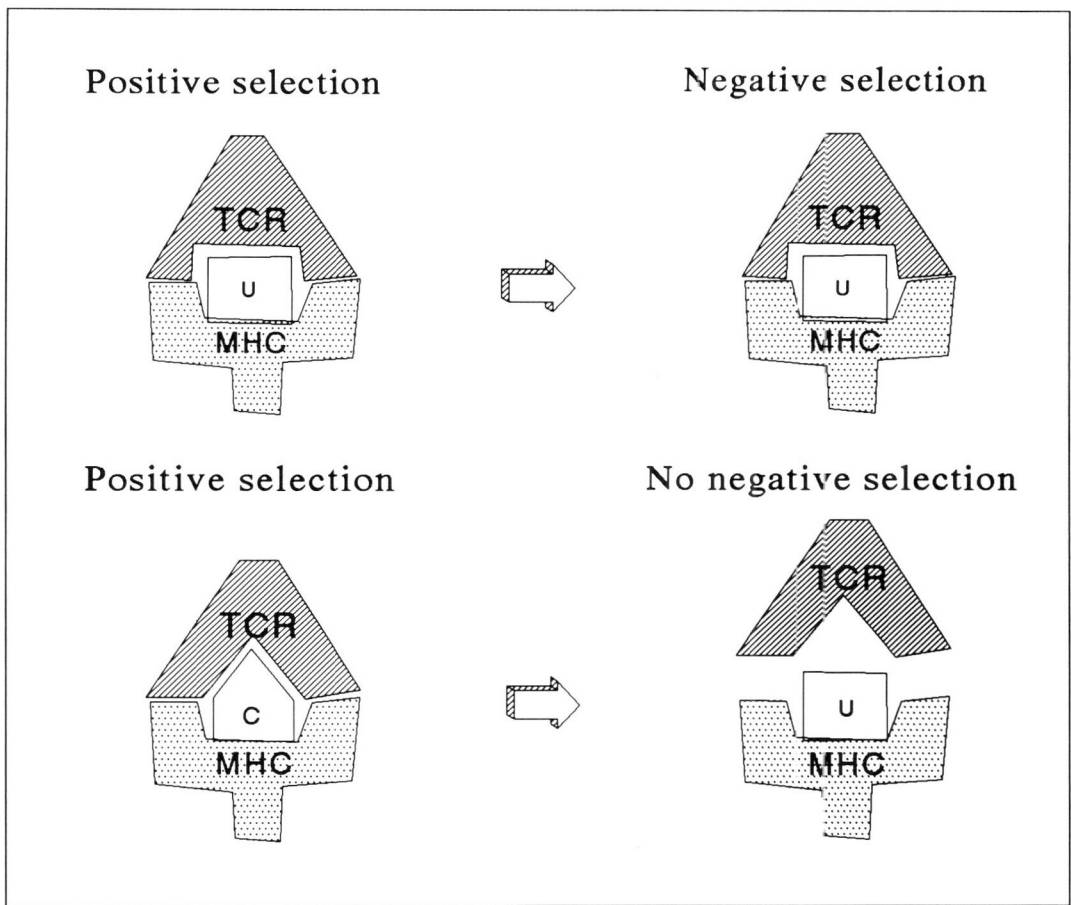

Fig. 3. The "unique peptide" model of intrathymic selection. This model also postulates that positive and negative selection have to occur in different compartments of the thymus.

prediction of this model was rendered very unlikely by the experiments of Pawlowski et al[30] and Hugo et al[31] showing that in vitro cultured fibroblasts can mediate positive selection. It is difficult to imagine why positively selecting self peptides would be shared between TEC and cultured fibroblast lines if TEC are supposed to be unique in this manner. As the authors of these studies conclude, this data means that the "special" peptide hypothesis is probably not correct. The only way to rescue the "special peptide" hypothesis would be to demonstrate that fibroblasts in the above experiments function by donating MHC molecules to resident TEC by shedding them in the thymus.

The "erroneous" peptide variant[27] of the "special peptide" hypothesis is more speculative, and therefore much more difficult to test. The idea that negative selection does not affect thymocytes that have been positively selected on "erroneous" peptides because identical errors in transcription/translation are extremely rare, is attractive. The major caveat is as follows: if identical errors are rare, as they probably are, how does a TEC then generate enough peptide to mediate positive selection? The authors answer this criticism in a most unusual manner. They postulate that a biological response, or at least positive selection, can occur on a *single* peptide:MHC complex, and that there is therefore no need to display more than a single "erroneous" peptide at the surface of

TEC. These authors conclude their argument by saying that, to their knowledge, no one has shown that a single peptide:MHC complex cannot mediate positive selection. Although one may be at odds with this line of reasoning, it is still very difficult to directly test this hypothesis. An indirect test came from the experiments of Hogquist et al[32] and Ashton-Rickardt et al[33] where positive selection was induced by synthetic peptides in a dose-dependent manner. This would suggest that a single peptide:MHC molecule, in the case of peptides used by these two groups, could probably not mediate positive selection. Together, neither variant of the "special peptide" hypothesis can be considered valid in light of the current experimental evidence.

THE "CONTEXT OF A SIGNAL" HYPOTHESIS

An extensive investigation of T-cell activation clarified the concept of two signals necessary for this process. As originally proposed by Bretscher and Cohn[34] and later experimentally proven by several groups,[35] TcR: (peptide:MHC) contact is not sufficient for sustained T-cell activation. In fact, in the absence of another signal this contact induces T-cell anergy . This signal, termed "second" or "costimulatory" signal, is induced by an interaction of a T-cell molecule and a corresponding APC molecule, and is not cognate (antigen-specific). The mechanism of action of costimulatory molecules is twofold. Firstly, they markedly contribute to the avidity of the contact between a T cell and an APC. This enhanced avidity promotes the interaction of a T cell and an APC over a longer period of time, thus allowing an exchange of signals between them. The net result is sustained activation of both cells. Most of the costimulatory molecules have been classified as cell adhesion molecules (CAM) and some can participate both in cell-cell contact and in cell contacts with the extracellular matrix. The second mechanism, established in several recent studies, involves signal transduction by these molecules (reviewed in ref. 35). The following examples illustrate this mechanism: LFA-1:ICAM-1 interaction seems to potentiate Ca^{++} mobilization and proliferation induced through TcR/CD3 or CD28; CD28 ligation induces tyrosine phosphorylation of a unique substrate, p100; the induction of transcription of a number of cytokines occurs via a unique CD28-response element in the promoter of the cytokine genes, etc.

An attractive idea is that similar interactions play a role in intrathymic selection, and actually regulate whether a cell is positively or negatively selected. According to this view, a thymocyte may be positively selected on the basis of the TcR specificity without costimulatory interactions. Costimulation would then play a role in negative selection. Alternatively, costimulatory interactions could regulate both positive and negative selection, and do so in a positive or negative fashion. In accordance with these lines of reasoning, TEC have been shown to poorly stimulate T-cell responses, in part owing to a lack of IL-1 production.[29] In another system, it was demonstrated that an in vitro propagated TEC line can mediate positive selection despite deficient APC function and a lack of the costimulatory molecule B7. Transfection of B7 into such a cell line restored APC function without altering positive selection (Vukmanovíc, S. et al, submitted).

The testing of this hypothesis has yielded inconclusive results so far. Among known accessory interactions, only that between LFA-1 and ICAM-1 has been shown to influence negative selection,[36] and the distribution of costimulatory molecules and their receptors is by no means restricted to the thymus. However, it is still possible that unknown costimulatory molecules participate in these events and actually regulate the balance between positive and negative selection. Molecules shared between thymocytes and thymic stromal cells could also subserve this function. In addition, it has been speculated that perhaps endogenous superantigens can participate in the process not only on the side of negative selection (as is well established) but also in positive selection. Experimental evidence on these issues, however, is scarce or nonexistent.

THE "STAGE OF DIFFERENTIATION" HYPOTHESES

These hypotheses postulate that thymocytes undergo a stage in development that is refractory to positive or negative selection, and therefore a cell can only be subject to one type of selection. The burden of deciding whether to be positively or negatively selected is thus alleviated by developmental programming. The most popular hypothesis of this type is known as a "dissociated receptor" hypothesis, and was put forward by Finkel et al (Fig. 4).[37-39] The experimental basis of this model was the observation that murine fetal day 17 thymocytes contain two populations of cells based on their susceptibility to deletion upon TcR/CD3 crosslinking. One could be induced to die with αCD3 mAb but not with αTcR$_\beta$ mAb, while the other was susceptible to both treatments. The authors concluded that the first

population was protected from deletion owing to a functional dissociation of the TcR and CD3 chains, and postulated that the first population is the one that is actually positively selected. Perhaps the major drawback of this hypothesis is that similar results have not been obtained in the adult.

The direct prediction of this hypothesis is that there is an orderly sequence of selection: positive precedes negative. This, however, appears not to be backed up by an increasing body of experimental evidence.[3,4,36] Several alternative explanations should be considered for the data of Finkel et al. Firstly, the stoichiometry of the TcR/CD3 complex could be such that two units of CD3$_\varepsilon$ chain, that was the target of αCD3 mAbs, may surround one unit of the TcR heterodimer.[40] In this case, a better sensitivity to the αCD3 mAb may be due to a superior binding and better signaling of this reagent. Still, differential

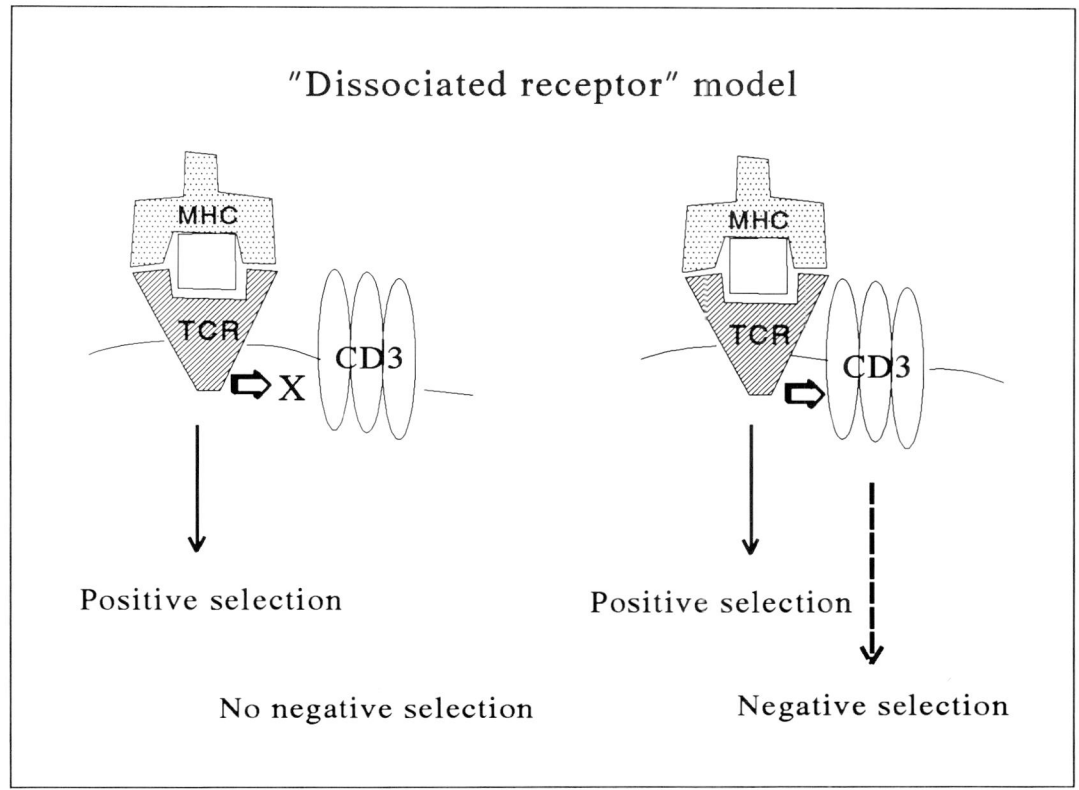

Fig. 4. The "dissociated receptor" model. X denotes a block in signal transduction. This model would permit the same peptide to mediate either positive or negative selection, depending on the developmental stage of the thymocyte.

sensitivity of two populations to αTcRβ mAb needs to be explained. A distinct possibility is that the phenomenon has to do with the development of this particular wave of thymocytes. This would fit well with an inability to document similar phenomenology in the adult. Along these lines, we[41] have recently discovered that in the fetal thymus Fas expression divides thymocytes almost precisely along the lines proposed by Finkel et al. A subset of day 17 DP cells does not express Fas. Such cells would be expected to be resistant to apoptosis. By contrast, all DP cells in the adult express Fas. These results could explain the data of Finkel by the fact that early Fas⁻ DP cells are resistant to apoptosis precisely due to a lack of this apoptosis-related antigen, and that this is the property of a first wave of fetal cells that is not duplicated in the adult. Further experiments should clarify this issue. Together, while the idea of this hypothesis remains viable, its present form is not supported by experimental results.

SUMMARY

The relationship between positive and negative selection remains the paradox that dominates thymic immunology. How do cells positively selected on self peptide:MHC avoid negative selection by the same self peptide and MHC? No definitive answers are as yet available, especially at the molecular and signaling levels. The most plausible hypothesis which has survived is one drawing upon the difference in affinity/avidity of TcR/T cell for the peptide:MHC complex. This hypothesis suggests that only thymocytes with an intermediate affinity/avidity towards the peptide:MHC complex would survive selection. Those with lower avidity would fail to be positively selected, whereas the ones having a high affinity/avidity would be negatively selected. This area promises much exciting experimentation and stimulating discussion for years to come.

REFERENCES

1. Lo D, Ron Y, Sprent J. Induction of MHC-restricted specificity and tolerance in the thymus. Immunol Res 1986; 5:221-232.

2. Sprent J, Webb SR. Function and specificity of T-cell subsets in the mouse. Adv Immunol 1987; 41:39-121.

3. Carlow DA, Teh S-J, Teh H-S. Altered thymocyte development resulting from expressing a deleting ligand on selecting thymic epithelium. J Immunol 1192; 148:2988-2995.

4. Spain LM, Berg LJ. Developmental regulation of thymocyte susceptibility to deletion by "self"-peptide. J Exp Med 1992; 176:213-223.

5. Ohashi PS, Pircher H, Burkl K et al. Distinct sequence of negative or positive selection implied by thymocyte T-cell receptor densities. Nature 1990; 346:861-863.

6. Davis MM, Chien Y-h. Topology and affinity of T-cell receptor mediated recognition of peptide-MHC complexes. Curr Opinion Immunol 1993; 5:45-49.

7. Matsui K, Boniface JJ, Reay PA et al. Low affinity interaction of peptide-MHC complexes with T-cell receptors. Science 1991; 254:1788-1791.

8. Weber S, Traunecker A, Oliveri F et al. Specific low-affinity recognition of major histocompatibility complex plus peptide by soluble T-cell receptor. Nature 1992; 356:793-795.

9. Williams AF, Beyers AD. T-cell receptors: at grips with interactions. Nature 1992; 356:746.

10. O'Rourke AM, Mescher MF. The roles of CD8 in cytotoxic T lymphocyte function. Immunol Today 1993; 14:183-188.

11. Teh H-S, Kishi H, Scott B et al. Deletion of autospecific T cells in T-cell receptor (TcR) transgenic mice spares cells with normal TcR levels and low levels of CD8 molecules. J Exp Med 1989; 169:795-806.

12. Robey EA, Ramsdell F, Kioussis D et al. The level of CD8 expression can determine the outsome of thymic selection. Cell 1992; 69:1089.

13. Lee NA, Loh DY, Lacy E. CD8 surface levels alter the fate of α/β T-cell receptor-expressing thymocytes in transgenic mice. J Exp Med 1992; 175:1013.

14. Kaye J, Ellenberger DL. Differentiation of an immature T-cell line: A model of thymic positive selection. Cell 1992; 71:423-435.

15. Bevan MJ. High determinant density may explain the phenomenon of alloreactivity. Immunol Today 1984; 5:128-130.

16. Demotz S, Grey HM, Sette A. The minimal number of class II MHC-antigen complexes needed for T-cell activation. Science 1990; 249:1028-1030.

17. Harding CV, Unanue ER. Quantitation of antigen-presenting cell MHC class II/peptide complexes necessary for T-cell stimulation. Nature 1990; 346:574-576.

18. Falk K, Rotzschke O, Deres K et al. Identification of naturally processed viral nonapeptides allows their quantification in infected cells and suggests an allele-specific T-cell epitope forecast. J Exp Med 1991; 174:425-434.

19. Schild H, Rotzchke O, Kalbacher H et al. Limit of T-cell tolerance to self proteins by peptide presentation. Science 1990; 247: 1587-1589.

20. Teh H-S, Kisielow P, Scott B et al. Thymic major histocompatibility complex antigens and the αβ T-cell receptor determine the CD4/CD8 phenotype of T cells. Nature 1988; 335:229.

21. Sha WC, Nelson CA, Newberry RD et al. Positive and negative selection of an antigen receptor on T cells in transgenic mice. Nature 1988;336:73-76.

22. Kaye J, Hsu M-L, Sauron M-E et al. Selective development of CD4+ T cells in transgenic mice expressing a class II MHC-restricted antigen receptor. Nature 1989; 341:746.

23. Berg LJ, Pullen AM, Fazekas de StGroth B et al. Antigen/MHC-specific T cells are preferentially exported from the thymus in the presence of their MHC ligand. Cell 1989; 58:1035.

24. Fraser JD, Straus D, Weiss A. Signal transduction events leading to T-cell lymphokine gene expression. Immunol Today 1993; 14:357-362.

25. Grossman Z, Paul WE. Adaptive cellular interactions in the immune system: The tunable activation threshold and the significance of subthreshold responses. Proc Natl Acad Sci USA 1992; 89:10365-10369.

26. Marrack P, Kappler J. The T-cell repertoire for antigen and MHC. Immunol Today 1988; 9:308-315.

27. Kourilsky P, Claverie J-M. MHC restriction, alloreactivity, and thymic education: a common link?. Cell 1989; 56:327-329.

28. Marrack P, McCormack J, Kappler J. Presentation of antigen, foreign major histocompatibility complex proteins and self by thymus cortical epithelium. Nature 1989; 338:503.

29. Lorenz RG, Allen P. Thymic cortical epithelial cells lack full capacity for antigen presentation. Nature 1989;340:557.

30. Pawlowski T, Elliott JD, Jaenisch R et al. Positive selection of T lymphocytes on firboblasts. Nature 1993;364:642.

31. Hugo P, Kappler JW, McCormack J et al. Fibroblasts can mediate thymocyte positive selection in vivo. Proc Natl Acad Sci USA 1993; in press.

32. Hogquist KA, Gavin MA, Bevan MJ. Positive selection of CD8+ T cells induced by major histocompatibility complex binding peptides in fetal thymic organ culture. J Exp Med 1993; 177:1469-1473.

33. Ashton-Rickardt PG, Van Kaer L, Schumacher TNM et al. Peptide contributes to the specificity of positive selection of CD8+ T cells in the thymys. Cell 1993; 73:1041-1049.

34. Bretscher P. The two-signal model of lymphocyte activation twenty-one years later. Immunol Today 1992; 13:74-76.

35. Liu Y, Linsley PS. Costimulation of T-cell growth Curr Opinion Immunol 1992; 4:265-270.

36. Carlow DA, Oers NSCvan, Teh S-J et al. Deletion of antigen-specific immature thymocytes by dendritic cells requires LFA-1/ICAM interactions. J Immunol 1992; 148:1595-1603.

37. Finkel TH, Kubo RT, Cambier JC. T-cell development and transmembrane signaling: changing biological response through an unchanging receptor. Immunol Today 1991;12:79.

38. Finkel TH, Cambier JC, Kubo RT et al. The thymus has two functionally distinct population of immature αβ+ T cells: one population is deleted by ligation of αβ TcR. Cell 1989;58:1047.

39. Finkel TH, Kappler JW, Marrack PC.

Immature thymocytes are protected from deletion early in ontogeny. Proc Natl Acad Sci USA 1992;89:3372-3374.

40. Wegener A-MK, Letourneur F, Hoeveler A et al. The T-cell receptor/CD3 complex is composed of at least two autonomous transduction modules. Cell 1992;68:83-95.

41. Andjelíc S, Drappa J, Lacy E et al. The onset of Fas expression parallels the acquisition of CD8 and CD4 in fetal and adult αβ thymocytes. Int Immunol 1994; 6. In press.

CHAPTER 11

CD4 AND CD8 ACCESSORY MOLECULES IN INTRATHYMIC T-CELL DEVELOPMENT

Sharon R. Seiler

Elizabeth Lacy

CD4 AND CD8

STRUCTURE: THE ROD AND THE BOX

C D4 and CD8 are glycoproteins displayed on the surface of T cells. Human CD4 (Fig. 1), sometimes known as T4 or Leu-3, and now notorious as the cellular binding site for the human immunodeficiency virus,[1] is a 55 kiloDalton (kD) monomer comprised of four immunoglobulin-like extracellular domains, a hydrophobic transmembrane sequence, and a short (38 amino acid), highly charged cytoplasmic tail.[2,3] Its two amino-terminal extracellular domains are linked by a shared β-strand to create an extended rigid structure,[4,5] and the structure of the third and fourth immunoglobulin-like domains mimics that of the first and second.[6] The extracellular domains of CD4 thus stack up to form a long bipartite rod rising from the cell surface.[7] Mouse CD4, also known as L3T4, is 55% identical to its human counterpart, and the cytoplasmic tails of the two molecules exhibit the highest degree of amino acid identity, 76%.[8]

Human CD8 (Fig. 1), also known as T8 and as Leu-2, is a disulfide-linked dimer, either an αα homodimer or an αβ heterodimer.[9-11] The α and β chains are similar in size (32-34 kD) and structure, although not in sequence. Each is comprised of a single amino-terminal immunoglobulin-like domain, an extended and highly glycosylated proline-rich linker region, a hydrophobic transmembrane region, and an intracellular domain. In the case of the α chain, the intracellular domain is 28 amino acids long and highly charged.[12-13] In the case of the β chain, intracellular domains of 16, 27, 49, or 52 amino acids can be produced by alternative splicing.[9-11,14]

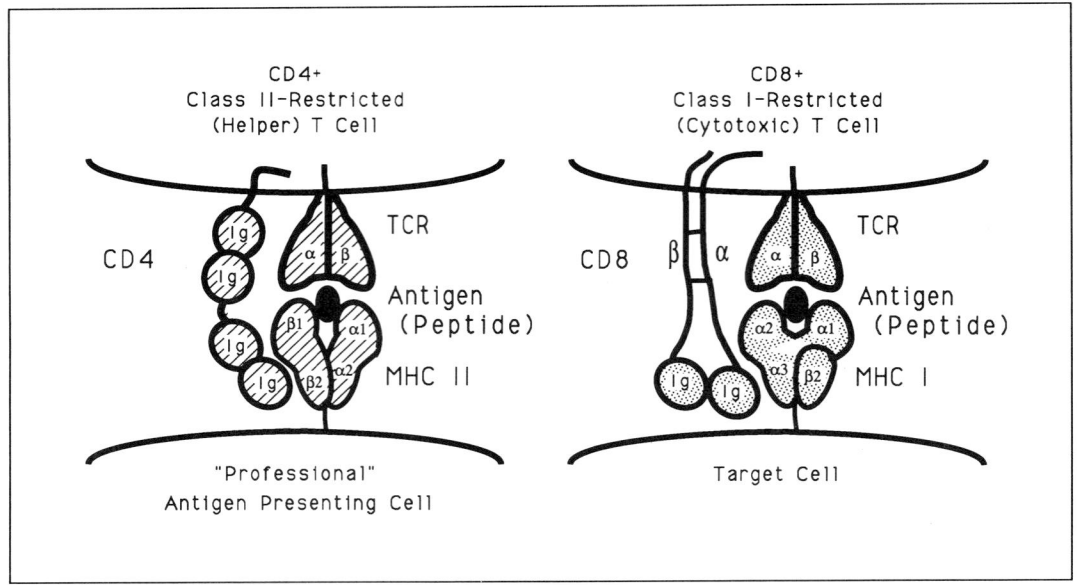

Fig. 1. Interactions of T cells and antigen-producing cells. All molecules are depicted schematically. The immunoglobulin-like domains of the CD4 and CD8 glycoproteins are denoted (Ig). CD8, the T-cell receptor (TcR), and the major histocompatibility complex (MHC) class I and class II molecules are heterodimers as indicated (α and β). The α subunit of the MHC class I molecule and the α and β subunits of the MHC class II molecule are comprised of distinct domains, as indicated (1,2,and 3). β₂ denotes the nonpolymorphic β₂-microglobulin chain of MHC class I. CD4 binds to a nonpolymorphic region of the β2 domain of MHC class II; CD8α binds to a nonpolymorphic region of the α3 domain of MHC class I. The highly polymorphic regions of both the MHC class I and class II molecules form clefts that bind peptide antigens. (The topography is similar to that of a hotdog and its bun.) A TcR binds to the surface that results when a peptide antigen binds in the cleft of an MHC molecule.

(See below.) X-ray crystallographic analysis of the amino-terminal domain of CD8α confirms that its three dimensional structure is identical to that of immunoglobulin variable domains and that CD8α homodimers, and presumably CD8 αβ heterodimers as well, are constructed in the same way as are antibody variable regions.[15] Thus CD8 can be pictured as a rounded box tethered to the cell surface by a slender, flexible stalk.[7,15] Murine CD8α, or Lyt-2, is 35-38 kD in size and shares 49% of its amino acids with its human counterpart. The transmembrane domain, which exhibits 76% amino acid identity, is the most highly conserved region of CD8α, while the cytoplasmic tails of mouse and human CD8α are 57% identical.[16] Murine CD8β, also known as Lyt-3, has a 16 amino acid cytoplasmic domain and a molecular weight of 28-30 kD.[17-19] It is

51% identical overall to its human homologue, and its cytoplasmic tail is 75% identical to the 16 amino acid form of the human cytoplasmic tail.[11]

SIGNIFICANCE: HELPERS OR KILLERS? A MATTER OF CLASS RESTRICTION

CD4 and CD8 first sparked the interest of immunologists when it became clear that their mutually exclusive expression defines two functionally distinct classes of mature, peripheral T cells (reviewed by Cantor and Boyse in 1977[20] and by Reinherz and Schlossman in 1980[21]). (In the parlance of immunologists anything outside the thymus is, by definition, peripheral.) Approximately 65% of peripheral T cells are CD4⁺ (and thus CD8⁻), while the remainder are CD8⁺ (and CD4⁻). CD4⁺ T cells are typically helper cells, which respond to antigenic stimulation by releasing a variety of soluble lymphokines required for induction of the inflammatory response and for the growth and differentiation of immune system cells, including B cells, macrophages, and additional T cells. By contrast, CD8[+] cells are usually cytotoxic cells, which respond to antigenic stimulation by lysing antigen-bearing "target" cells.

CD4 and CD8 and their role in T-cell differentiation became even more intriguing to researchers when it was recognized that a more stringent and far more profound distinction than their effector functions separates CD4[+] and CD8[+] T cells. All T cells recognize antigens in the form of peptide fragments bound to major histocompatibility complex (MHC) molecules on the surfaces of other cells. T cells that express CD4 recognize antigens presented by class II MHC molecules, the distribution of which is limited to "professional" antigen presenting cells, such as B cells and macrophages; CD8[+] T cells recognize antigens in association with class I MHC molecules, which are expressed on almost all somatic cells.[22] One consequence of this distinction is that CD4[+] (helper) cells respond primarily to extracellular antigens while CD8[+] (cytotoxic) cells target primarily intracellular antigens (reviewed by Germain and Margulies, 1993[23]). The absolute correlation between CD4/CD8 phenotype and MHC class specificity in mature T cells implies that the mechanisms underlying the determination of the CD4 and CD8 lineages and those underlying the selection of the T-cell repertoire are somehow linked during thymic ontogeny. (See below.) However, whether CD4/CD8 phenotype determines the MHC class specificity of a T cell or is itself determined by the MHC class specificity of the clonotypic αβ T-cell antigen/MHC receptor (TcR) was not immediately clear.

The heterogeneity of the T-cell population ordinarily confounds analyses of lineage determination. However, as a consequence of allelic exclusion, virtually all the T cells of TcR transgenic mice express a single TcR of defined specificity. Studies utilizing αβ TcR transgenic mice have established that the positive selection (see

below), maturation to functional competence, and CD4/CD8 phenotype of a given T cell are inextricably tied to each other and are absolutely dependent on the specificity of the αβ TcR for class II or class I MHC molecules (reviewed by von Boehmer in 1990[24] and by Loh in 1991[25]). Thus, in mice expressing a class II-restricted TcR transgene the majority of mature T cells are CD4[+] helper cells,[26,27] while in mice expressing a class I-restricted TcR transgene most peripheral T cells are CD8[+] and cytotoxic.[28-30]

CD4 AND CD8: THE MATURE T CELL

While CD4 and CD8 do provide a fantastically convenient system for the identification of MHC class II- and class I-restricted T cells by immunologists, there was, immediately, consensus among researchers that CD4 and CD8 must also play some biological role in the function and/or maturation of T cells. Initial experiments using both antibody blocking[31-35] and gene transfer[36-39] protocols provided strong evidence that CD4 and CD8 play a crucial role in the activation of peripheral T cells. Subsequent experiments have delineated two major roles for CD4 and CD8 in the function of mature T cells.

CD4 AND CD8 ARE ACCESSORY MOLECULES . . .

Cell adhesion assays demonstrate that CD4 and CD8α bind MHC molecules. CD4 binds to MHC class II molecules[40] and CD8α to MHC class I molecules (Fig. 1).[41,42] The ligand of CD4 is a nonpolymorphic determinant in the β_2 domain of MHC class II molecules.[43,44] Correspondingly, CD8α binds to a structurally analogous nonpolymorphic region within the α_3 domain of class I molecules.[45,46] CD8β appears to enhance the binding of CD8α to MHC class I molecules,[47,48] and, since CD8β is similar in structure to CD8α (see above), it is possible that the ligand for CD8β is a region of the monomorphic MHC class I β_2-microglobulin chain that is similar to the class I α_3 domain region bound by CD8α.[46,48,49]

Binding of CD4 to nonantigenic MHC class II molecules, or of CD8 to "bystander" class I molecules, augments the response of

T cells to antigenic stimulation,[38,39,50,51] presumably by increasing the overall avidity of the interaction between effector T cells and antigen-bearing cells. Thus CD4 and CD8 function, in part, as adhesion, or "accessory" molecules.

... AND CO-RECEPTORS

Antibody cross-linking experiments demonstrate that CD4 and CD8 also contribute directly to the process of signal transduction by the TcR during T-cell activation[52-56] and can thus be regarded as co-receptors.[57] Cross-linking of either CD4 or CD8 with the TcR elicits a far more robust T-cell response than does cross-linking of the TcR alone. The TcR contacts the bound peptide antigen and the highly polymorphic regions surrounding the peptide binding cleft at the top of MHC molecules,[49,58-60] while CD4 and CD8 bind MHC molecules via nonpolymorphic regions that support the peptide binding domains.[43,44,46] Therefore, it is possible that T-cell activation involves the formation of a complex in which CD4 or CD8 and the TcR co-engage the same MHC molecule on an antigen-bearing cell (Fig. 1). Antibody cross-linking of CD4 or CD8 and the TcR may therefore mimic a physiologically relevant event, the formation of a quaternary complex of CD4 or CD8 plus TcR and a single antigen-bearing MHC molecule. The formation of such quaternary complexes is completely consistent with the crystal structures of CD4[4-6] and MHC class II[60] and of CD8[15] and MHC class I.[49] In fact, antigen-dependent coordinate localization of CD4 and TcR has been demonstrated in T-cell clones.[61] Moreover, transfection studies have shown that binding of CD8 and the TcR to the same class I molecule is a critical factor in T-cell activation: Expression of an antigenically irrelevant MHC class I molecule bearing a functional CD8-binding α_3 domain does not rescue the T-cell activation function of an antigenic MHC molecule bearing a mutant, non-CD8-binding α_3 domain.[46]

The association of the cytoplasmic domains of both CD4 and CD8α with a src-related protein tyrosine kinase, p56[lck],[62,63]

suggests a pathway by which CD4 and CD8 might function in transmembrane signaling. Antibody cross-linking of either CD4 or CD8 induces the tyrosine kinase activity of p56[lck].[64-66] Conversely, CD4 and CD8 mutants lacking the cytoplasmic p56[lck] association domain, +•+•X•Cys•X•Cys•(Pro), where + is a basic amino acid,[67,68] are deficient in T-cell activation,[50,69,70] as are those T cells that lack functional p56[lck].[71,72]

So, the adhesive properties of CD4 or CD8 do potentiate the recognition of peptides presented by either MHC class II or class I molecules, respectively, but this effect is small by comparison to that of the co-receptor function induced when CD4 or CD8 and the TcR simultaneously engage a single MHC molecule and its bound peptide antigen, resulting in the juxtaposition of p56[lck] and cytoplasmic elements of the TcR complex.[50,70,73,74] Such engagement of CD4 or CD8 activates p56[lck] [64-66] which presumably then phosphorylates some cellular substrate(s) —in the currently popular model, one of the chains of the TcR complex— on tyrosine, initiating a cellular signaling cascade that is necessary for effective T-cell activation (reviewed by Samelson and Klausner in 1992[75] and by Weiss in 1993[76]). Other potential but thus far less widely celebrated substrates for p56[lck] include a 32 kD ras-like GTP-binding protein;[77,78] the 95 kD vav protein, a guanine nucleotide exchange factor expressed exclusively in hematopoietic cells;[79-81] and phospholipase C-γ1.[82]

CD4 AND CD8: THE IMMATURE T CELL

CD4 AND CD8 ARE MARKERS OF T-CELL ONTOGENY

Mature CD4+CD8- and CD4-CD8+ peripheral T cells arise from CD4-CD8- hematopoietic stem cells that migrate from fetal liver or from bone marrow and colonize the thymus. Although the complex sequence of events occurring during T-cell maturation in the thymus remains poorly understood, adoptive transfer experiments,[83-86] in vitro culture studies,[87,88] and kinetic analyses[89,90] have provided an outline (Fig. 2) of the major thymocyte subpopulations and their precursor-product relationships (reviewed by Nikolic-Zugic in 1991[91] and in von Boehmer, 1992[92]). In the αβ TcR lineage the differentiation of CD4⁻CD8⁻ thymocytes is dependent on the expression of the TcR β chain gene.[93] The immediate products of CD4⁻CD8⁻ precursors are CD4^{lo}CD8$^+$TcR^{lo} and/or CD4$^+$CD8^{lo}TcR^{lo} large thymocytes, most of which become CD4$^+$CD8$^+$TcR^{lo} within hours. The CD4$^+$CD8$^+$TcR^{lo} dividing blasts along with their small, mostly nondividing CD4$^+$CD8$^+$TcR$^+$ progeny constitute the vast majority (≥ 80%) of thymic T cells. Most of these CD4$^+$CD8$^+$TcR$^+$ cortical thymocytes die within a few days, but a small number (~1%) differentiate into the CD4$^+$CD8$^-$TcR^{hi} and CD4$^-$CD8$^+$TcR^{hi} mature medullary thymocytes that are exported from the thymus as functional T cells.

The thymic microenvironment is crucial not only to the differentiation of T cells, but also to determining the composition of the functional TcR repertoire. The essential immunological distinction between self and nonself is the result of a phenomenon known as thymic education. Thymocytes bearing TcRs that recognize foreign antigens in association with self-MHC molecules undergo positive selection in the thymus,[94,95] while those bearing potentially autoreactive TcRs are eliminated.[96-98] Consequently, only a subset of the TcRs expressed on thymocytes are found on mature T cells. The point(s) during thymocyte maturation at which selective mechanisms act are ill-defined, and the mechanisms by which positive and negative selection occur remain extremely perplexing. However, recent studies utilizing TcR transgenic mice have demonstrated that the fate of a CD4$^+$CD8$^+$TcR^{lo} thymocyte, once formed, is absolutely dependent on the specificity of its TcR and on the MHC and antigen composition of the thymus in which it finds itself (reviewed by von Boehmer in 1990[24] and by Loh in 1991[25]): If the TcR

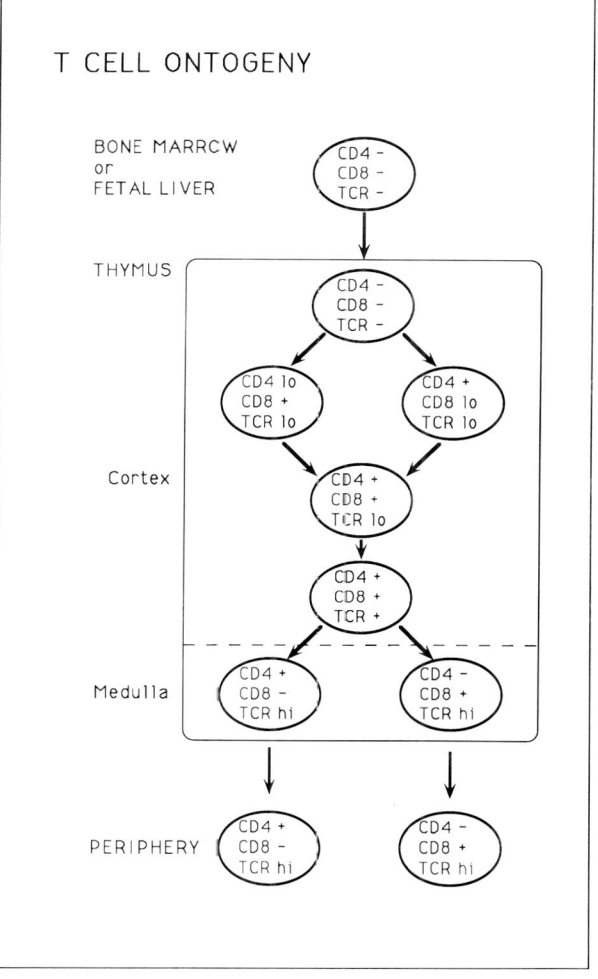

Fig. 2. Expression of CD4, CD8, and the TcR during T-cell ontogeny. See text and Chapter 3 (Phenotypic and Functional Stages of Intrathymic Development of TcR αβ Thymocytes) for details.

fails to bind any intrathymic ligand, the thymocyte dies a programmed cell death; if the TcR binds MHC complexed with antigenic self-peptide, presented largely by bone marrow-derived thymic dendritic cells, the cell is deleted immediately, apparently by apoptosis; if the TcR binds self MHC (complexed with nonantigenic self-peptide?)[99,100] on radiation-resistant thymic epithelial cells, the thymocyte escapes programmed cell death and matures to functional competence.

CD4 AND CD8 ARE REQUIRED FOR T-CELL DEVELOPMENT

CD4 and CD8 clearly play a crucial role in the selective events that shape the T-cell repertoire. Continuous perfusion of mice with anti-CD4 antibodies[101,102] blocks the development (positive selection) of CD4+CD8-TcR[hi] medullary thymocytes and prevents the clonal deletion (negative selection) of CD4-CD8+TcR[hi] medullary thymocytes bearing autoreactive TcRs. Conversely, continuous perfusion of mice with anti-CD8 antibodies[85] blocks the development of the mature CD4-CD8+TcR[hi] T-cell population. Experiments using mice carrying targeted deletions of the CD4[103,104] and CD8α[105,106] genes confirm that CD4 is specifically required for the development of class II-restricted CD4+CD8-TcR[hi] helper cells and CD8 for the positive selection of class I-restricted CD4-CD8+TcR[hi] cytolytic cells.

CD4-CLASS II AND CD8-CLASS I INTERACTIONS ARE REQUIRED FOR T-CELL DEVELOPMENT

How do CD4 and CD8 exert their effects on the establishment of MHC restriction by positive selection and the establishment of self-tolerance by negative selection? In thymocyte development, as in T-cell activation, CD4 function seems to require interaction with MHC class II molecules and CD8 function, interaction with MHC class I molecules. Antibody blockade of all MHC II class molecules[107,108] prevents the maturation of any CD4+CD8-TcR[hi] cells, but continuous perfusion of mice with haplotype-specific anti-MHC class II antibodies[109] prevents the maturation of only those CD4+CD8- helper cells bearing TcRs specific for the blocked molecules. Mice treated from birth with anti-MHC class I antibody lack all CD4-CD8+TcR[hi] cytotoxic T cells;[110] those similarly treated with haplotype-specific anti-MHC class I antibodies lack CD4CD8+TcR[hi] T cells restricted by molecules of the blocked haplotype.[111] Once again, gene targeting confirms the results achieved with antibody blocking protocols. MHC class I expression is all but obliterated by targeted mutation of the monomorphic

β_2-microglobulin chain. In the absence of MHC class I no CD4-CD8+TcR[hi] cells mature.[112,113] Mice lacking MHC class II molecules have been generated by targeted mutation of the I-Aβ locus in mice naturally lacking I-Eα. In such mice development of CD4+CD8-TcR[hi] cells is aborted.[114,115] In mice lacking both class I and class II MHC molecules all thymocyte development arrests at the CD4+CD8+ stage.[116]

In thymocyte development, as in T-cell activation, the most dramatic effects of CD4 and CD8 on the determination of cell fate are seen when CD4 or CD8 and the TcR interact with the same MHC molecule. Elegant genetic experiments have verified that coordinate engagement of MHC by TcR and CD8 is required for both positive and negative selection of class I-restricted cells. MHC class I molecules harboring mutations in their CD8-binding α3 domains (see above), but wild type for antigen presentation, were used to generate transgenic mice.[117-119] Even though endogenous MHC class I molecules that can bind CD8 are present in the thymuses of these mice, the mutant molecules neither positively nor negatively select T cells bearing receptors reactive with the corresponding wild type MHC class I molecules.

That the TcR and CD4 or CD8 must interact with the same MHC molecule to effect positive or negative selection directly, suggests that CD4 and CD8 must function as co-receptors in thymocytes as they do in peripheral T cells. Indeed, cross-linking of CD4 or CD8 with the TcR in thymocytes results in far greater increases in intracellular calcium concentration and tyrosine phosphorylation than does cross-linking of the TcR alone.[120,121] Comparison of T-cell development in transgenic mice expressing high (15-30x normal) levels of either full length or cytoplasmically truncated (tailless) CD4 suggests that the effects of CD4 on T-cell development are in fact mediated through its cytoplasmic tail.[122]

Based on its role in the activation of peripheral T cells, p56[lck] is one obvious candidate for transduction of CD4/CD8 signals during thymic education. p56[lck] is present in CD4+CD8+ thymocytes, and, as in mature

T cells, it is associated with CD4 and CD8 and activated by cross-linking of either molecule.[123] However, the molecular basis of signal transduction in thymocytes remains obscure at best. Cross-linking of CD4 or CD8 and the TcR results in the tyrosine phosphorylation of p56[lck] itself and of several additional and as yet unidentified cellular substrates.[121,123] However, in one experiment, specific inhibitors of protein tyrosine kinase failed to block negative selection of CD4+ CD8+ thymocytes in vitro.[124] Attempts to assess the role of p56[lck] in CD4/CD8 signal transduction by targeted mutation of the lck gene have been somewhat disappointing. Although the lck mutant mice do exhibit a dramatic arrest in T-cell development, their most striking phenotype is a pronounced thymic atrophy due to a drastic reduction in the number of CD4+CD8+ cells.[125] Consequently, the role of p56[lck] in mediating signals during later thymic selection events cannot be directly determined in these lck- mutants.

CD8-CLASS I (AND CD4-CLASS II?) INTERACTIONS SHAPE THE T-CELL REPERTOIRE

It is possible that CD4 and CD8 also influence the fate of thymocytes in more subtle ways. Both positive and negative selection depend on the interaction of CD4 or CD8 plus TcR with MHC plus peptide, and both processes apparently involve signaling through the TcR and either CD4 or CD8. Thus one of the most perplexing aspects of T-cell ontogeny is that apparently identical interactions seem to mediate both cell death and cell maturation. One way to resolve this paradox has been dubbed the "affinity model",[126,127] although it might be more accurately termed the avidity model. This model posits that the fate of a CD4+CD8+ thymocyte is determined by the overall avidity of its interaction with MHC molecules on thymic stromal cells: High avidity interactions lead to negative selection and lower avidity interactions to positive selection so that the mature T-cell repertoire consists of cells with low avidity for self MHC complexed with self-peptide (and high avidity for self MHC complexed with foreign peptide).

Experimental data support the affinity model. Thymocytes expressing a potentially autoreactive class I-restricted TcR, but only low levels of CD8, escape negative selection.[128] Conversely, thymocytes expressing a class-I restricted receptor and extremely elevated (6-10x normal) levels of CD8α are deleted under conditions where thymocytes expressing the same TcR and normal levels of CD8 are positively selected.[129] A similar transformation of otherwise positively selecting events into negatively selecting events is seen with more moderately elevated (2x normal) levels of CD8α and β together.[130] Thus increased levels of CD8 apparently can enhance interactions during thymocyte selection such that otherwise positively selecting events surpass the threshold required to trigger negative selection. Moderately elevated (2x normal) levels of the CD8αβ heterodimer seem to enhance positive selection as well,[131] although this effect cannot be replicated with elevated levels (2x, 3x, or 6-10x normal) of CD8α alone (N.A. Lee and E. Lacy, unpublished results). So it is possible that increased levels of CD8β also raise ordinarily nonselecting events past the threshold required for positive selection. Whether CD8 affects thymocyte-stromal cell interactions simply via its function as an adhesion molecule, binding bystander MHC molecules not involved in antigen presentation, or via its function as a co-receptor, binding the same MHC molecule as the TcR and transducing signals, or via both these mechanisms is not known. In unmanipulated systems, changes in the avidity of thymocyte-stromal cell interactions could be generated, in part, by increases in the level of TcR expression as thymocytes mature and/or by the increased density of MHC molecules on the dendritic cells of the thymic medulla relative to that on the epithelial cells of the thymic cortex.

LINEAGE COMMITMENT AND MHC CLASS RESTRICTION: INSTRUCTION OR SELECTION?

The determination of CD4/CD8 lineage is linked to positive selection during T-cell ontogeny (see above). Figuring out how CD4 gene expression, initially a feature of all thymocytes, becomes limited to those T cells expressing class II-restricted receptors while CD8 gene expression, likewise a hallmark of all immature thymocytes, becomes limited to those cells expressing class I-restricted TcRs is a fascinating problem in gene regulation and essential to understanding the molecular mechanisms underlying positive selection during T-cell ontogeny. Three models (Fig. 3) have been advanced to explain the developmental regulation of CD4/CD8 gene expression and its linkage to positive selection (refs. 57 and 132 and E. Lacy unpublished): The positive instruction model assumes that the CD4 and CD8 genes are initially transcribed only transiently and that either CD4 or CD8 is specifically re-activated during positive selection in response to signals transduced by either the TcR and CD8, in the case of cells bearing class I-restricted receptors, or the TcR and CD4, in the case of cells bearing class II-restricted receptors. The negative corollary of the instruction model assumes that the CD4 and CD8 genes are continuously transcribed in CD4⁺CD8⁺ thymocytes and that positive selection of cells bearing a class I-restricted TcR results in the inactivation of the CD4 gene; positive selection of cells bearing a class II-restricted TcR, in the inactivation of the CD8 gene. The stochastic/selection model also assumes that the CD4 and CD8 genes are continuously transcribed early in thymocyte development but proposes that one or the other is then turned off in each cell by a mechanism that acts independently of the MHC restriction of the TcR. In this model positive selection allows only those cells that express the appropriate combination of CD4 or CD8 and MHC-restricted TcR to mature to functional competence.

CD4 AND CD8: MOLECULAR BIOLOGY

Knowledge of the mechanisms controlling the expression of the CD4 and CD8 genes during T-cell development would be invaluable in elucidating the mechanisms linking positive selection and thymocyte differentiation. Data on CD4 and CD8 gene expression are, however, fragmentary at best.

STRUCTURE OF THE CD8 GENES

The molecular biology of the CD8 genes is surprisingly complex. In both mice[18,133] and humans[14,134] genes for CD8α and β are closely linked, with β lying approximately 25-35 kilobases (kb) upstream of α and in the same transcriptional orientation (Figs. 4 and 5A). The human locus spans approximately 100 kb on chromosome 2 and the mouse locus approximately 55 kb on the proximal portion of chromosome 6. In humans, the CD8β gene is not unique; a recent duplication event has generated a second gene, $CD8B_2$, presently unlinked to $CD8B_1$, but probably located on the same chromosome.[14,134]

The murine CD8α gene (Fig. 4) spans approximately 4.4 kb and consists of five exons, which correspond only roughly to the functional domains of the encoded protein.[135] Exon 1 encodes the leader peptide, the immunoglobulin-like amino-terminal domain, and about one-fourth of the linker domain; exon 2 encodes the central portion of the linker region; exon 3 encodes the membrane-proximal portion of the linker region and the entire transmembrane region; and exons 4 and 5 together encode the cytoplasmic tail. Alternative splicing of the murine CD8α transcript (Fig. 4) deletes exon 4 and changes the reading frame of exon 5 so that the resulting translation product, designated CD8α', has a 3 amino acid cytoplasmic tail instead of a 28 amino acid tail.[16,135,136]

The human CD8α gene (Fig. 5A) spans approximately 8 kb and is organized into 6 exons which do encode the separate functional domains of the protein. The first exon encodes the leader peptide; the second, the immunoglobulin-like amino-terminal domain; the third, the linker domain; the fourth, the transmembrane region; and the fifth and sixth, the cytoplasmic tail.[137] The human CD8α transcript is also alternatively spliced (Fig. 5B), but the alternatively spliced mRNA lacks not a cytoplasmic exon but the exon encoding the transmembrane region, and so gives rise to a secreted protein of 27-30 kD.[137,138]

In mouse, the single CD8β gene (Fig. 4) spans approximately 14 kb. Its exon/intron

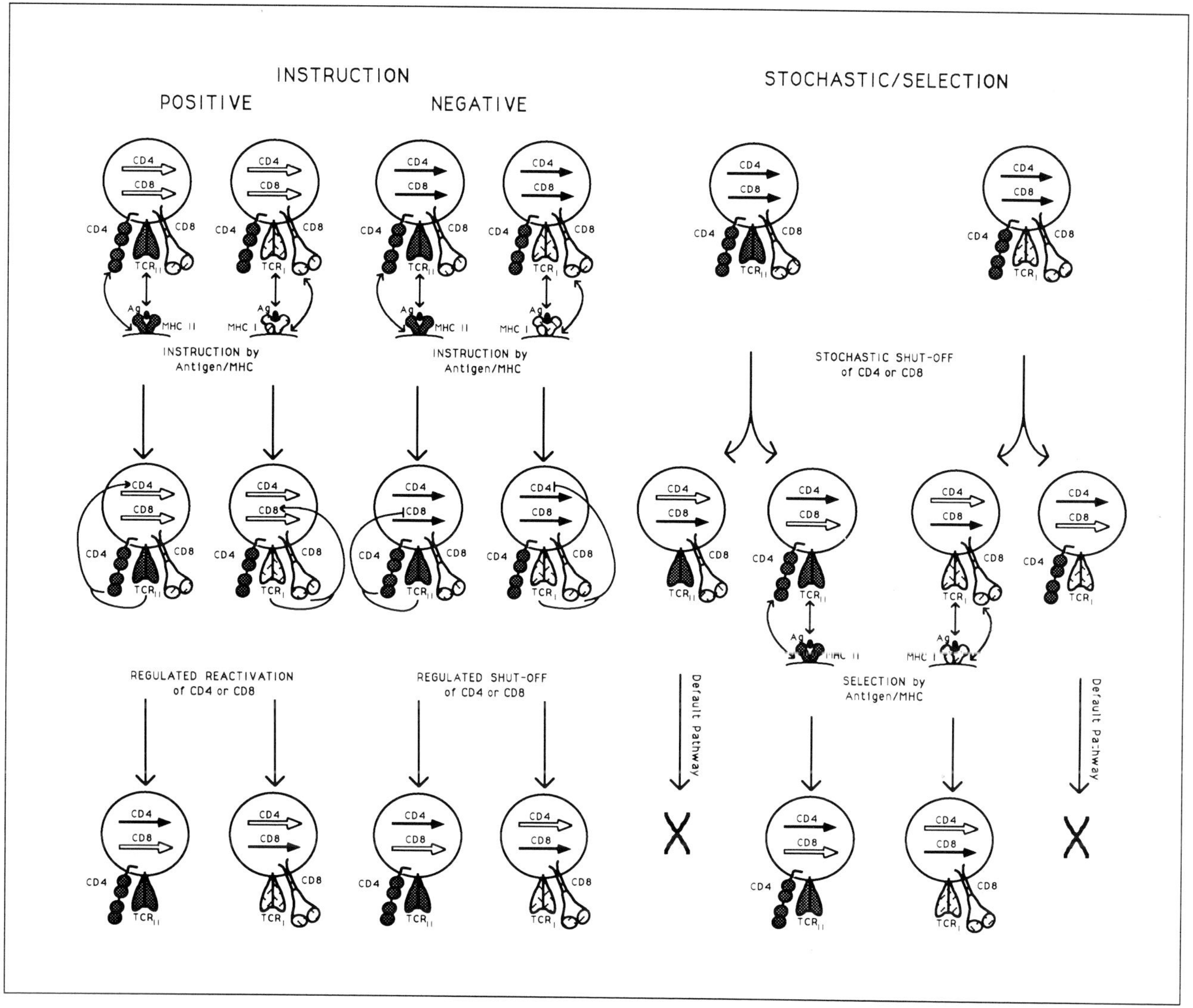

Fig. 3. Instruction or selection? Three models have been advanced to explain the developmental regulation of CD4/CD8 gene expression and its linkage to positive selection.

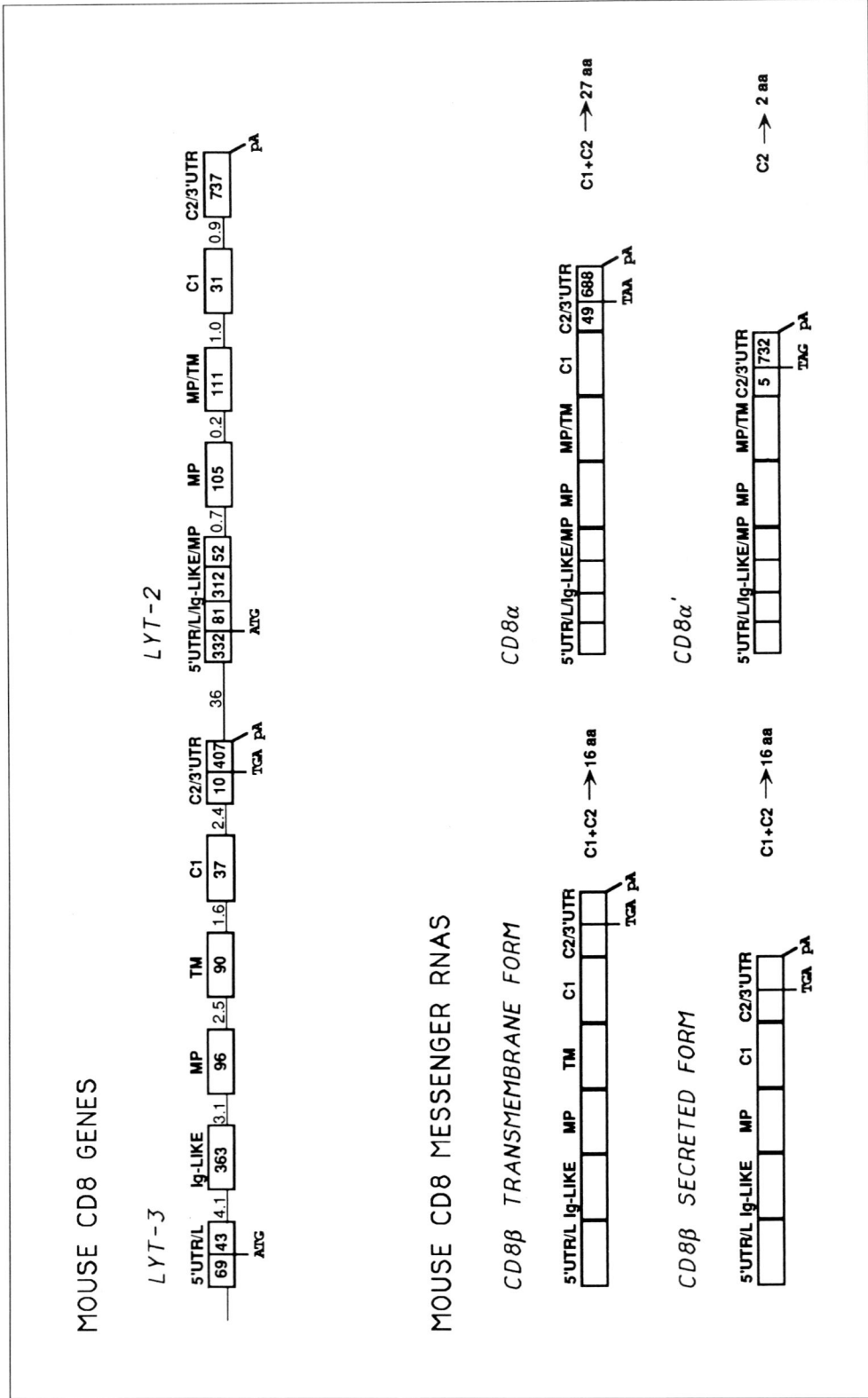

Fig. 4. The mouse CD8 genes and their messenger RNAs. Exons are depicted as rectangles; introns and extragenic regions by lines. Exon sizes are in basepairs (or bases); intron sizes and intergenic distance are in kilobasepairs. UTR denotes an untranslated region; Ig-like, the immunoglobulin-like domain; MP, the membrane-proximal linker region; TM, the transmembrane domain; and C, a cytoplasmic domain. ATG indicates the start codon. TAA, TGA, and TAG indicate the position of stop codons. pA indicates the position of polyadenylation signal sequences.

structure is completely analogous to that of the human CD8α gene, and it too gives rise to an alternatively spliced mRNA (Fig. 4) that encodes a secreted protein.[18,133]

The human *CD8B-1* gene (Fig. 5A) is spread over 50 to 70 kb and has three exons not yet characterized in the mouse gene.[14,134] One, designated S for secretory, is located upstream of and used as an alternative to the exon encoding the transmembrane region. It contains a translational stop as well as a polyadenylation sequence and encodes the 4 carboxy-terminal amino acids of a secreted protein. The exon encoding the transmembrane region can also be deleted by alternative splicing to produce mRNAs encoding a variety of longer secreted proteins. Two more exons are located 25 to 45 kb downstream of the two cytoplasmic exons, C1 and C2, previously identified in the mouse. Designated C3 and C4, both these exons have protein termination sequences and so can be independently utilized to provide distinct carboxy-terminal amino acid sequences. Exons C2 and C4 both contain polyadenylation signals. In addition, the human C2 exon has two possible splice acceptor sites. In toto, the *CD8B-1* gene could encode as many as 17 different products (Fig. 5B); 8 different membrane-bound proteins and 9 different secreted proteins. Thus far at least 8 different *CD8B-1* cDNAs have been cloned, and 4 of these code for membrane proteins.[9-11,14,134]

The human *CD8B-2* gene (Fig. 5A) spans 20 kb and represents a partial duplication of the *CD8B-1* gene that extends from at least 10 kb upstream of the first (leader) exon to approximately 8 kb downstream of the C2 exon. The homology between the *CD8B-1* and *CD8B-2* genes is very high (~99%) in both coding and noncoding regions.[134] At least one mRNA derived from the *CD8B-2* gene has been isolated,[14] so it is likely that both CD8β genes can be transcribed, although most mRNAs seem to originate from the *CD8B-1* gene.

EXPRESSION OF THE CD8 GENES

Northern analyses of CD4⁺CD8⁻ and CD4⁻CD8⁺ cells isolated from peripheral blood indicate that the expression of the CD8α gene is indeed transcriptionally controlled in mature T cells.[12] Although the tight linkage of the CD8α and β genes suggests that they could be coordinately controlled, the transcriptional activity of the CD8β gene in normal αβ TcR⁺ CD4⁺CD8⁻ cells has not been examined. Preliminary studies of a few T-cell leukemia lines imply that the CD8α and β genes are not invariably co-transcribed in αβ TcR T cells. Some (human) CD8⁺ αβ TcR⁺ lines express only the CD8α transcript,[9-11,139,140] while at least one (murine) CD4⁻CD8⁻ T-cell lymphoma line expresses CD8β transcripts in the absence of CD3α transcripts.[19] Transcriptional regulation of the CD8α and β genes in the various subpopulations of thymic T cells has not been studied.

Experiments in which either immature CD4^{lo}CD8⁻TcR^{lo} thymocytes or CD4⁻CD8⁺TcR^{hi} peripheral T cells were fused with a TcR⁻ variant of BW5147, a CD4⁻CD8⁻ thymoma line commonly used for the production of T-cell hybridomas,[141] emphasize that CD8α gene transcription is differentially regulated in these two cell populations: While T-cell hybrids derived from the fusion of BW5147 to mature CD8⁺ cells uniformly fail to express CD8α transcripts (reference 142 and J. Nikolic-Zugic and M.W. Moore personal communication), thymocyte hybrids express CD4 and the CD8α gene (Lyt-2.2 allele) derived from the thymocyte parent but not that (Lyt-2.1) derived from the BW fusion partner (Nikolic-Zugic and M.W. Moore personal communication). Thus, cellular factors that silence the transcription of CD8α in mature T cells, which have already undergone positive selection, are apparently without effect on transcription of CD8α in (unselected) thymocytes. This suggests that a cis-acting negative regulatory element that controls CD8α gene expression in mature T cells is activated during T-cell maturation. It is interesting to note that Carbone and co-workers[142] have shown that transcriptional downregulation by BW5147 is restricted to CD8α; that the 5' end of the CD8α gene is heavily methylated in CD8⁻ T cells, including the BW fusion partner, and

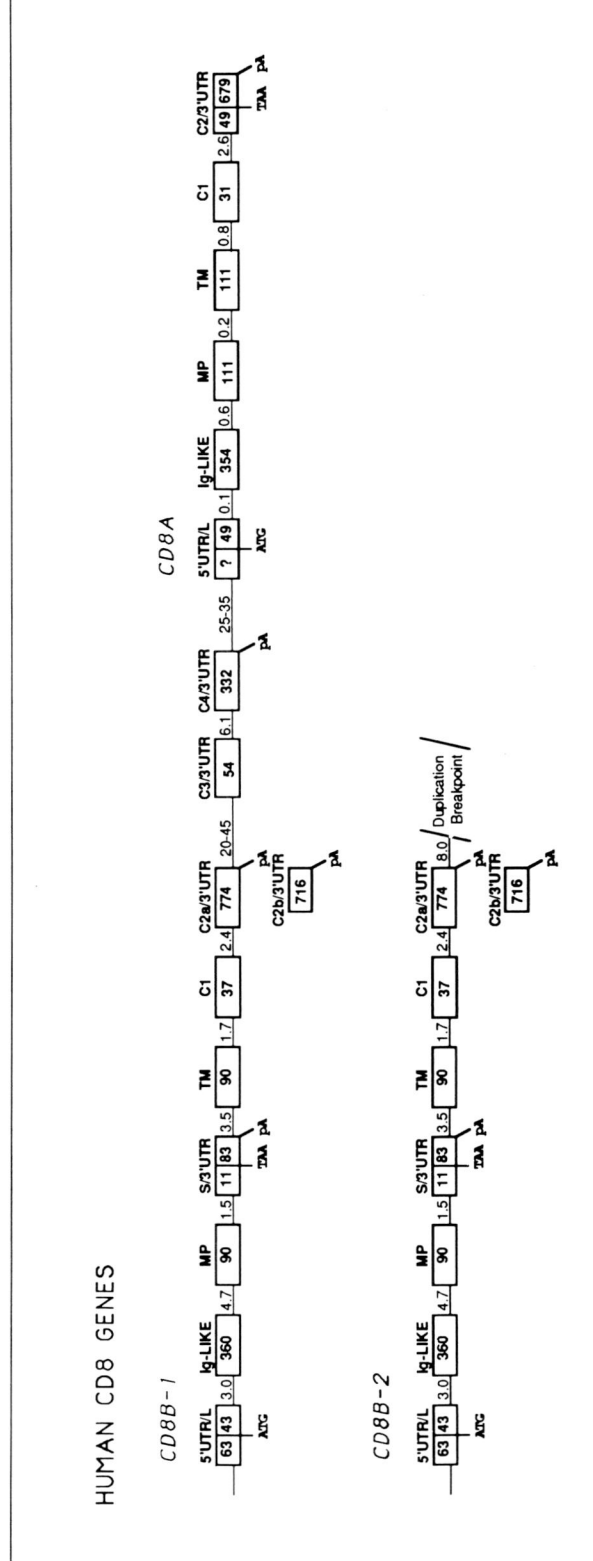

Fig. 5A. The human CD8 genes and their messenger RNAs. The structure of the human CD8 loci. Exons are depicted as rectangles; introns and extragenic regions by lines. Exon sizes are in basepairs; intron sizes and intergenic distance are in kilobasepairs. UTR denotes an untranslated region; Ig-like, the immunoglobulin-like domain; MP, the membrane-proximal linker region; S, the secretory domain; TM, the transmembrane domain; and C, a cytoplasmic domain. ATG indicates the start codon. TAA indicates the position of a stop codon. pA indicates the position of polyadenylation signal sequences. The C2a and C2b exons result from the alternative use of two splice acceptor sites. The size of the 5' untranslated region of the CD8α gene has been reported as 68, 84, 89, 121, 209, or >500 bp.[137,143]

hypomethylated in CD8+ T cells; and that the extinction of CD8α transcription in BW hybridomas correlates with re-methylation of the introduced CD8α gene. Nevertheless, the role, if any, of methylation in the regulation of CD8α gene transcription is unclear.

Recent analysis[143] indicates that a 146 base pair (bp) fragment located immediately upstream of the translational start site of human CD8α can direct expression of a reporter gene in CD8+ and CD8- T-cell lines as well as in non-T-cell lines. Promoter activity is dependent on the integrity of a 10 bp sequence that is bound in vitro by members of the cyclic AMP response element binding protein/activating transcription factor family. Fragments extending further upstream than 146 bp (to -234, -429, and -618 relative to the translation start) exhibit decreasing promoter activity and may contain negative regulatory elements. Since at least two of the transcriptional start sites identified in previous work lie upstream of -146, the physiologic role of the 146 bp promoter fragment is not entirely clear.

The CD8α and β genes generate alternatively spliced transcripts (Figs. 4 and 5B) encoding a variety of secreted and membrane-bound proteins (see above). The expression, stoichiometry, and function of the secreted CD8 proteins are complete mysteries. The multiple protein isoforms generated by the mouse CD8α and human CD8β genes have distinct intracellular domains which could be important in differential signaling during thymocyte development and/or T-cell activation. None of the CD8β membrane proteins, murine or human, can be efficiently expressed at the cell surface unless complexed with a CD8α molecule.[9,18,19] CD8α can be expressed efficiently as a cell surface homodimer in the absence of CD8β, but αβ heterodimers seem to predominate in normal αβ TcR peripheral T cells and thymocytes and in transfected cells.[18,19] The expression of the different CD8 isoforms during development has been carefully characterized only in the case of mouse CD8α:[144] Splicing and translation of the 28 amino acid cytoplasmic domain α and 3 amino acid cytoplasmic domain α' chains (Fig. 4) occur with equal

efficiency throughout T-cell development (~60:40 α:α'), but expression of CD8α' at the cell surface is tightly regulated. Although they comprise ~50% of intracellular α dimers, αα' dimers are never expressed on the cell surface. Additionally, although both αβ and α'β dimers are expressed with equal efficiency on the surface of immature T cells, α'β dimers are retained in the Golgi or a post-Golgi compartment in mature T cells so that only αβ dimers are expressed on the cell surface. Clearly, the post-translational mechanisms that regulate CD8 expression in mature (selected) T cells are different from those that regulate its expression in immature (unselected) cells.

STRUCTURE AND EXPRESSION OF THE CD4 GENE

The molecular biology of the CD4 gene is quite straightforward by comparison with that of the CD8 genes. The human CD4 gene is comprised of 10 exons[8,145] and spans approximately 50 kb on the short arm of chromosome 12.[145,146] The translational start site is located in exon 2, which encodes most of the hydrophobic signal sequence. The amino-terminal immunoglobulin-like domain is encoded by exons 3 and 4; the second, third, and fourth immunoglobulin-like domains by exons 5, 6, and 7, respectively. Exon 8 encodes the transmembrane region and part of the cytoplasmic tail. Exons 9 and 10 encode the remainder of the cytoplasmic domain. The human CD4 gene gives rise to a single mRNA of approximately 3 kb.[2,8,147]

The mouse CD4 gene is located on the distal segment of chromosome 6.[148] It spans approximately 40 kb,[149,150] and its exon/intron structure is virtually identical to that of the human CD4 gene.[149] The major mRNA product of the mouse CD4 gene is approximately 3.5 kb.[8,147,149,151] A minor CD4 mRNA of approximately 2.5 kb has been detected in mouse brain. It is apparently generated from a transcriptional start site within exon 6 and could encode a truncated protein that would lack a signal sequence and the amino-terminal 214 amino acids of the full length CD4 protein. However, the

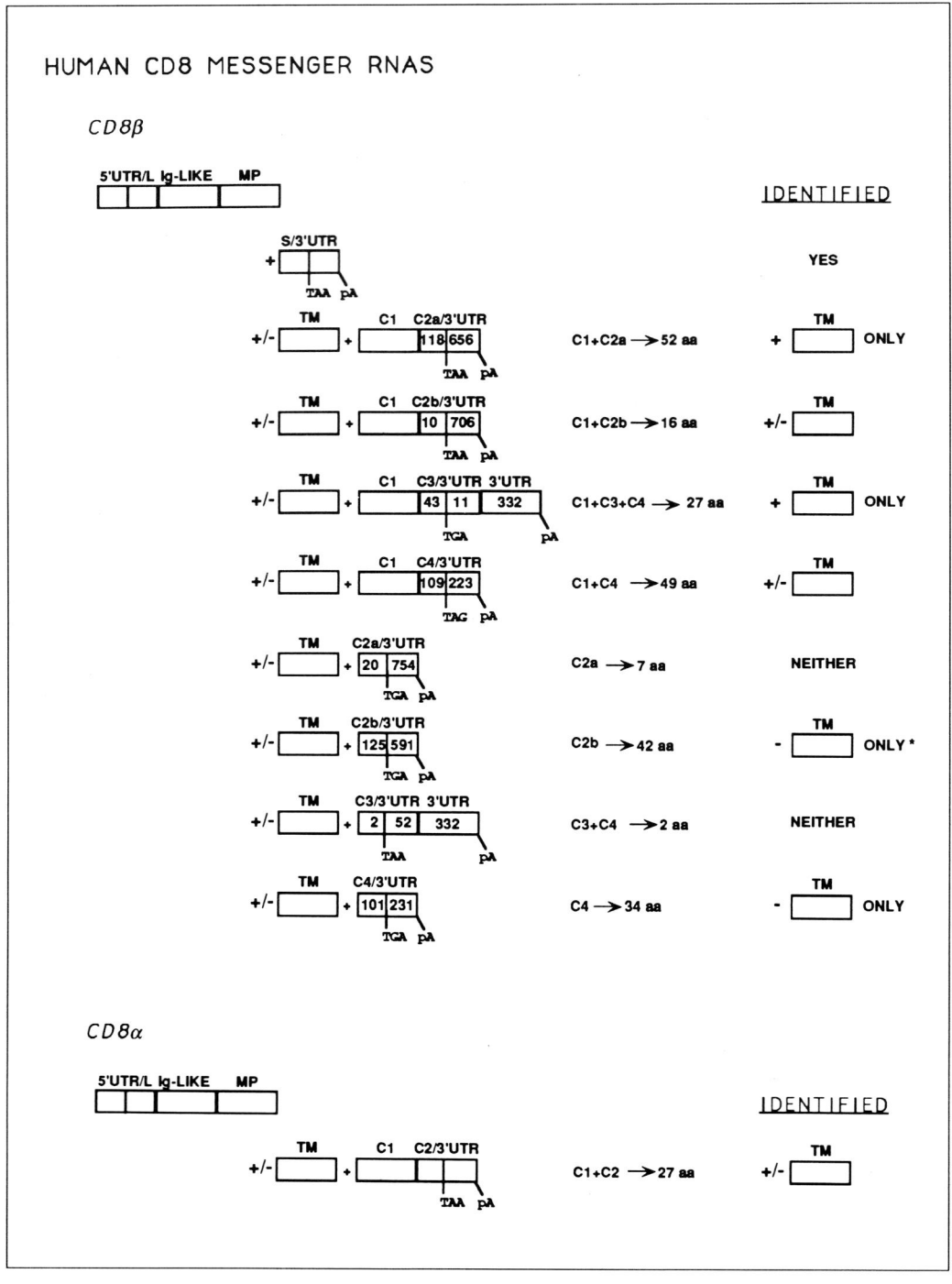

Fig. 5B. The human CD8 genes and their messenger RNAs. The structure of the human CD8 messenger RNAs. Exons are depicted as rectangles. Sizes are in bases. UTR denotes an untranslated region; Ig-like, the immunoglobulin-like domain; MP, the membrane-proximal linker region; S, the secretory domain; TM, the transmembrane domain; and C, a cytoplasmic domain. ATG indicates the start codon. TAA, TGA, and TAG indicate the position of stop codons. pA indicates the position of polyadenylation signal sequences. Except as indicated (*), all the CD8β mRNAs thus far identified are products of the CD8B-1 gene.

2.5 kb transcript is unlikely to be functional, and does not seem to be present in T cells.[8,147,149,151]

CD4, like CD8α, is transcriptionally regulated in peripheral T cells.[2] Expression studies in transfected cell lines and in transgenic mice have allowed dissection of some of the elements that regulate CD4 gene transcription during T-cell development.

The CD4 promoter itself may be a key component of the mechanism specifying subclass-specific expression of CD4 in mature (selected) T cells. A 172 bp fragment (-101 to +71 relative to the start site of transcription) containing the murine CD4 promoter is sufficient to drive expression of a reporter gene in mature CD4+CD8- but not CD4-CD8+ T-cell clones.[152] Similarly, a construct containing 3.5 kb of upstream sequence is sufficient to direct expression of the human CD4 gene, albeit at quite low levels, preferentially to peripheral CD4+CD8- cells in transgenic mice.[145]

The 172 bp murine CD4 promoter fragment has been studied extensively by Siu and co-workers.[152] Three specific complexes form when this fragment is incubated with nuclear extracts of mature CD4+ T-cell clones. Formation of one of these complexes is dependent on binding of a myb transcription factor to one or both of two myb binding sites located between -76 and -81 and between -88 and -93 relative to the transcriptional start. The factors responsible for the formation of the other two complexes have not been identified. It is important to note that although myb is critical for function of the CD4 promoter, it cannot be solely responsible for either the T-cell specific- or subclass-specific expression of CD4. Myb is expressed at high levels in a variety of hematopoietic cells where the CD4 promoter alone is inactive, including B cells and immature CD4+CD8+ cortical thymocytes. Additionally, mutations within the two myb binding sites of the CD4 promoter cause proportionate decreases in its activity in CD8+ and CD4+ T-cell clones.

Addition of a T-cell-specific enhancer element is necessary and sufficient to drive expression from the CD4 promoter in immature CD4+CD8+ thymoma cells in vitro[152] and in CD4+CD8+ thymocytes in vivo[104,145] as well as to reconstitute the efficient and subclass specific-expression of CD4 in mature T cells in transgenic mice.[104,145,153] In mice, a 339 bp fragment located about 13 kb upstream of the first CD4 exon functions as a T-cell-specific enhancer in vitro.[150] A 1.3 kb fragment located 6.5 kb upstream of the first exon is the human homologue of the CD4 enhancer.[145] Ligation of either a 4.5 kb fragment containing the murine enhancer[104] or a 1.3 kb fragment containing the human enhancer[145] to the human CD4 promoter results in the appropriate developmental regulation of a human CD4 transgene.

DNAase I footprint analysis identifies three protein binding sites within the 339 bp murine CD4 enhancer.[150] One site, CD4-2, binds a nuclear protein (known variously as TCF-1α or LEF-1) that also interacts with the TcR α chain enhancer and is expressed primarily in T cells and pre-B cells. However, mutations within this site effect enhancer activity only slightly. Sites CD4-1 and CD4-3 contain consensus binding sites for as yet unidentified basic helix-loop-helix proteins. While mutations within CD4-1 reduce enhancer activity only slightly, mutations within CD4-3 reduce enhancer activity by more than 90%. It is interesting to note that the sequence of the CD4-3 site is conserved in the human CD4 enhancer while the CD4-1 and CD4-2 sequences are not.[145] In fact, the CD4-3 site is embedded in a larger, 46 bp, region that is 83% conserved in the human enhancer. In addition, the region containing the greatest sequence homology (86% over 37 bp) does not contain any of the binding sites thus far defined for the mouse enhancer, so it is likely that the CD4 enhancer functions via the binding of a factor or factors absent from the nuclear extracts thus far examined.

That transcription of CD4 in thymocytes, but not in peripheral T cells, depends absolutely on the activity of a T-cell-specific enhancer[145,152] is consistent with the idea that the mechanisms that regulate the transcription of CD4 in immature (unselected) and mature (selected) T cells are not the same.

INSTRUCTION OR SELECTION? GENETIC APPROACHES

So, in their efforts to understand how CD4/CD8 lineage commitment is linked to positive selection, some researchers have now begun to focus their efforts on elucidating the molecular mechanisms underlying signal transduction by CD4 and CD8 and the TcR during thymocyte maturation and others on unraveling the complex developmental regulation of CD4 and CD8 gene expression. These biochemical and molecular approaches, although still in their infancy, show great promise. To date, however, most experiments probing the relationship between CD4/CD8 lineage commitment and positive selection have relied on genetically manipulated mice. The data generated by these genetic studies are not entirely consistent with the stochastic/selection model, nor are they entirely consistent with the instruction model (see above).[154]

The instruction model predicts that, even when a CD4 transgene is expressed in all thymocytes and T cells, positive selection of thymocytes that express a class II-restricted TcR will extinguish expression of CD8 so that only peripheral T cells bearing class I-restricted TcRs will express (endogenous) CD8 as well as the CD4 transgene. However, constitutive expression of a CD4 transgene in mice lacking expression of MHC class I molecules is sufficient to allow the maturation of CD8[+], but presumably class II-restricted, cytotoxic cells.[155] Similarly, expression of a CD4 transgene in all thymocytes rescues mature peripheral CD8[+], and presumably cytotoxic, T cells expressing a class II-restricted TcR transgene.[155] These results suggest that commitment to the CD8/cytotoxic lineage is independent of the MHC class specificity of the TcR and precedes positive selection; they are thus consistent with the stochastic/selection model. However, there are a number of caveats. Although physiologic levels of CD4 expression did permit maturation of some CD8[+] cells in mice lacking MHC class I molecules, efficient rescue required extremely high levels (15-30x normal) of CD4 expression. Additionally, the CD8[+] cells that are rescued when the CD4 and class II-restricted TcR transgenes are

simultaneously expressed at physiologic levels express only low levels of CD8; may express endogenous CD4; are, although abundant in the periphery, difficult to detect in the thymus and may or may not be functional. So it is possible that the peripheral population of CD8[+] cells in these double transgenic mice represents an unselected and/or immature population that is expanded as a result of extrathymic mechanisms.

The stochastic/selection model predicts that constitutive expression of a CD8 transgene in all thymocytes will permit CD4[+] MHC class I-restricted T cells to mature and exit the thymus. It does not seem to. Peripheral T cells that express both a CD8 transgene and (endogenous) CD4 are class II-restricted helper cells (ref. 156 and N.A. Lee and E. Lacy, unpublished results). Conversely, peripheral T cells that express a CD8 transgene and a class I-restricted TcR transgene are CD4[-].[129,131,156] Thus expression of CD8 is not sufficient to rescue CD4[+] MHC class I-restricted thymocytes, nor does the presence of CD8 interfere with the maturational program of CD4[+] class II-restricted helper T cells. These results suggest that positive selection of a thymocyte bearing a class I-restricted TcR is invariably accompanied by the termination of CD4 expression and that signaling via CD8 in a thymocyte bearing a class II-restricted TcR is either impossible or without effect; they are thus consistent with the instruction model for thymocyte maturation. However, it is important to note the possibility that a form of CD8 crucial for selective signaling in thymocytes may be lacking in the transgenic mice utilized for these experiments: Two groups generated lines of mice transgenic for CD8α alone.[129,156] The third group generated mice transgenic for both CD8α and β,[131] but it is not inconceivable that the two additional cytoplasmic exons identified in the human CD8β gene (see above) are also present in the mouse gene but absent from the CD8β transgenic construct, which contained only 10 kb of sequence 3' to exon C2. These "extra" exons could encode at least four additional membrane-bound forms of CD8β, any or all of which might be necessary for proper

CD8 function in thymocytes.

Some additional observations also tend to cast doubt on the validity of the stochastic/selection model. Intrinsic to the stochastic/selection model is the notion that the commitment of a thymocyte to the CD4 or CD8 lineage is independent of the MHC class restriction of its TcR and thus necessarily precedes positive selection. However, while CD4+CD8- thymocytes bearing class I-restricted TcRs have been documented in TcR transgenic mice[157] and in mice lacking MHC class II molecules,[116] there is little convincing evidence for the existence of their counterparts, CD4-CD8+ thymocytes bearing class II-restricted TcRs.[116] Furthermore, expression of a hybrid transgene consisting of the CD8 extracellular domains fused to the CD4 transmembrane and cytoplasmic domains in thymocytes bearing a class I-restricted TcR results in the appearance of peripheral T cells that co-express endogenous CD4 and endogenous CD8.[158] Although it is not clear that these CD4+CD8+ T cells are functional or mature, their existence is more consistent with the idea that selective events act on CD4+CD8+ thymocytes than with the idea that such events affect CD4+CD8- or CD4-CD8+ thymocytes. Finally, while the stochastic/selection model posits that commitment to the CD4 or CD8 lineage is random, CD4+CD8+TcR^hi thymocytes, which give rise to both CD4+CD8- and CD4-CD8+ cells upon intrathymic transplantation, give rise only to CD4-CD8+ cells in culture,[159] suggesting that lineage commitment is not actually a stochastic process.

Aesthetically, the instruction model is perhaps easier to accept than the stochastic/selection model, which requires the invocation of a separate preselection mechanism that dictates random commitment to the CD4/helper differentiation pathway or the CD8/cytotoxic pathway. Why bother with a CD4+CD8+ intermediate at all? By contrast, the instruction model requires only that signaling through CD4 and CD8 in thymocytes be different. Since CD4 and CD8 are, despite their common associations with p56^lck, demonstrably different in their signaling behavior,[160] this requirement is easily met.

A NEW MODEL: INSTRUCTION BY CD8/SELECTION OF CD4

In toto, the results of T-cell maturation studies in genetically manipulated mice indicate that positive selection via CD8 and a class I-restricted TcR instructs thymocytes to maintain expression of CD8, extinguish expression of CD4, and differentiate into cytotoxic cells, whereas positive selection via CD4 and a class II-restricted TcR simply allows thymocytes to mature but has no effect on their expression of CD8 or on their effector phenotype. This pattern of T-cell maturation suggests that neither the instruction nor the stochastic/selection model is correct for all thymocytes, but it can be reconciled with another model in which co-engagement of CD8 and a class I-restricted TcR instructs, while co-engagement of CD4 and a class II-restricted TcR simply selects.

The CD8 instruction/CD4 selection model (Fig. 6) posits that instructional signaling via CD8 and a class I-restricted TcR in CD4+CD8+TcR+ thymocytes initiates a differentiation program that generates CD4-CD8+ cytotoxic T cells; that in the absence of such an instructional signal, CD4+CD8+TcR+ thymocytes continue on a default pathway in which CD8 expression is extinguished and expression of CD4 maintained; and that signaling via co-engagement of CD4 and a class II-restricted TcR is required to rescue CD4+TcR+ thymocytes from the ultimate default pathway, programmed cell death, and perhaps to activate the expression of genes required for helper function.

This model abrogates the requirement that commitment to either the CD4/helper lineage or the CD8/cytotoxic lineage occur at random. It explains why CD4+CD8- thymocytes bearing class I-restricted TcRs can be easily detected,[116,157] while a reciprocal population of CD4-CD8+ thymocytes with class II-restricted TcRs cannot be. It is completely consistent with experiments in which the expression of a CD8 transgene neither rescues CD4+ cells that express class I-restricted TcRs nor interferes with the maturation of CD4+ helper cells expressing class II-restricted TcRs.[129,131,156] Although the CD8 instruction/CD4 selection model is not

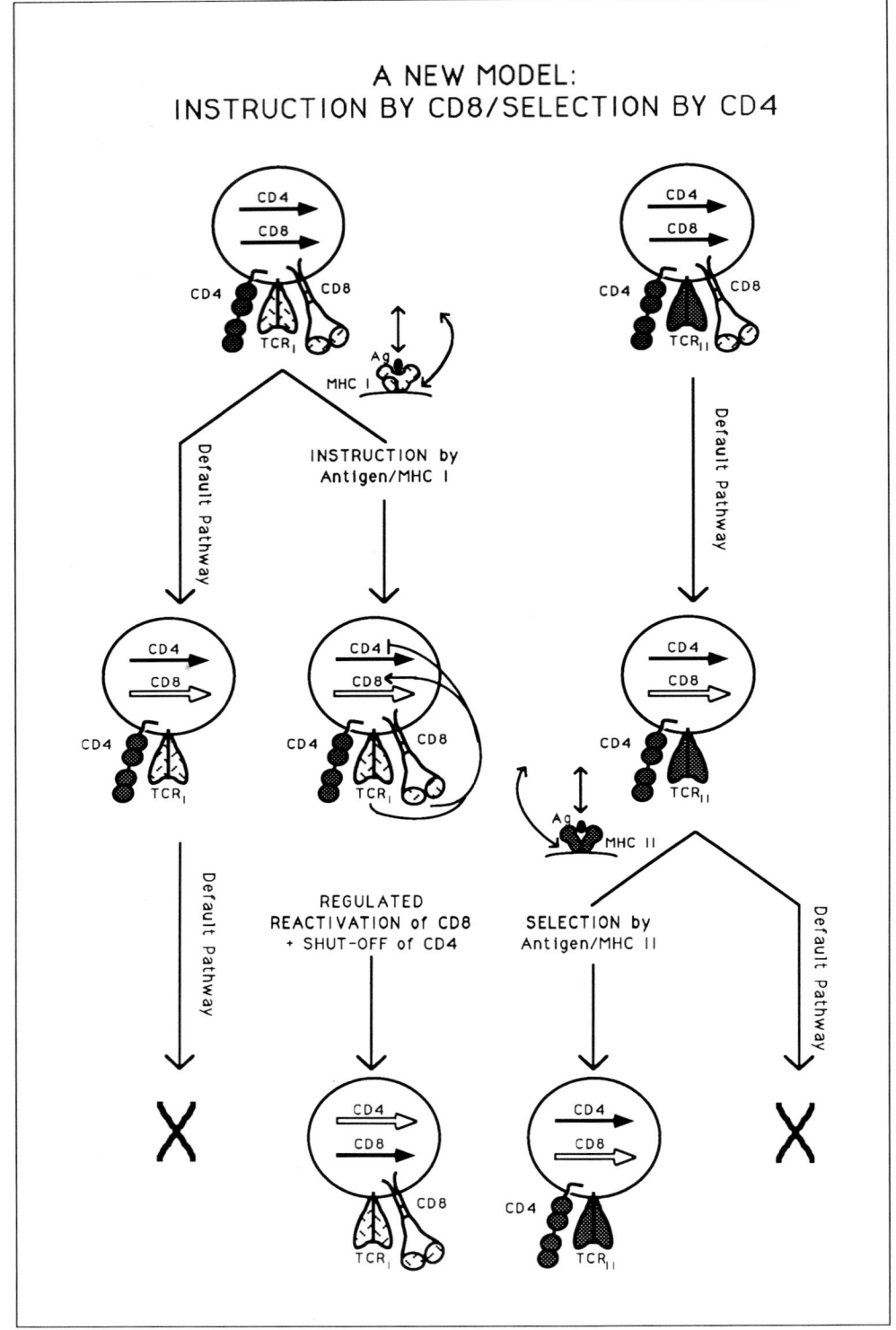

Fig. 6. A new model: Instruction by CD8/Selection by CD4. A new model explains the developmental regulation of CD4/CD8 gene expression and its linkage to positive selection.

consistent with the rescue of CD8$^+$ cytotoxic cells by a CD4 transgene in mice lacking class I molecules,[155] it is possible that the high levels of CD4 required for efficient rescue somehow mimic the effects of signaling via CD8. Furthermore, the CD8 instruction/CD4 selection model suggests that the CD8$^+$ cells rescued in mice transgenic for CD4 and a class II-restricted TcR[155] are unlikely to be functional cytotoxic cells.

Based on the results of T-cell fusion experiments (J. Nikolic-Zugic and M.W. Moore personal communication; see above)[142] it is possible to imagine that a factor required to maintain the CD8 gene(s) in a transcriptionally active state decays away in thymocytes and that signaling through a class I-restricted TcR and a CD8 co-receptor instructs the thymocyte to synthesize more of this CD8 anti-silencer factor. Since continued expression of CD8 is almost always linked to the expression of genes required for cytolytic activity and since the CD8 ligand, MHC class I, is expressed on virtually all somatic cells, it makes sense that commitment of thymocytes to the CD8 lineage should be very stringently controlled.

SUMMARY

CD4 and CD8 function as co-receptors in mature peripheral T cells, under conditions where antigen/MHC specificity and the nature of the T-cell response are predetermined. These molecules function as co-receptors in immature T cells as well, and not surprisingly, the ligands that trigger signaling in thymocytes are the same as those that trigger signaling in mature cells, MHC class II in the case of CD4, and MHC class I in the case of CD8. Signaling through CD4 and/or CD8 in immature T cells shapes the composition of the functional TcR repertoire and ultimately dictates the nature of any immune response. However, the response of individual thymocytes to signals transduced by CD4 and/or CD8 remains unclear. The model most consistent with the data now available is one in which signaling through CD8 (and a class I-restricted TcR) on CD4$^+$CD8$^+$TcR$^+$ cells is instructive and commits thymocytes to the CD4$^-$CD8$^+$ cytotoxic

lineage while signaling through CD4 (and a class II-restricted TcR) merely allows the functional maturation of cells that have already defaulted to a CD4$^+$ helper pathway. Ongoing studies to elucidate the molecular mechanisms underlying regulation of CD4 and CD8 gene expression and to define the nature of the signals transduced in thymocytes will perhaps clarify our understanding of how CD4 and CD8 function during T-cell development.

REFERENCES

1. Maddon PJ, Dalgleish AG, McDougal JS et al. The T4 gene encodes the AIDS virus receptor and is expressed in the immune system and the brain. Cell 1986; 47:333-348.
2. Maddon PJ, Littman DR, Godfrey M et al. The isolation and nucleotide sequence of a cDNA encoding the T-cell surface protein T4: A new member of the immunoglobulin gene family. Cell 1985; 42:93-104.
3. Clark SJ, Jefferies WA, Barclay AN et al. Peptide and nucleotide sequences of rat CD4 (W3/25) antigen: Evidence for derivation from a structure with four immunoglobulin-related domains. Proc Natl Acad Sci 1987; 84:1649-1653.
4. Wang J, Yan Y, Garrett TPJ et al. Atomic structure of a fragment of human CD4 containing two immunoglobulin-like domains. Nature 1990; 348:411-418.
5. Ryu S-E, Kwong PD, Truneh A et al. Crystal structure of an HIV-binding recombinant fragment of human CD4. Nature 1990; 348:419-426.
6. Brady RL, Dodson EJ, Lange G et al. Crystal structure of domains 3 and 4 of rat CD4: Relation to the NH$_2$-terminal domains. Science 1993; 260:979-983.
7. Parham P. The box and the rod. Nature 1992; 357:538-539.
8. Maddon PJ, Molineaux SM, Maddon DE et al. Structure and expression of the human and mouse T4 genes. Proc Natl Acad Sci 1987; 84:9155-9159.
9. DiSanto JP, Knowles RW, Flomenberg N. The human Lyt-3 molecule requires CD8 for cell surface expression. EMBO J 1988; 7:3465-3470.
10. Norment AM, Littman DR. A second

subunit of CD8 is expressed in human T cells. EMBO J 1988; 7:3433-3439.

11. Shiue L, Gorman SD, Parnes JR. A second chain of human CD8 is expressed on peripheral blood lymphocytes. J Exp Med 1988; 168:1993-2005.

12. Littman DR, Thomas Y, Maddon PJ et al. The isolation and sequence of the gene encoding T8: A molecule defining functional classes of T lymphocytes. Cell 1985; 40:237-246.

13. Sukhatme VP, Sizer KC, Vollmer AC et al. The T-cell differentiation antigen Leu-2/T8 is homologous to immunoglobulin and T-cell receptor variable regions. Cell 1985; 40:591-597.

14. DiSanto JP, Smith D, de Bruin D et al. Transcriptional diversity at the duplicated human CD8β loci. Eur J Immunol 1993; 23:320-326.

15. Leahy DJ, Axel R, Hendrickson WA. Crystal structure of a soluble form of the human T-cell coreceptor CD8 at 2.6 Å resolution. Cell 1992; 68:1145-1162.

16. Zamoyska R, Vollmer AC, Sizer KC et al. Two Lyt-2 polypeptides arise from a single gene by alternative splicing patterns of mRNA. Cell 1985; 43:153-163.

17. Nakauchi H, Shinkai Y-I, Okumura K. Molecular cloning of Lyt-3, a membrane glycoprotein marking a subset of mouse T lymphocytes: Molecular homology to immunoglobulin and T-cell receptor variable and joining regions. Proc Natl Acad Sci 1987; 84:4210-4214.

18. Gorman SD, Sun YH, Zamoyska R et al. Molecular linkage of the Ly-3 and Ly-2 genes: Requirement of Ly-2 for Ly-3 surface expression. J Immunol 1988; 140:3646-3653.

19. Blanc D, Bron C, Gabert J et al. Gene transfer of the Ly-3 chain gene of the mouse CD8 molecular complex: Co-transfer with the Ly-2 polypeptide gene results in detectable cell surface expression of the Ly-3 antigenic determinants. Eur J Immunol 1988; 18:613-619.

20. Cantor H, Boyse EA. Regulation of cellular and humoral immune responses by T-cell subclasses. Cold Spring Harbor Symp Quant Biol 1977; 41:23-32.

21. Reinherz EL, Schlossman SF. The differentiation and function of human T lymphocytes. Cell 1980; 19:821-827.

22. Swain SL. T-cell subsets and the recognition of MHC class. Immunol Rev 1983; 74:129-142.

23. Germain RN, Margulies DH. The biochemistry and cell biology of antigen processing and presentation. Ann Rev Immunol 1993; 11:403-450.

24. von Boehmer H. Developmental biology of T cells in T-cell-receptor transgenic mice. Ann Rev Immunol 1990; 8:531-556.

25. Loh DY. Molecular requirements for cell fate determination during T lymphocyte development. New Biol 1991; 3:924-932.

26. Kaye J, Hsu M-L, Sauron M-E et al. Selective development of CD4+ T cells in transgenic mice expressing a class II MHC-restricted antigen receptor. Nature 1989; 341:746-749.

27. Berg LJ, Pullen AM, Fazekas de St. Groth B et al. Antigen/MHC-specific T cells are preferentially exported from the thymus in the presence of their MHC ligand. Cell 1989; 58:1035-1046.

28. Teh HS, Kisielow P, Scott B et al. Thymic major histocompatibility complex antigens and the αβ T-cell receptor determine the CD4/CD8 phenotype of T cells. Nature 1988; 335:229-233.

29. Sha WC, Nelson CA, Newberry RD et al. Selective expression of an antigen receptor on CD8-bearing T lymphocytes in transgenic mice. Nature 1988; 335:271-274.

30. Pircher H, Bürki K, Lang R et al. Tolerance induction in double specific T-cell receptor transgenic mice varies with antigen. Nature 1989; 342:559-561.

31. MacDonald HR, Thiernesse N, Cerottini J-C. Inhibition of T-cell-mediated cytolysis by monoclonal antibodies directed against Lyt-2: Heterogeneity of inhibition at the clonal level. J Immunol 1981; 126:1671-1675.

32. Landegren U, Ramstedt U, Axberg I et al. Selective inhibition of human T-cell cytotoxicity at level of target recognition or initiation of lysis by monoclonal OKT3 and Leu-2a antibody. J Exp Med 1982; 155:1579-1584.

33. Hollander N. Effects of anti-Lyt antibodies on T-cell function. Immunol Rev 1982;

68:43-66.

34. Swain SL, Dialynas DP, Fitch FW et al. Monoclonal antibody to L3T4 blocks the function of T cells specific for class 2 major histocompatibility complex antigens. J Immunol 1984; 132:1118-1123.

35. Rogozinski L, Bass A, Glickman E et al. The T4 surface antigen is involved in the induction of helper function. J Immunol 1984; 132:735-739.

36. Dembic Z, Haas W, Zamoyska R et al. Transfection of the CD8 gene enhances T-cell recognition. Nature 1987; 326:510-511.

37. Gabert J, Langlet C, Zamoyska R et al. Reconstitution of MHC class I specificity by transfer of the T-cell receptor and Lyt-2 genes. Cell 1987; 50:545-554.

38. Gay D, Maddon P, Sekaly R et al. Functional interaction between human T-cell protein CD4 and the major histocompatibility complex HLA-DR antigen. Nature 1987; 328:626-629.

39. Ratnofsky SE, Peterson A, Greenstein JL et al. Expression and function of CD8 in a murine T-cell hybridoma. J Exp Med 1987; 166:1747-1757.

40. Doyle C, Strominger JL. Interaction between CD4 and class II MHC molecules mediates cell adhesion. Nature 1987; 330:256-259.

41. Norment AM, Salter RD, Parham P et al. Cell-cell adhesion mediated by CD8 and MHC class I molecules. Nature 1988; 336:79-81.

42. Rosenstein Y, Ratnofsky S, Burakoff SJ et al. Direct evidence for binding of CD8 to HLA class I antigens. J Exp Med 1988; 169:149-160.

43. König R, Huang L-Y, Germain RN. MHC class II interaction with CD4 mediated by a region analogous to the MHC class I binding site for CD8. Nature 1992; 356:796-798.

44. Cammarota G, Scheirle A, Takacs B et al. Identification of a CD4 binding site on the β_2 domain of HLA-DR molecules. Nature 1992; 356:799-801.

45. Potter TA, Rajan TV, Dick RF II et al. Substitution at residue 227 of H-2 class I molecules abrogates recognition by CD8-dependent, but not CD8-independent, cytotoxic T lymphocytes. Nature 1989;

337:73-75.

46. Salter RD, Benjamin RJ, Wesley PK et al. A binding site for the T-cell co-receptor CD8 on the α_3 domain of HLA-A2. Nature 1990; 345:41-46.

47. Wheeler CJ, von Hoegen P, Parnes JR. An immunological role for the CD8 β-chain. Nature 1992; 357:247-249.

48. Karaki S, Tanabe M, Nakauchi H et al. β-chain broadens range of CD8 recognition for MHC class I molecule. J Immunol 1992; 149:1613-1618.

49. Bjorkman PJ, Saper MA, Samraoui B et al. Structure of the human class I histocompatibility antigen, HLA-A2. Nature 1987; 329:506-512.

50. Miceli MC, von Hoegen P, Parnes JR. Adhesion versus coreceptor function of CD4 and CD8: Role of the cytoplasmic tail in coreceptor activity. Proc Natl Acad Sci 1991; 88:2623-2627.

51. O'Rourke AM, Mescher MF. The roles of CD8 in cytotoxic T lymphocyte function. Immunol Today 1993; 14:183-188.

52. Emmrich F, Strittmatter U, Eichmann K. Synergism in the activation of human CD8 T cells by cross-linking the T-cell receptor complex with the CD8 differentiation antigen Proc Natl Acad Sci 1986; 83:8298-8302.

53. Eichmann K, Jönsson J-I, Falk I et al. Effective activation of resting T lymphocytes by cross-linking submitogenic concentrations of the T-cell antigen receptor with either Lyt-2 or L3T4. Eur J Immunol 1987; 17:643-650.

54. Owens T, Fazekas de St. Groth B, Miller JFAP. Coaggregation of the T-cell receptor with CD4 and other T-cell surface molecules enhances T-cell activation. Proc Natl Acad Sci 1987; 84:9209-9213.

55. Boyce NW, Jönsson J-I, Emmrich F et al. Heterologous crosslinking of Lyt-2 (CD8) to the αβ-T-cell receptor is more effective in T-cell activation than homologous αβ-T-cell receptor cross-linking. J Immunol 1988; 141:2832-2888.

56. Jönsson J-I, Boyce NW, Eichmann K. Immunoregulation through CD8 (Lyt-2): State of aggregation with the αβ/CD3 T-cell receptor controls interleukin-2

dependent T-cell growth. Eur J Immunol 1989; 19:253-260.

57. Janeway CA Jr. Accessories or coreceptors? Nature 1988; 335:208-210.

58. Bjorkman PJ, Saper MA, Samraoui B et al. The foreign antigen binding site and T-cell recognition regions of class I histocompatibility antigens. Nature 1987; 329:512-518.

59. Garrett TPJ, Saper MA, Bjorkman PJ et al. Specificity pockets for the side chains of peptide antigens in HLA-Aw68. Nature 1989; 342:692-696.

60. Brown JH, Jardetzky TS, Gorga JC et al. Three-dimensional structure of the human class II histocompatibility antigen HLA-DR1. Nature 1993; 364:33-37.

61. Kupfer A, Singer SJ, Janeway CA Jr. et al. Coclustering of CD4 (L3T4) molecule with the T-cell receptor is induced by specific direct interaction of helper T cells and antigen-presenting cells. Proc Natl Acad Sci 1987; 84:5888-5892.

62. Veillette A, Bookman MA, Horak EM et al. The CD4 and CD8 T-cell surface antigens are associated with the internal membrane tyrosine-protein kinase p56^{lck}. Cell 1988; 55:301-308.

63. Rudd CE, Trevillyan JM, Dasgupta JD et al. The CD4 receptor is complexed in detergent lysates to a protein-tyrosine kinase (pp58) from human T lymphocytes. Proc Natl Acad Sci 1988; 85:5190-5194.

64. Veillette A, Bookman MA, Horak AM et al. Signal transduction through the CD4 receptor involves the activation of the internal membrane tyrosine-protein kinase p56^{lck}. Nature 1989; 338:257-259.

65. Veillette A, Bolen JB, Bookman MA. Alterations in tyrosine protein phosphorylation induced by antibody-mediated cross-linking of the CD4 receptor of T lymphocytes. Mol Cell Biol 1989; 9:4441-4446.

66. Luo K, Sefton BM. Cross-linking of T-cell surface molecules CD4 and CD8 stimulates phosphorylation of the *lck* tyrosine protein kinase at the autophosphorylation site. Mol Cell Biol 1990; 10:5305-5313.

67. Shaw AS, Chalupny J, Whitney JA et al. Short related sequences in the cytoplasmic domain of CD4 and CD8 mediate binding

to the amino-terminal domain of the p56^{lck} tyrosine protein kinase. Mol Cell Biol 1990; 10:1853-1862.

68. Turner JM, Brodsky MH, Irving BA et al. Interaction of the unique N-terminal region of tyrosine kinase p56^{lck} with cytoplasmic domains of CD4 and CD8 is mediated by cysteine motifs. Cell 1990; 60:755-765.

69. Zamoyska R, Derham P, Gorman SD et al. Inability of CD8α' polypeptides to associate with p56^{lck} correlates with impaired function *in vitro* and lack of expression *in vivo*. Nature 1989; 342:278-281.

70. Glaichenhaus N, Shastri N, Littman DR et al. Requirement for association of p56^{lck} with CD4 in antigen-specific signal transduction in T cells. Cell 1991; 64:511-520.

71. Straus DB, Weiss A. Genetic evidence for the involvement of the lck tyrosine kinase in signal transduction through the T-cell antigen receptor. Cell 1992; 70:585-593.

72. Karnitz L, Sutor SL, Torigoe T et al. Effects of p56^{lck} deficiency on the growth and cytolytic effector function of an interleukin-2-dependent cytotoxic T-cell line. Mol Cell Biol 1992; 12:4521-4530.

73. Fazekas de St. Groth B, Gallagher PF, Miller JFAP. Involvement of Lyt-2 and L3T4 in activation of hapten-specific Lyt-2$^+$, L3T4$^+$ T-cell clones. Proc Natl Acad Sci 1986; 83:2594-2598.

74. Jones B, Khavari PA, Conrad PJ et al. Differential effects of antibodies to Lyt-2 and L3T4 on cytolysis by cloned, Ia-restricted T cells expressing both proteins. J Immunol 1987; 139:380-384.

75. Samelson LE, Klausner RD. Tyrosine kinases and tyrosine-based activation motifs: Current research on activation via the T-cell antigen receptor. J Biol Chem 1992; 267:24913- 24916.

76. Weiss A. T-cell antigen receptor signal transduction: A tale of tails and cytoplasmic protein-tyrosine kinases. Cell 1993; 73:209-212.

77. Telfer JC, Rudd CE. A 32-kD GTP-binding protein associated with the CD4-p56^{lck} and CD8-p56^{lck} T-cell receptor complexes. Science 1991; 254:439-441.

78. Schraven B, Schirren A, Kirchgessner H et al. Four CD45/p56lck-associated phospho-

proteins (pp29-pp32) undergo alterations in human T-cell activation. Eur J Immunol 1992; 22:1857-1863.

79. Adams JM, Houston H, Allen J et al. The hematopoietically expressed *vav* proto-oncogene shares homology with the *dbl* GDP-GTP exchange factor, the *bcr* gene and a yeast gene (*CDC24*) involved in cytoskeletal organization. Oncogene 1992; 7:611-618.

80. Bustelo XR, Ledbetter JA, Barbacid M. Product of *vav* proto-oncogene defines a new class of tyrosine protein kinase substrates. Nature 1992; 356:68-71.

81. Gulbins E, Coggeshall KM, Baier G et al. Tyrosine kinase-stimulated guanine nucleotide exchange activity of vav in T-cell activation. Science 1993; 260:822-825.

82. Weber JR, Bell GM, Han MY et al. Association of the tyrosine kinase LCK with phospholipase C-γ1 after stimulation of the T-cell antigen receptor. J Exp Med 1992; 176:373-379.

83. Fowlkes BJ, Edison L, Mathieson BJ et al. Early T lymphocytes: Differentiation in vivo of adult intrathymic precursor cells. J Exp Med 1985; 162:802-822.

84. Crispe IN, Moore MW, Husmann LA et al. Differentiation potential of subsets of CD4⁻CD8⁻ thymocytes. Nature 1987; 329:336-339.

85. Smith L. CD4⁺ murine T cells develop from CD8⁺ precursors *in vivo*. Nature 1987; 326:798-800.

86. Nikolic-Zugic J, Bevan MJ. Thymocytes expressing CD8 differentiate into CD4⁺ cells following intrathymic injection. Proc Natl Acad Sci 1988; 85:8633-8637.

87. Nikolic-Zugic J, Moore MW, Bevan MJ. Characterization of the subset of immature thymocytes which can undergo rapid *in vitro* differentiation. Eur J Immunol 1989; 19:649-653.

88. Nikolic-Zugic J, Moore MW. T-cell receptor expression on immature thymocytes with *in vivo* and *in vitro* precursor potential. Eur J Immunol 1989; 19:1957-1960.

89. Egerton M, Scollay R, Shortman K. Kinetics of mature T-cell development in the thymus. Proc Natl Acad Sci 1990; 87:2579-2582.

90. Shortman K, Vremec D, Egerton M. The kinetics of T-cell antigen receptor expression by subgroups of CD4⁺CD8⁺ thymocytes: Delineation of CD4⁺CD8⁺3²⁺ thymocytes as post-selection intermediates leading to mature T cells. J Exp Med 1991; 173:323-332.

91. Nikolic-Zugic J. Phenotypic and functional stages in the intrathymic development of αβ T cells. Immunol. Today 1991; 12:65-70.

92. von Boehmer H. Thymic selection: A matter of life and death. Immunol Today 1992; 13:454-458.

93. Mombaerts P, Clarke AR, Rudnicki MA et al. Mutations in T-cell antigen receptor genes α and β block thymocyte development at different stages. Nature 1992; 360:225-231.

94. Zinkernagel RM, Callahan GN, Althage A et al. On the thymus in the differentiation of "H-2 self-recognition" by T cells: Evidence for dual recognition? J Exp Med 1978; 147:882-896.

95. Fink P, Bevan MJ. H-2 antigens of the thymus determine lymphocyte specificity. J Exp Med 1978; 149:766-775.

96. Kappler JW, Roehm N, Marrack PC. T-cell tolerance by clonal elimination in the thymus. Cell 1987; 49:273-280.

97. Kappler JW, Staerz UD, White J et al. Self-tolerance eliminates T cells specific for Mls-modified products of the major histocompatibility complex. Nature 1988; 332:35-40.

98. MacDonald RH, Schneider R, Lees RK et al. T-cell receptor V_β use predicts reactivity and tolerance to *Mlsᵃ*-encoded antigens. Nature 1988; 332:40-45.

99. Nikolic-Zugic J, Bevan MJ. Role of self-peptides in positively selecting the T-cell repertoire. Nature 1990; 334:65-67.

100. Ashton-Rickardt PG, Van Kaer L, Schumacher TNM et al. Peptide contributes to the specificity of positive selection of CD8⁺ T cells in the thymus. Cell 1993; 73:1041-1049.

101. Fowlkes BJ, Schwartz RH, Pardoll DM. Deletion of self-reactive thymocytes occurs at a CD4⁺8⁺ precursor stage. Nature 1988; 334:620-623.

102. MacDonald HR, Hengartner H, Pedrazzini T. Intrathymic deletion of self-reactive cells prevented by neonatal anti-CD4 antibody treatment. Nature 1988; 335:174-176.

103. Rahemtulla A, Fung-Leung W-P, Schilham MW et al. Normal development and

function of CD8[+] cells but markedly decreased helper cell activity in mice lacking CD4. Nature 1991; 353:180-184.

104. Killeen N, Sawada S, Littman DR. Regulated expression of human CD4 rescues helper T-cell development in mice lacking expression of endogenous CD4. EMBO J 1993; 12:1547-1553.

105. Fung-Leung W-P, Schilham MW, Rahemtulla A et al. CD8 is needed for development of cytotoxic T cells but not helper T cells. Cell 1991; 65:443-449.

106. Fung-Leung W-P, Wallace VA, Gray D et al. CD8 is needed for positive selection but differentially required for negative selection of T cells during thymic ontogeny. Eur J Immunol 1993; 23:212-216.

107. Kruisbeek AM, Fultz MJ, Sharrow SO et al. Early development of the T-cell repertoire: In vivo treatment of neonatal mice with anti-Ia antibodies interferes with differentiation of I-restricted T cells but not K/D-restricted T cells. J Exp Med 1983; 157:1932-1946.

108. Kruisbeek AM, Mond JJ, Fowlkes BJ et al. Absence of the Lyt-2[-], L3T4[+] lineage of T cells in mice treated neonatally with anti-I-A correlates with absence of intrathymic I-A-bearing antigen-presenting cell function. J Exp Med 1985; 161:1029-1047.

109. Marrack P, Kushnir E, Born W et al. The development of helper T-cell precursors in mouse thymus. J Immunol 1988; 140:2508-2514.

110. Marusic-Galesic S, Stephany DA, Longo DL et al. Development of CD4[-]CD8[+] cytotoxic T cells requires interactions with class I MHC determinants. Nature 1988; 333:180-183.

111. Zuñiga-Pflücker JC, Longo DL, Kruisbeek AM. Positive selection of CD4[-]CD8[+] T cells in the thymus of normal mice. Nature 1989; 338:76-78.

112. Zjilstra M, Bix M, Simister NE et al. β2-microglobulin deficient mice lack CD4[-]CD8[+] cytolytic T cells. Nature 1990; 344:742-746.

113. Koller BH, Marrack P, Kappler JW et al. Normal development of mice deficient in β$_2$m, MHC class I proteins, and CD8[+] T cells. Science 1990; 248:1227-1230.

114. Cosgrove D, Gray D, Dierich A et al. Mice lacking MHC class II molecules. Cell 1991; 66:1051-1066.

115. Grusby MJ, Johnson RS, Papaioannou VE et al. Depletion of CD4[+] T cells in major histocompatibility complex class-II deficient mice. Science 1991; 253:1417-1420.

116. Chan SH, Cosgrove D, Waltzinger C et al. Another view of the selective model of thymocyte selection. Cell 1993; 73:225-236.

117. Aldrich CJ, Hammer RE, Jones-Youngblood S et al. Negative and positive selection of antigen-specific cytotoxic T lymphocytes affected by the α3 domain of MHC I molecules. Nature 1991; 352:718-721.

118. Ingold AL, Landel C, Knall C et al. Coengagement of CD8 with the T-cell receptor is required for negative selection. Nature 1991; 352:721-723.

119. Killeen N, Moriarty A, Teh H-S et al. Requirement for CD8-major histocompatibility complex class I interaction in positive and negative selection of developing T cells. J Exp Med 1992; 176:89-97.

120. Deusch K, Daley JF, Levine H et al. Differential regulation of Ca^{2+} mobilization in human thymocytes by coaggregation of surface molecules. J Immunol 1990; 144:2851-2858.

121. Gilliland LK, Teh H-S, Uckun FM et al. CD4 and CD8 are positive regulators of T-cell receptor signal transduction in early T-cell differentiation. J Immunol 1991; 146:1759-1765.

122. van Oers NSC, Garvin AM, Davis CB et al. Disruption of CD8-dependent negative and positive selection of thymocytes is correlated with a decreased association between CD8 and the protein tyrosine kinase, p56[*lck*]. Eur J Immunol 1992; 22:733-743.

123. Veillette A, Zuñiga-Pflücker JC, Bolen JB et al. Engagement of CD4 and CD8 expressed on immature thymocytes induces activation of intracellular tyrosine phosphorylation pathways. J Exp Med 1989; 170:1671-1680.

124. Nakayama K, Loh DY. No requirement for p56[*lck*] in the antigen-stimulated clonal deletion of thymocytes. Science 1992; 257:94-96.

125. Molina TJ, Kishihara K, Siderovski DP et al. Profound block in thymocyte development

in mice lacking p56^{lck}. Nature 1992; 357:161-164.

126. Sprent J, Lo D, Gao E-K et al. T-cell selection in the thymus. Immunol Rev 1988; 101:173-190.

127. Schwartz RH. Acquisition of immunologic self-tolerance. Cell 1989; 57:1073-1081.

128. Teh H-S, Kishi H, Scott B et al. Deletion of autospecific T cells in T-cell receptor (TcR) transgenic mice spares cells with normal TcR levels and low levels of CD8 molecules. J Exp Med 1989; 169:795-806.

129. Lee NA, Loh DY, Lacy E. CD8 surface levels alter the fate of α/β T-cell receptor-expressing thymocytes in transgenic mice. J Exp Med 1992; 175:1013-1025.

130. Robey EA, Ramsdell F, Kioussis D et al. The level of CD8 expression can determine the outcome of thymic selection. Cell 1992; 69:1089-1096.

131. Robey EA, Fowlkes BJ, Gordon JW et al. Thymic selection in CD8 transgenic mice supports an instructive model for commitment to a CD4 or CD8 lineage. Cell 1991; 64:99-107.

132. Robey E, Axel R. CD4: Collaborator in immune recognition and HIV infection. Cell 1990; 60:697-700.

133. Nakayama K-I, Shinkai Y-I, Okumura K et al. Isolation and characterization of the mouse CD8 β-chain (Ly-3) genes: Absence of an intervening sequence between V- and J-like gene segments. J Immunol 1989; 142:2540-2546.

134. Nakayama K-I, Kawachi Y, Tokito S et al. Recent duplication of the two human CD8 β-chain genes. J Immunol 1992; 148:1919-1927.

135. Liaw CW, Zamoyska R, Parnes JR. Structure, sequence, and polymorphism of the Lyt-2 T-cell differentiation antigen gene. J Immunol 1986; 137:1037-1043.

136. Tagawa M, Nakauchi H, Herzenberg LA et al. Formal proof that different-size Lyt-2 polypeptides arise from differential splicing and post-transcriptional regulation. Proc Natl Acad Sci 1986; 83:3422-3426.

137. Norment AM, Lonberg N, Lacy E et al. Alternatively spliced mRNA encodes a secreted form of human CD8α: Characterization of the human CD8α gene. J Immunol 1989; 142:3312-3319.

138. Giblin P, Ledbetter JA, Kavathas P. A secreted form of the human lymphocyte cell surface molecule CD8 arises from alternative splicing. Proc Natl Acad Sci 1989; 86:998-1002.

139. Johnson P. A human homolog of the mouse CD8 molecule, Lyt-3: Genomic sequence and expression. Immunogenetics 1987; 26:174-177.

140. Terry LA, DiSanto JP, Small TN et al. Differential expression and regulation of the human CD8α and CD8β chains. Tissue Antigens 1990; 35:82-91.

141. White J, Blackman M, Bill J et al. Two better cell lines for making hybridomas expressing specific T-cell receptors. J Immunol 1989; 143:1822-1825.

142. Carbone AM, Marrack P, Kappler JW. Remethylation at sites 5' of the murine Lyt-2 gene in association with shutdown of Lyt-2 expression. J Immunol 1988; 141:1369-1375.

143. Gao M-H, Kavathas PB. Functional importance of the cyclic AMP response element-like decamer motif in the CD8α promoter. J Immunol 1993; 150:4376-4385.

144. Zamoyska R, Parnes JR. CD8 polypeptide that is lost after passing the Golgi but before reaching the cell surface: A novel sorting mechanism. EMBO J 1988; 7:2359-2367.

145. Blum MD, Wong GT, Higgins KM et al. Reconstitution of the subclass-specific expression of CD4 in thymocytes and peripheral T cells of transgenic mice: Identification of a human CD4 enhancer. J Exp Med 1993; 177:1343-1358.

146. Isobe M, Huebner K, Maddon PJ et al. The gene encoding the T-cell surface protein T4 is located on human chromosome 12. Proc Natl Acad Sci 1986; 83:4399-4402.

147. Lonberg N, Gettner SN, Lacy E et al. Mouse brain CD4 transcripts encode only the COOH-terminal half of the protein. Mol Cell Biol 1988; 8:2224-2228.

148. Field EH, Tourvieille B, D'Eustachio P et al. The gene encoding the mouse T-cell differentiation antigen L3T4 is located on chromosome 6. J Immunol 1987; 138:1968-1970.

149. Gorman SD, Tourvieille B, Parnes JR. Structure of the mouse gene encoding CD4

and an unusual transcript in brain. Proc Natl Acad Sci 1987; 84:7644-7648.

150. Sawada S, Littman DR. Identification and characterization of a T-cell-specific enhancer adjacent to the murine CD4 gene. Mol Cell Biol 1991; 11:5506-5515.

151. Tourvieille B, Gorman SD, Field EH et al. Isolation and sequence of L3T4 complementary DNA clones: Expression in T-cells and brain. Science 1986; 234:610-614.

152. Siu G, Wurster AL, Lipsick JS et al. Expression of the CD4 gene requires a myb transcription factor. Mol Cell Biol 1992; 12:1592-1604.

153. Gillespie FP, Doros L, Vitale J et al. Tissue-specific expression of human CD4 in transgenic mice. Mol Cell Biol 1993; 13:2952-2958.

154. von Boehmer H, Kisielow P. Lymphocyte lineage commitment: Instruction versus selection. Cell 1993; 73:207-208.

155. Davis CB, Killeen N, Crooks MEC et al. Evidence for a stochastic mechanism in the differentiation of mature subsets of T lymphocytes. Cell 1993; 73:237-247.

156. Borgulya P, Kishi H, Müller U et al. Development of the CD4 and CD8 lineage of T cells: Instruction versus selection. EMBO J 1991; 10:913-918.

157. Crompton T, Pircher H, MacDonald HR. CD4+CD8- thymocytes bearing major histocompatibility complex class I-restricted T-cell receptors: Evidence for homeostatic control of early stages of CD4/CD8 lineage development. J Exp Med 1992; 176:903-907.

158. Seong RH, Chamberlain JW, Parnes JR. Signal for T-cell differentiation to a CD4 cell lineage is delivered by CD4 transmembrane region and/or cytoplasmic tail. Nature 1992; 356:718-720.

159. Petrie HT, Strasser A, Harris AW et al. CD4+CD8- mature thymocytes require different post-selection processing for final development. J Immunol 1993; 151:1273-1279.

160. Julius M, Maroun CR, Haughn L. Distinct roles for CD4 and CD8 as co-receptors in antigen receptor signaling. Immunol. Today 1993; 14:177-183.

CHAPTER 12

SIGNAL TRANSDUCTION IN DEVELOPING THYMOCYTES

Janko Nikolić-Žugić

Sofija Andjelić

Which intracellular signal transduction pathways do thymocytes use during intrathymic development? While this question is at the cutting edge of thymocyte research, the topic of signal transduction in thymocytes is less well understood than any other topic covered in this monograph. There are several reasons for this. Signal transduction is a rapidly expanding discipline that progressed considerably in a relatively short period of time. However, the sheer complexity and enormous redundancy of signaling pathways makes it very difficult to integrate all available information into a coherent model that would link a stimulus and a cellular response. To reduce the complexity, and to obtain enough material for biochemical assays, most investigators tend to work with transformed cell lines. Since transformation itself results from aberrant regulation of cell cycling, such lines may often display signaling abnormalities that are not shared by normal cells. Moreover, although many signaling concepts are shared between lower eukaryotes and mammals, extrapolations from one to another organism and tissue are potentially misleading. An additional conceptual problem lies in the tendency to view signaling pathways in a linear, unidimensional fashion. Interactions between different pathways and feedback loops existing within and between pathways are poorly understood. The picture of signal transduction is therefore necessarily fragmented, and contains many assumptions and extrapolations.

The general problems outlined above hold true for the area of T-cell signaling (Fig. 1 and please don't run away). However, in the area of thymocyte signaling, the confusion is near-complete. Thymocytes respond to stimulation very differently from mature T cells, usually by dying rather than dividing. Moreover, thymocytes are notoriously fragile outside the thymus, and even in vivo are subject to cell death at an extraordinarily high rate. The phenotypic and functional heterogeneity of thymocytes often correlates with their heterogenous response to stimulation. Our current information on signaling in thymocytes originates from studying unseparated

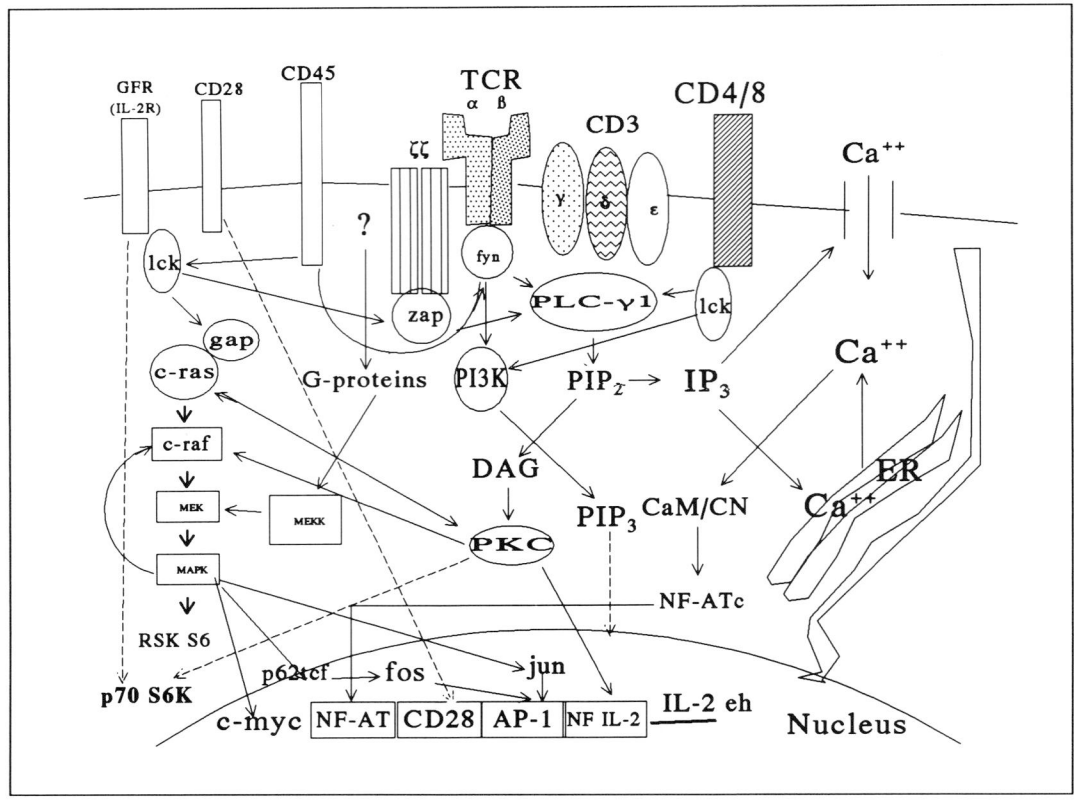

Fig. 1. Signal transduction in T lymphocytes. Solid arrows connecting different molecules denote direct activation. Bidirectional arrows implicate feedback loops or an uncertain order of activation. Broken arrows denote activation that most likely involves one or more unknown intermediates. MAP kinases most likely translocate to the nucleus before acting on transcription factors. ER - endoplasmic reticulum. ? - uncertain beginning of the pathway. This figure is broken in three smaller, more detailed and more intelligible figures shown later in the text.

thymocytes or T-cell hybridomas generated by fusing a developmentally arrested thymoma with mature peripheral T cells. The first approach essentially measures and extrapolates the results to the response of DP cells that make up 80% or more of all thymocytes, but this approach is very vulnerable to artifacts due to the possible vigorous responses of less numerous subsets. The strategy of using hybridomas has the disadvantage of not being able to discern whether a signaling pathway originates from the mature or the immature parent, or from a combination occurring in a heterokaryon. More recently, several groups resorted to genetic manipulations of signal-associated molecules in transgenic animals. Although these studies have contributed to our understanding of the function

of some molecules, we still know very little on the developmental stage specific signaling changes in maturing thymocytes.

For reasons outlined above, we shall start this chapter by describing the known aspects of signal transduction in mature T lymphocytes, and then follow with a discussion of these pathways in thymocytes. The scope of this review is such that detailed attention cannot be paid to all aspects of signaling, especially not to the full description of all experimental findings. For the full description of various signaling pathways in T and non-T cells, and especially for detailed references, the reader is encouraged to peruse the recent reviews by Perlmutter et al,[1] Blenis,[2] Schreiber and Crabtree,[3] Cambier[4] and Berridge.[5]

SIGNALING EVENTS IN MATURE T LYMPHOCYTES

The TcR is the key structure that initiates signaling events in T cells upon recognizing a cognate peptide associated with the restricting MHC molecule. TcR is a multimolecular signal transducing unit that consists of clonotypic α and β (or γ and δ) chains (TcR proper, or the TcR heterodimer), three chains of the CD3 complex (γ, δ and ε chains), and ζ chain homodimers (or ζη heterodimers). TcR proper recognizes the peptide:MHC complex, while CD3 and ζ chains facilitate signal transduction. Upon TcR: ligand interaction, a cascade of biochemical events transduces the signal to the nucleus, causing gene transcription and translation that culminate in cellular activation, proliferation and lymphokine secretion.

During the past decade, extensive research has been aimed at dissecting early biochemical changes following T-cell activation. Using peptide:MHC complexes, anti-TcR antibodies and mitogenic lectins as TcR agonists, it was observed that T cells undergo a rapid increase in intracellular Ca^{++} levels shortly after stimulation.[6] This observation was followed by the finding that TcR ligation induces hydrolysis of phosphatidylinositides (PI), presumably via the activation of the PI-specific phospholipase Cγ1 (PLCγ1) (reviewed in ref. 7). PI breakdown generates at least two second messengers: diacylglycerol (DAG) and inositol phosphates such as IP_3 (reviewed in ref. 8). DAG is the activator of a family of Ca^{++}- and phosphoinositide-dependent serine/threonine protein kinase enzymes known as protein kinase C (PKC). DAG increases the affinity of PKC for Ca^{++} and phospholipids, thus permitting its activation at resting intracellular Ca^{++} levels. Inositol triphosphate (IP_3) regulates the Ca^{++} content in the cell by inducing its influx from intracellular (chiefly ER) and extracellular sources (reviewed in ref. 7). Most importantly, a combination of pharmacological agents that induce PKC activation (tumor-promoting phorbol esters) and calcium influx (Ca^{++} ionophores) bypasses the TcR and stimulates the resting T cells.[6,8] Furthermore, phorbol esters are also necessary for a full T-cell response to anti-CD3 mAb or mitogens in the absence of accessory cells (reviewed in ref. 9). These results are consistent with the two-signal model for optimal T-cell activation. According to this model, TcR occupancy (signal 1) in the absence of the APC-derived costimulatory signal (signal 2) is not sufficient for T-cell activation. Rather, such stimulation renders the cell unresponsive to further stimulation by inducing anergy (reviewed in ref. 9). The TcR-induced Ca^{++} influx and the initial activation of PKC (as well as other intracellular changes) would correspond to signal 1, whereas the PMA-mediated sustained activation of PKC (and, perhaps, other substrates) might correspond to signal 2. It thus appeared that the backbone of the key TcR-mediated signaling pathway in T cells was solved. Questions remained, however, on the exact connection between the TcR engagement and the PI breakdown, as well as on the mediators of nuclear activation downstream of PKC and Ca^{++}.

More recent biochemical studies demonstrated that several TcR complex subunits become rapidly phosphorylated on tyrosine residues upon activation.[10] It became clear that an additional protein tyrosine kinase (PTK) pathway lies between, and most likely couples, the TcR and the PI turnover. Indeed, the activation of nonreceptor tyrosine kinases, including those that belong to the Src family of PTK is the first biochemical event detectable upon T-cell activation.[11] Tyrosine phosphorylation was found to be both necessary and sufficient for T-cell activation.[12] We shall therefore discuss the putative key players in T-cell signaling starting from the PTK (Fig. 2) and moving towards the nuclear activators.

PROTEIN TYROSINE KINASES (PTK)

SRC FAMILY OF PTK

This family of enzymes was named by its first member, Src, which was shown to be the oncogenic factor of the transforming Rous sarcoma virus. All kinases from the Src family are myristoylated (to facilitate membrane attachment) and all contain a highly conserved catalytic domain and very similar SH2

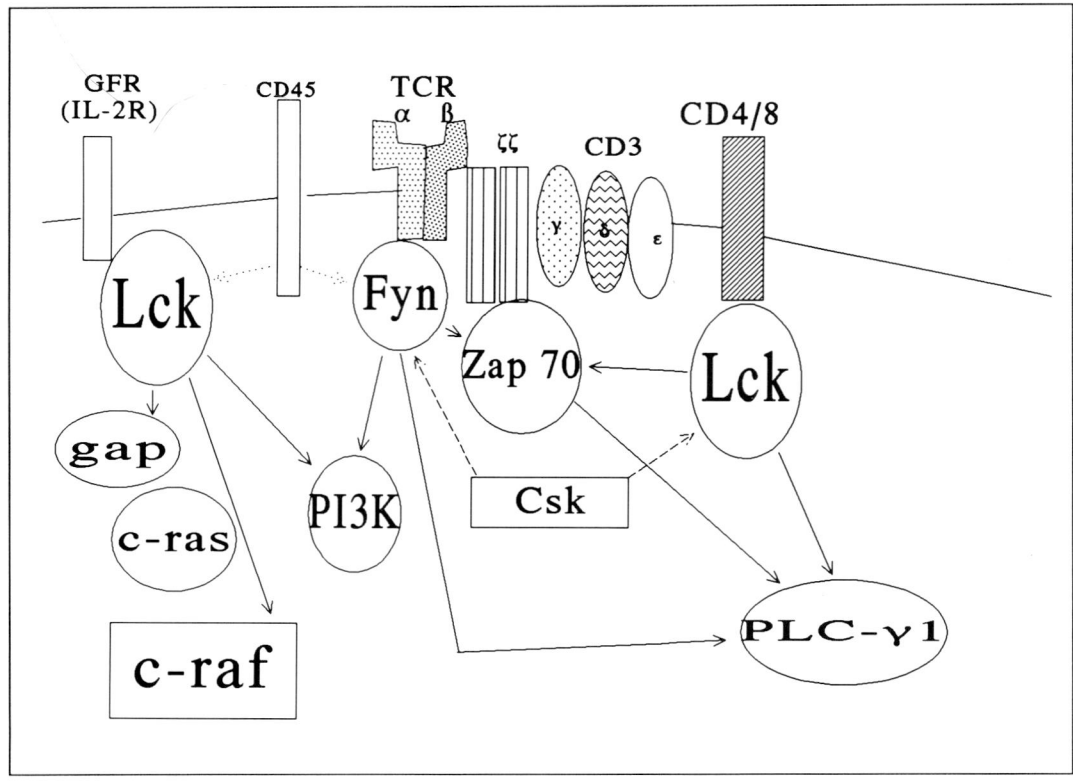

Fig. 2. Protein-tyrosine phosphorylation and dephosphorylation in T cells. Solid arrows - activating phosphorylation. Dashed arrows - inhibitory phosphorylation. Dotted arrows - activating dephosphorylation.

and SH3 domains. Seventy amino-terminal residues, however, are polymorphic, and this part of the molecule probably interacts with different cell surface receptors (reviewed in ref. 1). SH2 and SH3 domains are modular structures that behave rather independently of the other parts of the enzyme (except that the SH2 domain can bind to the C-terminal regulatory phosphotyrosine of the kinase domain), very much like certain transcription factors. These domains can also be found in other non-PTK molecules. A proposed role of the SH2 domain is to bind phosphotyrosine-containing proteins and recruit them to the site of activation. SH3 domain could, directly or via adapters, bind guanine nucleotide-release factors, providing a potential hook to p21 GTP-binding proteins. Another important common feature shared by the members of the Src family is the C-terminal regulatory tyrosine residue.

This tyrosine is believed to be the target site for the regulators of PTK activity (see below).[1]

Two enzymes from the Src family have been implicated in T-cell activation: p56Lck and p59Fyn. p56Lck is a T-cell specific member of the Src tyrosine kinases family that binds to intracellular tails of CD4 and CD8 accessory/coreceptor molecules.[13] mAb crosslinking of the TcR and CD4 or CD8 augments T-cell activation, and this co-activation increases in vitro kinase activity of p56Lck.[13] Yet, only about 50% of cellular Lck is bound to CD8 or CD4 molecules (perhaps more to the latter—Lck may have a higher affinity for the CD4 molecule than for CD8) (reviewed in ref. 14). Lck also binds to the IL-2 receptor (IL-2R) β chain via its catalytic domain, and increases the IL-2R phosphorylation in vitro.[15] Evidence that Lck is essential for normal signal transduction through the TcR came from the study of the Lck⁻ mutant of the Jurkat T-cell line.[16] Lck⁻ Jurkat cells exhibit defective tyrosine phosphorylation, Ca⁺⁺ mobilization and lymphokine production. Restoration of Lck expression completely corrects these defects. It has been proposed that the recognition of the peptide:MHC complex results in the co-aggregation of CD4/CD8 and the TcR complex that would lead to juxtaposition of the Lck kinase and the elements of the TcR complex. This would facilitate the interaction of Lck with its substrates and with other kinases bound to the TcR complex. However, recent experiments by Xu and Littman[17] have demonstrated that the kinase portion of p56Lck is not necessary for T-cell activation via the chimeric CD4/Lck protein. By contrast, an intact SH2 domain of the molecule is critical for T-cell activation. Therefore, p56Lck significantly contributes to T-cell activation by aggregating with other components of the signaling machinery. A possible mode of action in the latter case could be the recruitment of other signaling molecules via the SH2 (and, perhaps, SH3) domain.

Of the two isoforms of p59Fyn (resulting from alternative splicing), one, p59FynT, is predominant in T cells.[18] The T-cell form of Fyn interacts directly with the TcR αβ heterodimer,[19] but its mechanism of action in T-cell activation is still quite obscure. Given the p59Fyn-TcR association, it was expected that enzymatic action of Fyn would be regulated directly through the TcR. However, the catalytic activity of p59Fyn is not enhanced upon TcR stimulation in vitro. An overexpression of p59Fyn in a T-cell hybridoma and in thymocytes of transgenic (tg) mice resulted in enhanced signal transduction through the TcR complex,[20] but an in vivo targeted disruption of the *fyn* gene resulted in only minor signaling defects in peripheral T cells.[21]

A critical issue in judging the role of p56Lck and p59Fyn in early signaling events is the identification of their downstream targets. Among putative substrates identified so far are the PLCγ1, rasGAP (will be discussed separately, together with p21Ras), the phosphatidylinositol 3 kinase (PI3K), Raf and

MAP kinases. As mentioned above, the activation of PLC induces PI breakdown and generation of the second messengers: DAG and IP_3. In coimmunoprecipitation assays, PLC was found to associate with TcR, but only after the TcR was itself phosphorylated.[22] The significance of this association is not clear. p56Lck was also found to coprecipitate with PLC in a T-cell line.[23]

The PI3 kinase plays the key role in transducing signals from various receptor tyrosine kinases such as PDGFR, EGFR and the insulin receptor (reviewed in 24). The p85 subunit of PI3K interacts with phosphotyrosine residues on the receptors or receptor substrates through one or both of its SH2 domains.[25] It was found that p59Fyn coprecipitates significant levels of PI3 kinase in IL-2 deprived CTLL-2 cells.[26] When stimulated with IL-2, these cells showed an increase in p59Fyn-associated PI3K activity. Precipitation studies revealed that the PI3K p85 subunit binds to the SH3 domain of Fyn and that anti-CD3 stimulation can increase the level of Fyn-SH3 associated PI3 kinase activity. PI3K also coprecipitates with CD4-p56Lck complexes in human CD4⁺ T-cell clones.[27]

p56Lck was shown to phosphorylate and activate MAP kinases[28] in vitro, and this could represent an important link between proximal and distal phosphorylation events during T-cell activation. If relevant in vivo, this activity is unlikely to reflect the direct physiological action of Lck. It is more likely that such an activation can occur via p21Ras and/or PKC pathways.

SYK FAMILY OF PTK

The first member of this family, p72Syk, is a dominant kinase in B cells, and probably plays little or no role in T-cell signaling.[1] However, Weiss and colleagues have identified a novel PTK, associated with the phosphorylated form of the TcR complex ζ chain.[29] This enzyme, named ZAP 70 ζ-associated protein of 70 kD), belongs to the Syk family and is phosphorylated on tyrosine following TcR stimulation. Another 70 kD protein associated with the CD3 complex was detected after TcR stimulation, but it is not clear whether this protein is identical or homologous to ZAP 70.[30] Recent experiments on Jurkat cells transfected with chimeric constructs bearing the extracellular/transmembrane domain of CD16/CD7 chimera fused to tyrosine kinases from Syk and Src families suggested that Syk kinases may act more directly on the signaling machinery of T cells than kinases from the Src family.[31] Aggregation of either of the two Syk kinases, but not that of the Src (Lck and Fyn) kinases, led to Ca^{++} influx in cells lacking a TcR. In other experiments from the same study, ZAP 70 acted synergistically with a Src family kinase in mediating cellular responses. This finding is consistent with the model by Weiss: ZAP 70 would be triggered by Fyn and/or Lck upon TcR ligation, and would be instrumental in relaying signals downstream.[30] By contrast, a recently published study using COS-1 nonlymphoid cells showed that p59Fyn may link ζ directly to the PLC-γ1 activation pathway without the requirement for ZAP 70.[32] These studies illustrate how the variability of results obtained from diverse experimental system can easily lead to controversies, and underline how poor our knowledge is of the exact mechanisms of signaling through the TcR.

REGULATION OF PTK ACTIVATION

In a variety of signaling systems, kinases act in balance with protein tyrosine phosphatases (PTP). Indeed, dephosphorylation of a negative regulatory tyrosine of the Src kinases results in the augmentation of the kinase activity.[27] A candidate regulator of PTK activity in T cells is CD45, a transmembrane receptor phosphotyrosine phosphatase.[33] The CD45 molecule is present on most hematopoietic cells; it exists in multiple isoforms generated by the alternative splicing of three exons (A,B and C) encoding the membrane-distal part of the extracellular domain. The intracellular portion of the CD45 molecule is responsible for the phosphatase activity and is invariant. CD45 was shown to dephosphorylate the C-terminal tyrosine of Src kinases and enhance their kinase activity in vitro. Furthermore, defects in TcR-mediated Ca^{++} mobilization in CD45⁻

mutant cells can be restored by transfection of CD45. Although several groups showed that cross-linking of anti-CD45 and anti-CD3 antibodies results in inhibition of CD3 induced T-cell activation, these results can be explained by experimental artifacts.[33] The extracellular portion of the CD45 molecule is not necessary for the TcR-mediated signal transduction.[34] But a targeted disruption of CD45 in vivo essentially abrogates both B and T-cell activation.[35] Together, the case for the involvement of CD45 in the regulation of PTK activation during T-cell signal transduction is quite strong. Along these lines, one should be reminded of the existence of CD45 isoforms, since it is possible that different isoforms may bind to different ligands and/or have a different function.

Another newly discovered kinase, p50Csk (C-terminal src kinase), was found to phosphorylate the C-termini of all Src kinases tested, but not other substrates.[36] p50Csk is expressed ubiquitously, with the highest levels in the thymus, the spleen and the neonatal brain.[37] The development of Csk-deficient mice was arrested at an early embryonic stage. These embryos exhibited several-fold higher Src-type kinase activity (p60c-Src, p59Fyn, p53/56Lyn).[37] It was suggested that p50Cskmay be the unique and specific in vivo negative regulator of all Src kinases. Indeed, Csk was shown to negatively regulate TcR-mediated signaling.[38] When overexpressed in a T-cell line, Csk leads to an inhibition of tyrosine phosphorylation and downregulation of lymphokine secretion. This effect is dependent upon the intact kinase domain of Csk.[38] It is thus possible that CD45 and Csk antagonize each other in regulating activation of PTKs.

OTHER PTKS

The IL-2 inducible T-cell kinase, Itk,[39] and a T-cell specific kinase, Tsk,[40] have recently been cloned. Both bear some homology to the Src family, and both have only been initially characterized. An interesting feature of Tsk is that it is developmentally regulated in a similar fashion as Lck: Tsk mRNA levels are 5-10 fold higher in thymocytes than in peripheral T cells, and increase in the thymus during the neonatal development. Tsk was also found in day 14 fetal thymus, suggesting a role in early T lymphocyte development.

DAG EFFECTORS

As mentioned previously, activation of PLC generates two second messengers: DAG and IP$_3$. The key mediator of the DAG-initiated signaling cascade is the protein kinase C (PKC). Members of the PKC family of serine-threonine kinase isozymes share extensive sequence homology and, presumably, similar function, but have different tissue-specific distribution (reviewed in refs. 8 and 41). The finding that T-cell activation can be mimicked by a combination of the PKC activator phorbol-myristate acetate (PMA) and a calcium ionophore ionomycin (Iono)

has prompted extensive research on the role of PKC in T lymphocyte activation. The majority of these experiments were performed using PMA as the PKC activator. However, caution should be used when interpreting the results: PMA has pleiotropic effects, and some of the effects may have been mediated by molecules other than PKC. PMA also can lead to an exhaustion of PKC activity by continuous, chronic stimulation. However, most studies described below were performed by acute PMA treatment and are thus due to PKC stimulation.

PKC

PKC (Fig. 3) is thought to mediate its effects at two levels: by phosphorylating and/ or indirectly regulating the membrane-bound molecules and by relaying signals into the

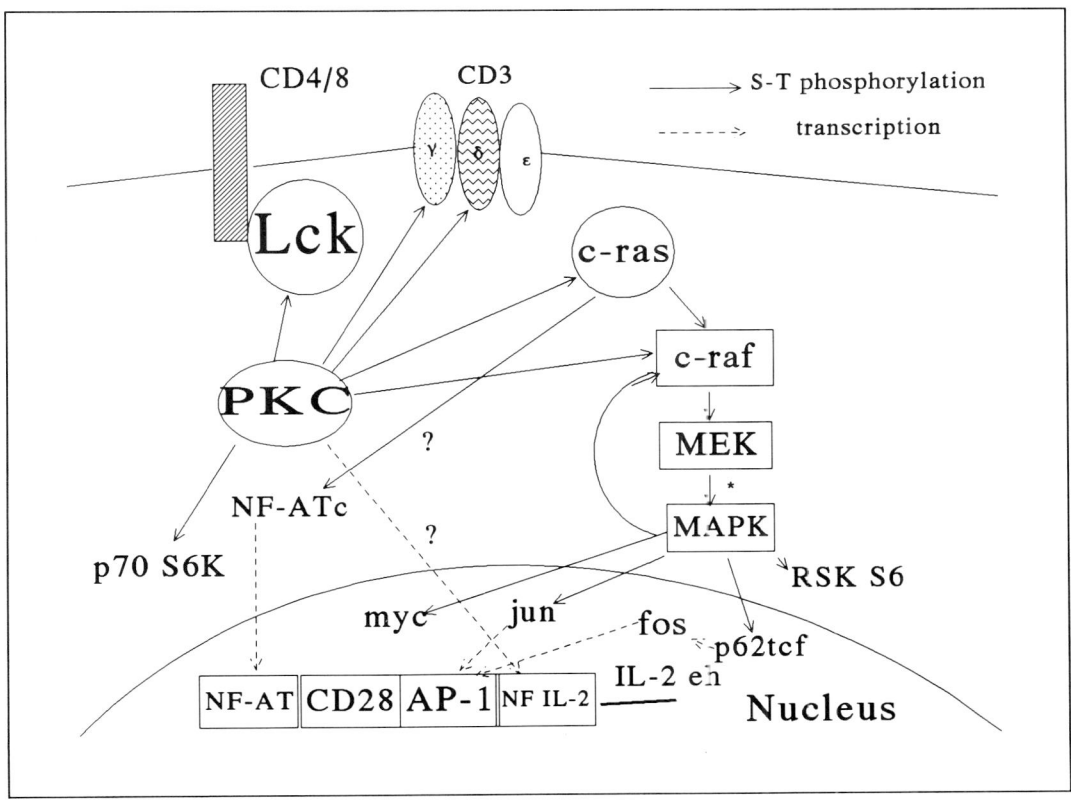

Fig. 3. Serine-threonine phosphorylation in T cells. Solid lines and dotted lines represent phosphorylation and transcription, respectively. * - this reaction involves both tyrosine and serine-threonine phosphorylation. ? - other intermediates are probably present. Note: the mechanism of Ras action is not known, but it does not involve phosphorylation; it is possible that Ras brings other molecules in proximity with P-Y and P-S/T kinases.

nucleus. This division may be misleading, due to the fact that some of the membrane-bound PKC substrates/effectors, e.g., p21ras, could in turn mediate nuclear activation and cell cycle progression. At the membrane level, PKC can downregulate surface expression of the TcR complex and induce phosphorylation of CD3 δ and γ polypeptides.[42] PMA-activated PKC can also induce the dissociation of p56Lck from CD4, and concomitant CD4 internalization.[43] These events are accompanied by phosphorylation of both Lck and CD4. Furthermore, in a recent study PMA treatment led to CD8/CD4 mRNA downregulation at the posttranscriptional level in fetal thymocytes.[44]

In addition to its effects on membrane-bound proteins, PMA- and TcR-induced PKC activation conveys signals to the nucleus via an insufficiently defined pathway. DNA sequences that act as the PKC response elements upon T-cell activation have been identified within the transcription control regions of the IL-2 gene.[45,46] The PMA response element within the IL-2 enhancer was found to bind transcription factors AP-1 and NF-κB. Two other TcR response elements bind NFAT-1 and NFIL-2, respectively, and PKC activation was shown to induce NFIL-2. Inasmuch as PKC is not likely to activate the transcription factors directly, the question of paramount interest is: which PKC substrates may function in downstream signal transduction? The candidates for such effectors are the MAP kinases, Raf, p21ras and the p70 ribosomal S6 kinase (Rsk).[2] The last enzyme is specifically induced by IL-2 and could play a role in translation. p70 S6 kinase can also be activated by Src kinases, G proteins and other stimuli, and its IL-2—mediated activation is specifically blocked by the immunosuppressant rapamycin.[2]

MAP KINASES

Mitogen activated protein (MAP) kinases, also known as extracellularly regulated kinases (erk), can be activated in many cell types by a variety of stimuli including insulin, the epidermal growth factor and phorbol esters.[2] They belong to a group of protein serine-threonine kinases (PS-TK) that require phosphorylation on both tyrosine and threonine residues to be activated.[47] These enzymes could thus integrate signals transmitted by both PTK and PS-TK. One pathway probably operates via the serine-threonine kinase p72Raf and its substrate MEK kinase {MAP/Erk kinase (MEK) kinase}. The latter enzyme is capable of phosphorylating both tyrosine and serine-threonine residues[48,49] and can directly activate MAP kinases (Fig. 3). Interestingly, Raf is a candidate substrate for MAP kinases, suggesting the existence of a feedback loop in this pathway. At the upstream end, Raf was shown to bind directly to p21Ras by its N-terminal domain, suggesting a role for Raf as the bridging molecule between Ras and MEK.[50] To make this part of the signaling pathway even more complex, Raf was also shown to be the substrate for the CD4/p56Lck receptor system.[51] One possibility here would be that Ras acts by recruiting Raf to the site of action of CD4/Lck.

On the other hand, PKC was shown to activate Raf by direct phosphorylation in vivo and in vitro. PKC can also activate Ras (see below). PKC can, therefore, theoretically activate the MAP kinase pathway at least two distinct points. It is possible, but not yet proven, that the emphasis and relative importance of these "subpathways" of activation of MAP kinases by PKC may vary in different cell types. [MAP kinases can also be activated through the serpentine receptors, e.g., the acetylcholine receptor, via heterotrimeric G proteins and an enzyme named (somewhat unfortunately) MEKK kinase.[49] The existence and potential importance of this pathway in T cells is not established.]

Several substrates of MAP kinases are transcription factors or molecules that are known to regulate the cell cycle. In addition to Raf, MAP kinases can phosphorylate and/or indirectly activate the AP-1 nuclear factor encoded by *c-fos* and *c-jun* genes, the *c-myc* gene product,[1] the transcription factor p62Tcf and the 90kD *rsk*.[2] For example, MAP kinase-activated p62Tcf forms a complex with the *c-fos* promoter, and may induce its transcription. Along with Jun (another substrate of MAP kinases), Fos forms the AP-1 transcription factor that is involved in the formation of the transcription complex that regulates the IL-2 promoter (Figs. 1 and 3). Myc was implicated in cell cycle progression[52] and apoptosis,[53] and p90Rsk S6K could play a role in regulating translation. The last enzyme is specifically induced upon TcR stimulation.

P21RAS

The product of the *c-ras* protooncogene is a GTP-binding protein that regulates cell growth in many cell types. The GDP-bound form of the enzyme is inactive, and the enzyme is activated by the exchange of GDP for free cytosolic GTP.[54] The GTPase activity of p21ras is controlled by GTPase activating proteins (GAPs); p120GAP is the best characterized protein from this group.[55] GAP could be activated in vitro by tyrosine phosphorylation; the phosphorylated form of GAP binds p56Lck.[56] However, it is not clear whether GAP is regulated by Lck, or vice versa. Extensive studies indicate that both receptor and nonreceptor tyrosine kinases function upstream from Ras, and use Ras in downstream signaling. Recent experiments from non-T-cell systems showed that the central role in this interaction belongs to adaptor molecules such as Grb2.[57] Grb2 is a bifunctional factor: it binds to mSos proteins through its SH3 domains, and to tyrosine kinases (such as Shc), or their substrates, via its SH2 domain.[58] mSos (murine homologue of the *Drosophila* protein Son of sevenless) is a GTP-exchange factor. Grb2 thus serves as the adaptor protein linking tyrosine kinases to Ras, and, perhaps, to other small G-proteins.[59] This pathway is yet to be confirmed in T lymphocytes.

Activation of human peripheral blood T lymphocytes via the TcR caused a prolonged stimulation of p21ras.[60] TcR triggering was found to inactivate the RasGAP activity, and thus prevent the hydrolysis of the GTP-Ras complex. PKC activators, such as phorbol esters and diacylglycerols, also activate Ras, suggesting that Ras may be among the PKC substrates. But there is evidence that the TcR can use another, PKC-independent, activation pathway, possibly through a tyrosine kinase[60] (Fyn, Lck or another, unknown kinase?).

One of the putative roles for p21Ras in T cells would be to couple membrane receptors to intracellular signaling machinery that controls the expression of the activation-induced genes (such as the IL-2). Indeed, in the murine thymoma line, Ras induced the transcription factor NF-AT, that binds to a DNA sequence within the IL-2 enhancer.[61] In these experiments, effects of Ras activation synergized with the Ca^{++} activation pathway, leading to the augmentation of NF-AT expression. As discussed below, Ca^{++}-controlled signals can induce the expression of transcription factors. Potential synergy between Ras-induced signals and Ca^{++} effectors may thus be important for the integration of T-cell responses to stimuli that act through distinct intracellular pathways.

CA++ EFFECTORS

For a long time, calmodulin was known as the primary cytosolic receptor for Ca^{++}.[62] In murine splenocytes the major enzyme that binds calmodulin is the protein phosphatase calcineurin (Fig. 4).[63] Calcineurin is the target for the immunosuppressive drugs cyclosporin A (CsA) and FK 506.[64] These immunosuppressants were previously known to inhibit T-cell activation by interfering with the activation of IL-2 transcription factors NF-AT and NF-IL2A.[3] Overexpression of murine calcineurin in Jurkat T cells leads to an augmentation of both NF-AT- and NF-IL2A-dependent transcription in response to elevated intracellular Ca^{++}.[65] Calcineurin acts on the NF-AT by mediating activation and translocation of its cytoplasmic component, $NF-AT_c$, into the nucleus. Together, these results confirm that calcineurin is one of the key enzymes in T-cell activation.

SIGNAL TRANSDUCTION IN THYMOCYTES

Signaling processes during the intrathymic differentiation of T cells are poorly defined. The key challenge in the area of thymocyte signaling is to elucidate stage-specific signaling patterns. Understanding signal transduction at various stages of development holds the keys to a number of

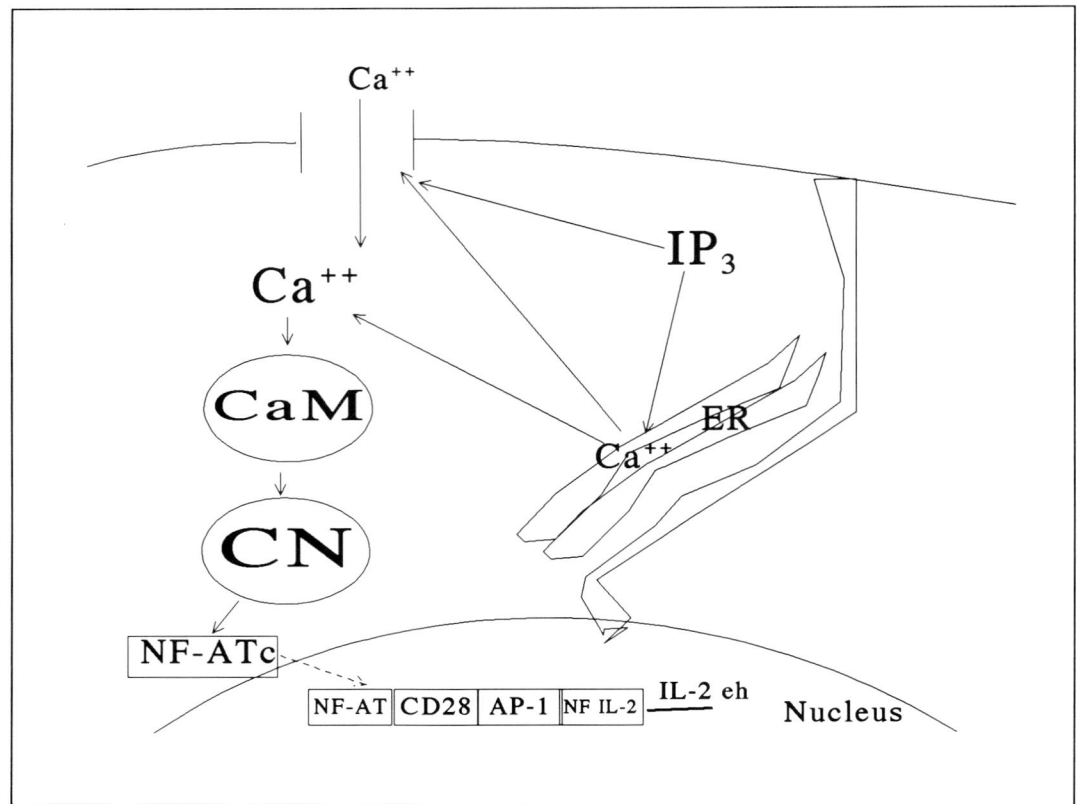

Fig. 4. Ca⁺⁺-induced signal transduction in T cells. Solid arrows - activation; Broken arrows - transcription. CaM - calmodulin; CN - calcineurin; eh - enhancer.

questions concerning thymocyte biology. In our opinion, the following are among the most intriguing: 1. What governs the migration and the commitment of a multipotent precursor to the T-cell lineage? 2. What signals induce TcR rearrangement, accessory molecule expression and thymocyte expansion? 3. What signals mediate positive selection? 4. How is apoptosis regulated in negatively selected and nonselected cells? 5. How do cells chose to express CD8 or CD4? and 6. What signals participate in terminal maturation and emigration?

SIGNALING AND EARLY DEVELOPMENT

MIGRATION AND COMMITMENT OF A LYMPHOID PRECURSOR; EARLY PROLIFERATION AND TcR REARRANGEMENT

Very little is known on what induces the migration of T-cell precursors to the thymus and what signals lead them to commit to the T-cell lineage. The early years of thymology were dominated by the idea that the thymus functions by producing soluble factors (thymic hormones) that induce the proliferation and/or maintenance of lymphocytes.[66] Even as these ideas were discarded in light of experimental evidence, the hypothesis that the thymus may secrete chemotactic peptides that would attract precursors remained attractive. To date, there is no evidence to support this hypothesis. A putative chemoattractant, identical to the β_2-microglobulin, was identified by Dargemont et al.[67] However, experimentally induced deficiency of this molecule does not affect T-cell development.[68,67] Alternatively, immigration could be guided by homing molecules. Indeed, thymocyte precursors express homing molecules such as CD44 and Mel-14, and these molecules may be instrumental in guiding uncommitted precursors to the thymus.

The key committing event to the T-cell lineage is the rearrangement of TcR genes. As discussed in Chapter 3, it is completely unknown what may induce this thymus-dependent event. It is also not known how a T cell decides to rearrange and assemble αβ or γδ TcR. One possibility is that the silencers in the α gene[69] can extinguish the transcription/rearrangement of the γ/δ loci. The activity of silencers in non-T-cell lines also suggests that lineage commitment may be initiated by the relief from silencing. But initial signals that would activate the recombination and/or regulate the silencers are obscure. A cytokine, a combination of cytokines or a combination of cell contacts and cytokines may be involved in this process, since a number of cytokines and cytokine receptors are expressed by early thymocytes (see Chapter 4).

The best characterized parameter of immunocompetence in mature T cells, the production of cytokines (in particular of IL-2), has been used to test the responsiveness of thymocytes. By this criterion, overall responsiveness of early thymocytes to activation is quite remarkable (for details, see Chapter 4 and 5). In fact, until the onset of the expression of CD8 and CD4 (or, perhaps, the onset of TcR rearrangement) the activity of the IL-2 enhancer in early thymocytes in response to TcR agonists (PMA and ionomycin) and lymphokines, e.g., IL-1, is comparable to, or greater than, that in mature T cells.[70,71] Thereafter, the production of transcription factors NF-AT, AP-1, and NF-κB ceases and is not reactivated until the cell reaches the SP stage.[70] This loss of inducibility of the IL-2 gene correlates with other signaling changes that appear to facilitate apoptosis.

The development of TN thymocytes is not overtly affected by the germline disruption of CD45[35], TcR ζ[72], lck[73] or fyn[21] genes, although a more detailed analysis of the early T-cell development is necessary before any firm conclusions can be made. Lck⁻ mice display a block in progression from a TN to TL and DP stages (see Chapter 3), perhaps suggesting that the expression of CD8 and CD4 molecules could be regulated via this kinase. By contrast, tg mice overexpressing a constitutively active form of Lck exhibit a selective defect of TcRβ recombination,[74] suggesting a specific role for Lck in mediating the allelic exclusion of β genes. In either case, the kinase would have to mediate its effects independently of CD8 and CD4 molecules, because the accessory molecules are not expressed at the stage at which the defects in development are observed. In fact, a mutant form of Lck that cannot associate to CD4/8 is as effective in preventing TcRβ rearrangement as the wild-type molecule.[75] The effects of Lck during the early development could thus be mediated by the enzyme bound to IL-2Rβ or to another, presently unknown molecule.

The other event implicated in the regulation of CD8 and CD4 expression is TcRβ rearrangement (discussed in Chapter 3). However, it is unlikely that the rearrangement of β chain alone is responsible for the onset of accessory molecule expression, because a thymocyte subset that has rearranged the β locus (CD25⁺ TN cells) still cannot express CD8 and CD4 without the help of thymic epithelium. The most recent results from von Boehmer's group identified a novel glycoprotein, p33, that pairs with the β chain in immature, but not mature thymocytes [H. von Boehmer, personal communication]. This chain could be instrumental in early thymocyte signaling and the onset of CD4/8 expression.

INTERMEDIATE DEVELOPMENT AND POSITIVE SELECTION

Once thymocytes initiate the expression of CD8 and CD4, they become DP in a matter of hours. DP cells express TcR at low levels, and undergo continuous α rearrangement in order to maximize the production of selectable TcRs (see Chapters 3 and 6). TcR complexes on DP thymocytes contain few ζ chains and low amounts of Fyn kinase.[76,77] For these and other reasons, e.g., a lack of IL-2 inducibility, DP cells exhibit profound defects in responsiveness to stimulation: these cells do not proliferate and do not secrete lymphokines. Nevertheless,

DP cells do undergo positive selection in response to TcR-induced stimuli, and it is critically important to elucidate the signaling pathways that mediate this process.

TYROSINE PHOSPHORYLATION IN DP THYMOCYTES

It was shown that thymocytes undergoing positive selection display higher Lck and Fyn kinase activity than nonselected thymocytes.[78] DP thymocytes also undergo phosphorylation of the ζ chain and tyrosine kinase activation in response to the intrathymic engagement of TcR and CD8/4 molecules.[76] However, in one recent study,[79] a compelling case was made that Lck does not play a role in positive selection of CD8$^+$ cells. The coupling of Lck to CD8 was disrupted in these experiments by mutating the cytoplasmic tail of CD8. This manipulation had no effect on positive selection of CD8$^+$ CTL. This finding is in agreement with the idea that the primary role for Lck may be in early development, rather than in selection, although Lck still could be important for positive selection of CD4$^+$ cells. A recent study showed that 60-70% of TcR complexes on immature DP thymocytes are coupled to tyrosine-phosphorylated proteins.[80] The extent of TcR coupling to phosphotyrosine proteins was found to inversely correlate to the signaling capacities of these TcRs; upon in vitro incubation, the extent of such coupling decreased, leading to an enhanced expression of TcR molecules and the TcR-associated ζ chain and to improved Ca^{++} mobilization. These findings support the concept that phosphorylation may serve as a negative regulatory modification of TcR bound proteins.[27]

The targeted germline disruption of the *fyn* gene induced a profound block in TcR stimulation of mature thymocytes, but peripheral T cells exhibited only slight hyporesponsiveness.[21] Otherwise, no defects in thymocyte development were found. These data argue that the action of p59Fyn can probably be compensated by another tyrosine kinase. Thus, at present, there is no evidence that either Lck or Fyn play a major role in positive selection.

The ζ-deficient mouse[72] provided the opportunity for the direct evaluation of ζ-transduced signals during thymocyte maturation, and, indirectly, for the possible role of the associated kinase ZAP 70. Since the presence of the ζ chain is required for an efficient cell surface expression of the TcR complex, one would expect that thymocytes in mice lacking this chain should exhibit defects in TcR expression with a concomitant arrest of T-cell development at an early stage. ζ^- mice have small thymuses with severely reduced thymocyte numbers and slightly lower percentages of DP thymocytes. Together, these mice have a tenfold reduction of absolute numbers of DP cells compared to control values. The generation of SP cells is heavily impaired, but not completely abrogated. TcR complexes are expressed at very low levels on both thymic and peripheral SP cells. The origin, signaling characteristics and immunocompetence of these SP cells have not been established. The defects in thymocyte maturation of these mice were thus clearcut, but not absolute.

The targeted germline disruption of the exon 6 of the CD45 gene led to heavily impaired thymocyte development, with an arrest at the transition between DP and SP stages.[35] TcR expression by a few "leaky" SP cells is extremely low, and it was not clear whether thymic or extrathymic mechanisms are responsible for the existence of these cells. The straightforward conclusion from these studies is that the CD45 phosphatase must play a major role in T-cell selection. Disruption of CD2[81] and CD28[82] costimulatory molecules had no discernible effects on thymocyte maturation.

NEGATIVE SELECTION AND APOPTOSIS

Thymocytes that fail positive selection, as well as those that undergo negative selection by clonal deletion, will die by apoptosis. Apoptotic cell death is an active process that requires transcription and translation, is characterized by membrane blebbing, nuclear condensation and fragmentation of DNA into oligonucleosomal units and is encountered in most tissues at some stage of their development (reviewed in ref. 83). The key difference between apoptosis and the necrotic cell death is that apoptosis is "clean:" dead cells are rapidly removed by phagocytes, there is no spilling of intracellular contents into the local environment, and therefore no inflammatory response. Apoptosis is thus an ideal tool for the modeling of tissues during development. Apoptosis can be induced in thymocytes by a variety of physical and chemical stimuli, the best studied of which is the effect of corticosteroids.[84,85] Whatever the stimulus, the ultimate effector of apoptotic DNA fragmentation is believed to be a Ca^{++}-dependent endogenous endonuclease.

Although both nonselected and negatively selected thymocytes die by apoptosis, these two categories of cells probably use different initial signals and perhaps different signaling machinery. Namely, nonselected cells undergo a true programmed cell death—they will die unless rescued by positive selection. By contrast, negatively selected cells undergo an "active" form of apoptosis. Apoptosis due to clonal deletion is more correctly termed activation-induced cell death (AICD)—the stimulus that signals death is ligation of the TcR. Of the two, apoptosis in AICD is a much better defined process, and we shall discuss it first.

Studies of apoptosis in thymocytes begun with the realization that for the majority of thymocytes, TcR ligation induces cell death, rather than proliferation and lymphokine secretion.[86] Apoptosis could be induced in vitro and in vivo by stimulation of thymocytes with αCD3 mAb.[86,87] Confirmation that apoptosis is the mechanism of death during clonal elimination was obtained by injecting cognate peptide antigens into TcR transgenic mice[88] (see the Exp. model #2, Table 2, Chapter 8): DP thymocytes isolated from such mice displayed cellular changes typical of apoptosis. Apoptotic death could also be induced in a TcR-independent manner using a calcium ionophore, and calcium chelators can inhibit both TcR- and ionophore-induced apoptosis.[86,87] Calcium is therefore considered the key intracellular mediator of apoptosis.

How is the TcR linked to Ca^{++} during negative selection? The usual axis involving PTKs and PLC would seem a logical guess. However, PTK inhibitors did not block

clonal deletion of autoreactive cells in a TcR tg model.[89] In addition, a dissociation of CD8 and Lck did not affect negative selection of class I restricted TcR tg thymocytes.[79] Fyn "knockout" had no effect either,[21] while the effects of ζ and CD45 disruption have not been evaluated as yet. Our initial question thus remains unanswered at present.

Finkel et al[90,91,92] measured Ca^{++} mobilization and clonal deletion in immature fetal thymocytes following stimulation through CD3 or through TcR. They identified a subset of fetal DP thymocytes which was resistant to αTcR mAb- and superantigen (SAG)-mediated deletion and which did not flux Ca^{++} when stimulated through the $\alpha\beta$ heterodimer. Based on these results, they proposed that incomplete coupling of the TcR and the downstream signaling machinery protected a subset of immature thymocytes from deletion and that these cells may represent a subset capable of undergoing only positive and not negative selection. Further, the authors proposed that the incomplete coupling of the TcR components was caused by a disproportionally low expression of the ζ chain in these cells.[93] These results were never supported by comparable results from the adult mice nor by adequate biochemical data. An alternative explanation for these results, based on the expression of Fas on fetal thymocytes,[94] is discussed in Chapter 10.

How does Ca^{++} transmit apoptotic signals to the nucleus? The only known Ca^{++} effector pathway in T cells acts via calmodulin (CaM), calcineurin (CN) and NF-AT (Fig. 4), and is inhibitable by CsA and FK506 (reviewed in 3). CsA was shown to inhibit clonal deletion of MMTV-reactive thymocytes in vivo,[95,96] supporting the importance of the CaM/CN pathway in clonal deletion. By contrast, CsA could inhibit apoptosis in vitro in some, but not other models.[97-99] In general, CsA was less effective when a deleting signal consisted only of TcR ligation or Ca^{++} elevation, and it has been proposed that this immunosuppressant only acts when apoptosis is induced by two signals.[98] Given that the inhibition of calcineurin by CsA may not be the only mechanism of action by this drug, additional experiments are necessary to

establish the importance of calmodulin/
calcineurin pathway. The lack of CsA inhibition of Ca^{++}-induced apoptosis clearly indicates that Ca^{++} may use another, calcineurin-independent and/or CsA-resistant pathway, to induce apoptosis. For example, the addition of Ca^{++} (but not Mg^{++}) ions to isolated thymocyte nuclei can by itself cause DNA fragmentation,[99-101] raising the possibility that Ca^{++} elevation in the nucleus may directly activate endonuclease and cause apoptosis. Alternatively, other unidentified mediators could transmit Ca^{++}-induced signals to the nucleus.

Corticosteroids cause apoptosis by binding to a nuclear receptor consisting a zinc-finger protein that in turn binds to a specific DNA sequence and induces transcription of new genes.[22] The steroid-induced apoptosis pathway most likely does not involve cytosolic signaling molecules. Corticosteroid- and TcR-induced signals antagonize each other in T-cell hybridomas,[102] again suggesting the existence of distinct, but connected pathways. It is not clear at which level the pathways could be connected (the endogenous endonuclease is one candidate), and whether steroids, at physiological levels, play a role in normal thymocyte development, selection and/or apoptosis.

Recently, several molecules have been associated with apoptosis. Among them, the protooncogene product Bcl-2 has been studied in great detail. Bcl-2 was shown to protect T and B cells from apoptosis in both cell lines and transgenic animals.[103] In "knockout" mice lacking Bcl-2,[104] the immune system develops normally, but cells, especially mature ones, exhibit decreased viability in vitro. This decrease in viability can be circumvented by TcR stimulation. However, at or around four weeks of age, both T and B cells disappear, perhaps due to a combined impaired generation of precursors and shorter lifespan of mature lymphocytes. Bcl-2 is a cytosolic protein bound to the intracellular membranes, and its mode of action is at present unknown. It is likely that the action of Bcl-2 is balanced by other proteins that dimerize with it, since at least three proteins that potentiate or antagonize

Bcl-2 have been isolated and cloned.[105,106]

We recently showed that susceptibility of early thymic subsets to Ca^{++} induced apoptosis varied with the developmental stage of the cell, while susceptibility to steroid-induced apoptosis remains constant.[99] This variation correlates to the expression of Bcl-2 mRNA: Bcl-2 mRNA is present in resistant TN CD25$^+$ cells and absent in Ca^{++} sensitive TL CD25$^-$ thymocytes. TL subset is the first thymocyte subset to express low levels of the TcR and costimulatory CD8/4 molecules.[107,108] Bcl-2 expression may thus serve as a protection mechanism that enables early thymocyte subsets to proceed safely to the stage at which they express TcR and undergo selection.

p53 is the tumor suppressor gene implicated in the regulation of apoptosis.[109] Immature thymocytes from mice homozygous for p53 deletion undergo apoptosis in response to stimulation via the TcR or by steroids, but are resistant to apoptosis induced by ionizing radiation.[110,111] These studies indicate that irradiation induces apoptosis by yet another mechanism, distinct from that used by TcR and steroids.

Fas is the cell surface glycoprotein that transduces apoptotic signals when ligated with mAbs. The Fas gene is disrupted by the insertion of a retrotransposon (Etn)[112,113] in mice harboring the *lpr* mutation,[114] and this defect leads to generalized autoimmunity by an unknown mechanism. A deregulation of cell death in thymocytes and lymphocytes of *lpr* animals was demonstrated recently.[115,116] We completed a study on Fas expression during thymocyte ontogeny in normal mice.[94] Our data suggests that the onset of the Fas expression parallels the appearance of CD8/4 and TcR molecules on developing thymocytes. Fas upregulation on DP thymocytes may facilitate the elimination of cells that failed to undergo positive selection. It is possible that positive selection can induce the downregulation of Fas. This would protect useful, positively selected cells from apoptosis. However, at present there is no experimental evidence to support these speculations.

LATE THYMOCYTES AND THE CONTROL OF EMIGRATION

Signals and signal transduction at the final stages of thymocyte maturation are obscure. It is believed that most thymocytes at this stage only finish maturation and differentiation in response to stimuli received earlier in development. However, several studies have challenged this view,[117-119] indicating that post-DP thymocytes may still require intrathymic signals for terminal maturation. Our own studies, described in Chapter 3 (Late development) show thymocytes as advanced in development as the SP TcR^{hi} stage, to still require the thymic microenvironment. Unfortunately, the nature of this late intrathymic contact/factor is not known.

Concomitant with complete downregulation of one of the accessory molecule, TcR^{hi}SP thymocytes regain inducibility of the IL-2 gene.[70] Whether the late intrathymic contact mentioned above plays a role in this process or whether the IL-2 gene becomes inducible in response to a signal received at an earlier stage of development is not known.

A complete mystery surrounds T-cell emigration from the thymus. Again, chemotaxis, homing receptors (or a loss thereof) or a combination of the two could regulate this process. In addition, the signaling characteristics of recent emigrants, although tested to some degree, deserve another critical examination.

SUMMARY

Signals that govern the development of T cells and pathways of their transduction to the nucleus are poorly defined. It is likely that cytokine signals regulate the expansion of early thymocytes, and, perhaps, even the onset of the TcR rearrangement. The function of several enzymes implicated in TcR-mediated signal transduction has been tested in thymocytes. These experiments suggest that the protein-tyrosine kinase Lck plays an important role in early development (including, but perhaps not limited to, the regulation of TcR β allelic exclusion) at a pre-DP stage via an unknown mechanism. Neither Lck nor Fyn seem to play a major role in positive and negative selection. By contrast, the CD45 phosphatase, as well as the ζ chain

of the TcR complex, appear to be necessary for the selection events.

Clonal deletion is regulated by a Ca^{++}-mediated apoptotic pathway that could use the calmodulin/calcineurin axis to transmit signals to the nucleus. Apoptosis is modulated by a number of molecules including Bcl-2, Fas and Myc. Nothing is known on the mechanism of action of these molecules. Signals that influence the terminal maturation and the release of thymocytes into the periphery are poorly understood.

REFERENCES

1. Perlmutter RM, Levin SD, Appleby MW et al. Regulation of lymphocyte function by protein phosphorylation. Annu Rev Immunol 1993; 11:451-499.

2. Blenis J. Signal transduction via the MAP kinases: Proceed at your own RSK. Proc Natl Acad Sci USA 1993; 90:5889-5892.

3. Schreiber SL, Crabtree GR. The mechanism of action of cyclosporin A and FK506. Immunol Today 1992; 13:136-142.

4. Cambier JC. Signal transduction by T- and B-cell antigen receptors: converging structures and concepts. Curr Opinion Immunol 1992; 4:257-264.

5. Berridge MJ. Inositol trisphosphate and calcium signalling. Nature 1993; 361:315-324.

6. Weiss A, Imboden J, Shoback D et al. Role of T3 surface molecules in human T-cell activation: T3-dependent activation results in an increase in cytoplasmic free calcium. Proc Natl Acad Sci USA 1984; 81:4169-4173.

7. Gardner P. Calcium and T lymphocyte activation. Cell 1989; 59:15-20.

8. Nishizuka Y. Intracellular signaling by hydrolysis of phospholipids and activation of protein kinase C. Science 1992; 258:607-614.

9. Schwartz RH. A cell culture model for T lymphocyte clonal anergy. Science 1990; 248:1349.

10. Samelson LE, O'Shea JJ, Luong H et al. T-cell antigen receptor phosphorylation induced by an anti-receptor antibody. J Immunol 1987; 139:2708-2714.

11. June CH, Fletcher MC, Ledbetter JA et al. Increases in tyrosine phosphorylation are detectable before phospholipase C activation

after T-cell receptor stimulation. J Immunol 1990; 144:1591-1599.

12. June CH, Fletcher MC, Ledbetter JA et al. Inhibition of tyrosine phosphorylation prevents T-cell receptor-mediated signal transduction. Proc Natl Acad Sci USA 1990; 87:7722-7726.

13. Veillette A, Bookman MA, Horak EM et al. The CD4 and CD8 T-cell surface antigens are associated with the internal membrane tyrosine proteine kinase p56Lck. Cell 1988; 55:301.

14. Julius M, Maroun CR, Haughn L. Distinct roles for CD4 and CD8 as coreceptor in antigen receptor signalling. Immunol Today 1993; 14:177-182.

15. Hatakeyama M, Kono T, Kobayashi N et al. Interaction of the IL-2 receptor with the src family kinase p56Lck identification of novel intermolecular association. Science 1991; 252:1523-1528.

16. Straus DB, Weiss A. Genetic evidence for the involvement of the Lck tyrosine kinase in signal transduction through the T-cell antigen receptor. Cell 1992; 70:585-593.

17. Xu H, Littman DR. A kinase-independent function of Lck in potentiating antigen-specific T-cell activation. Cell 1993; 74:633-643.

18. Cooke MP, Perlmutter RM. Expression of a novel form of the Fyn proto-oncogene in hematopoietic cells. New Biol 1989; 1:66.

19. Samelson LE, Phillips AF, Luong ET et al. Association of the Fyn protein tyrosine kinase with the T-cell antigen receptor. Proc Natl Acad Sci USA 1990; 87:4358-4362.

20. Cooke MP, Abraham KM, Forbush KA et al. Regulation of T-cell receptor signalling by a src family protein-tyrosine kinase (p59Fyn). Cell 1991; 65:281-291.

21. Stein PL, Lee H-M, Rich S et al. pp59Fyn mutant mice display differential signalling in thymocytes and peripheral T cells. Cell 1992; 70:741-750.

22. Weiss A, Koretzky G, Schatzman RC et al. Functional activation of the T-cell antigen receptor induces tyrosine phosphorylation of phospholipase C_c1. Proc Natl Acad Sci USA 1991; 88:5484-5488.

23. Weber JR, Bell GM, Han MY et al. Association of the tyrosine kinase LCK with phospholipase C-γ1 after stimulation of the T-cell antigen receptor. J Exp Med 1992; 176:373-379.

24. Ullrich A, Schlessinger J. Signal transduction by receptors with tyrosine kinase activity. Cell 1990; 61:203-212.

25. McGlade CJ, Ellis C, Reedijk M et al. SH2 domains of the p85α subunit of phosphatidylinositol 3-kinase regulate binding to growth factor receptors. Mol Cell Biol 1992; 12:991-997.

26. Augustine JA, Sutor SL, Abraham RT. Interleukin 2- and polyomavirus middle T antigen-induced modification of phosphatidylinositol 3-kinase activity in activated T lymphocytes. Mol Cell Biol 1991; 11:4431-4440.

27. Rudd CE. CD4, CD8 and the TcR-CD3 complex: a novel class of protein-tyrosine kinase receptor. Immunol Today 1990; 11:400-406.

28. Ettehadieh E, Sanghera JS, Pelech SL et al. Tyrosyl phosphorylation and activation of MAP kinases by p56lck. Science 1992; 255:853-855.

29. Chan AC, Irving BA, Fraser JD et al. The ζ chain is associated with a tyrosine kinase and upon T-cell antigen receptor stimulation associates with ZAP 70, a 70-kDa tryosine phosphoprotein. Proc Natl Acad Sci USA 1991; 88:9166-9170.

30. Weiss A. T-cell antigen receptor signal transduction: a tale of tails and cytoplasmic protein-tyrosine kinases. Cell 1993; 73:209-212.

31. Kolanus W, Romeo C, Seed B. T-cell activation by clustered tyrosine kinases. Cell 1993; 74:171-183.

32. Hall CG, Sancho J, Terhorst C. Reconstitution of T-cell receptor ζ-mediated calcium mobilization in nonlymphoid cells. Science 1993; 261:915-917.

33. Alexander D, Shiroo M, Robinson A et al. The role of CD45 in T-cell activation— resolving the paradoxes?. Immunol Today 1992; 13:477-481.

34. Volarevic S, Niklinska BB, Burns CM et al. Regulation of TcR signaling by CD45 lacking transmembrane and extracellular domains. Science 1993; 260:541-544.

35. Kishihara K, Penninger J, Wallace VA et al. Normal B lymphocyte development but

impaired T-cell maturation in CD45-Exon6 protein tyrosine phosphatase-deficient mice. Cell 1993; 74:143-156.

36. Cooper JA, Howell B. The when and how of Src regulation. Cell 1993; 73:1051-1054.

37. Nada S, Yagi T, Takeda H et al. Constitutive activation of Src family kinases in mouse embryos that lack csk. Cell 1993; 73:1125-1135.

38. Chow ML, Fournel M, Davidson D et al. Negative regulation of T-cell receptor signalling by tyrosine protein kinase p50csk. Nature 1993; 365:156-160.

39. Siliciano JD, Morrow TA, Desiderio SV. Itk, a T-cell-specific tyrosine kinase gene inducible by interleukin 2. Proc Natl Acad Sci USA 1992; 89:11194-11198.

40. Heyeck SD, Berg LJ. Developmental regulation of a murine T-cell-specific tyrosine kinase gene, Tsk. Proc Natl Acad Sci USA 1993; 90:669-673.

41. Coussens L, Parker PJ, Rhee L et al. Multiple, distinct forms of bovine and human protein kinase C suggest diversity in cellular signaling pathways. Science 1986; 233:859-866.

42. Cantrell DA, Davies AA, Crumpton MJ. Activators of protein kinase C down-regulate and phosphorylate the T3/T-cell antigen receptor complex of human T lymphocytes. Proc Natl Acad Sci USA 1985; 82:8158-8162.

43. Acres BB, Conlon PJ, Mochizuki DY et al. Rapid phosphorylation and modulation of the T4 antigen on cloned helper T cells induced by phorbol myristate acetate or antigen. J Biol Chem 1986; 261:16210-16214.

44. Takahama Y, Singer A. Post-transcriptional regulation of early T-cell development by T-cell receptor signals. Science 1992; 258: 1456-1462.

45. Fraser JD, Straus D, Weiss A. Signal transduction events leading to T-cell lymphokine gene expression. Immunol Today 1993; 14:357-362.

46. Crabtree GR. Contingent genetic regulatory events in T lymphocyte activation. Science 1989; 243:355-361.

47. Anderson NG, Maller JL, Tonks NK et al. Requirement for integration of signals from two distinct phosphorylation pathways for activation of MAP kinase. Nature 1990;

343:651-653.

48. Kyriakis JM, App H, Zhang H-f. Raf-1 activates Map kinase-kinase. Nature 1992; 358:417-421.

49. Lange-Carter CA, Pleiman CM, Gardner AM et al. A divergence in the MAP kinase regulatory network defined by MEK kinase and Raf. Science 1993; 260:315-319.

50. Vojtek AB, Hollenberg SM, Cooper JA. Mammalian ras interacts directly with the serine/threonine kinase raf. Cell 1993; 74:205-214.

51. Thompson PA, Ledbetter JA, Rapp UR et al. The Raf-1 serine-threonine kinase is a substrate for the p56lck protein tyrosine kinase in human T-cells. Mol Cell Biol 1991; 2:609-617.

52. Cole MD. The myc oncogene: Its role in transformation and differentiation. Blood 1991; 77:1025-1032.

53. Shi Y, Glynn JM, Guilbert LJ et al. Role for c-myc in activation-induced apoptotic cell death in T-cell hybridomas. Science 1992; 257:212-214.

54. Sigal, I.S., D'Alonzo, J.S., Ahern, J.D. et al. The ras oncogene protein as a G-protein. In: Advances in Second Messenger and Phosphoprotein Research, Vol. 21, edited by Adelstein R, Klee C and Rodbell M. New York: Raven Press Ltd. 1988, p. 193-214.

55. Hall A. Signal transduction through small GTPases—A tale of two GAPs. Cell 1992; 69:389-391.

56. Amrein KE, Flint N, Panholzer B et al. Ras GTPase-activating protein: A substrate and a potential binding protein of the protein-tyrosine kinase p56lck. Proc Natl Acad Sci USA 1992; 89:3343-3346.

57. Lowenstein EJ, Daly RJ, Batzer AG et al. The SH2 and SH3 domain-containing protein GRB2 links receptor tyrosine kinases to ras signaling. Cell 1992; 70:431-442.

58. Li N, Batzer A, Daly R et al. Guanine-nucleotide-releasing factor hSos1 binds to Grb2 and links receptor tyrosine kinases to Ras signalling. Nature 1993; 363:85-88.

59. Egan SE, Giddings BW, Brooks MW et al. Association of Sos Ras exchange protein with Grb2 is implicated in tyrosine kinase signal transduction and transformation. Nature

1993; 363:45-51.

60. Downward J, Graves J, Cantrell D. The regulation and function of p21ras in T cells. Immunol Today 1992;13:89-92.

61. Rayter SI, Woodrow M, Lucas SC et al. p21ras mediates control of IL-2 gene promoter function in T-cell activatioin. The EMBO J 1992; 12:4549-4556.

62. Means AR, Dedman JR. Calmodulin—an intracellular calcium receptor. Nature 1980; 285:72-77.

63. Kincaid RL, Takayama H, Billingsley ML et al. Differential expression of calmodulin-binding proteins in B, T lymphocytes and thymocytes. Nature 1987; 330:176-178.

64. Liu J, Farmer JD, Lane WS et al. Calcineurin is a common target of cyclophilin-cyclosporin A and FKBP-FK506 complexes. Cell 1991; 66:807-815.

65. O'Keefe SJ, Tamura J, Kincaid RL et al. FK-506- and CsA-sensitive activation of the interleukin-2 promoter by calcineurin. Nature 1992; 357:692-69.

66. Davies AJ. The tale of T cells. Immunol Today 1993; 14:137-140.

67. Dargemont C, Dunon D, Deugnier M-A et al. Thymotaxin, a chemotactic protein, is identical to β_2-microglobulin. Science 1989; 246:803-806.

68. Zijlstra M, Li E, Sajjadi F et al. Germ-line transmission of a disrupted β_2-microglobulin gene procued by homologous recombination in embryonic stem cells. Nature 1989; 342:435-438.

69. Winoto A, Baltimore D. $\alpha\beta$ Lineage-specific expression of the α T-cell receptor gene by nearby silencers. Cell 1989; 59:649-655.

70. Rothenberg EV. The development of functionally responsive T cells. Adv Immunol 1992; 51:85-214.

71. Zuniga-Pflucker JC, Schwartz HL, Lenardo MJ. Gene transcription in differentiating immature T-cell receptor[neg] thymocytes resembles antigen-activated mature T cells. J Exp Med 1993; 178:1139-1149.

72. Love PE, Shores EW, Johnson MD et al. T-cell development in mice that lack the ζ chain of the T-cell antigen receptor complex. Science 1993; 261:918-921.

73. Molina TJ, Kishihara K, Siderovski DP et al. Profound block in thymocyte development

in mice lacking p56lck. Nature 1992; 357:161-164.

74. Abraham KM, Levin SD, Marth JD et al. Thymic tumorigenesis induced by over-expression of p56lck. Proc Natl Acad Sci USA 1991; 88:3977-3981.

75. Levin SD, Abraham KM, Anderson SJ et al. The protein tyrosine p56Lck regulates thymocyte development independently of its interaction with CD4 and CD8 coreceptors. J Exp Med 1993; 178:245-255.

76. Nakayama R, Samelson LE, Nakayama Y et al. Ligand-stimulated signaling events in immature CD4+CD8+ thymocytes expressing competent T-cell receptor complexes. Proc Natl Acad Sci USA 1991; 88:9949-9953.

77. Sancho J, Silverman LB, Castigli E et al. Developmental regulation of transmembrane signaling via the T-cell antigen receptor/CD3 complex in human T lymphocytes. J Immunol 1992; 148:1315-1321.

78. Carrera AC, Baker C, Roberts TM et al. Tyrosine kinase triggering in thymocytes undergoing positive selection. Eur J Immunol 1992; 22:2289-2294.

79. Chan IT, Limmer A, Louie MC et al. Thymic selection of cytotoxic T cells independent of CD8α-lck association. Science 1993; 261:1581-1584.

80. Nakayama T, Springer A, Hsi ED et al. Intrathymic signalling in immature CD4+ CD8+ thymocytes results in tyrosine phosphorylation of the TcR ζ chain. Nature 1989; 341:651-654.

81. Killeen N, Stuart SG, Littman DR. Development and function of T cells in mice with a disrupted CD2 gene. EMBO J 1992; 11:4329-4340.

82. Shahinian A, Pfeffer K, Lee KP et al. Differential T-cell costimulatory requirements in CD28-deficient mice. Science 1993; 261:609-612.

83. Raff MC. Social controls on cell survival and cell death. Nature 1992; 356:397.

84. Cohen JJ. Apoptosis. Immunol Today 1993; 14:126-130.

85. Cohen JJ. Programmed cell death in the immune system. Adv Immunol 1991; 50:55.

86. Smith CA, Williams GT, Kingston E et al. Antibodies to CD3/T-cell receptor complex

induce death by apoptosis in immature T cells in thymic cultures. Nature 1989; 337:181.

87. Shi Y, Bissonnette RP, Parfrey N et al. In vivo administration of monoclonal antibodies to the CD3 T-cell receptor complex induces cell death (apoptosis) in immature thymocytes. J Immunol 1991; 146:3340.

88. Murphy KM, Heimberger AB, Loh DY. Induction by antigen of intrathymic apoptosis of CD4⁺8⁺ TcRlo thymocytes in vivo. Science 1990; 250:1720.

89. Nakayama K-I, Loh DY. No requirement for p56lck in the antigen-stimulated clonal deletion of thymocytes. Science 1992; 257:94-96.

90. Finkel TH, Cambier JC, Kubo RT et al. The thymus has two functionally distinct population of immature αβ⁺ T cells: one population is deleted by ligation of αβ TcR. Cell 1989; 58:1047.

91. Finkel TH, Marrack P, Kappler JW et al. aBT-cell receptor and CD3 transduce different signals in immature T cells: implications for selection and tolerance. J Immunol 1989; 142:3006.

92. Finkel TH, Kappler JW, Marrack PC. Immature thymocytes are protected from deletion early in ontogeny. Proc Natl Acad Sci USA 1992; 89:3372-3374.

93. Finkel TH, Kubo RT, Cambier JC. T-cell development and transmembrane signaling: changing biological response through an unchanging receptor. Immunol Today 1991; 12:79.

94. Andjelic S, Drappa J, Lacy E et al. The onset of Fas expression parallels the acquisition of CD8 and CD4 in fetal and adult αβ thymocytes. Int Immunol 1994; 7:(In Press)

95. Gao E, Lo D, Cheney R et al. Abnormal differentiation of thymocytes in mice treated with CsA. Nature 1989; 336:176.

96. Jenkins MK, Schwartz RH, Pardoll DM. Effects of CsA on T-cell development and clonal deletion. Science 1988; 241:1655.

97. Vasquez N, Kaye J, Hedrick SM. In vivo and in vitro clonal deletion of double-positive thymocytes. J Exp Med 1992; 175:1307.

98. Ucker DS, Meyers J, Obermiller PS. Activation-driven T-cell death. II. Quantitative differences distinguish stimuli triggering nontransformed T-cell proliferation or death. J Immunol 1992; 149:1583.

99. Andjelic S, Jain N, Nikolic-Zugic J. Immature thymocytes become sensitive to calcium-mediated apoptosis with the onset of CD3,CD4, and the T-cell receptor exoression: A role for bcl-2. J Exp Med 1993; 178. In press.

100. Cohen JJ, Duke RC. Glucocorticoid activation of a calcium-dependent endonuclease in thymocyte nuclei leads to cell death. J Immunol 1984; 132:38-42.

101. Ramakrishnan N, Catravas GN. N-(2-mercaptoethyl)-1,3-propanediamine (WR-1065) protects thymocytes from programed cell death. J Immunol 1992; 148:1817-1821.

102. Zacharchuk CM, Mercep M, Chakraborti PK et al. Programmed T lymphocyte death: Cell activation- and steroid-induced pathways are mutually antagonistic. J Immunol 1990; 145:4037-4045.

103. Korsmeyer SJ. Bcl-2: a repressor of lymphocyte death. Immunol Today 1992; 13:285-287.

104. Nakayama K-i, Nakayama K, Negishi I et al. Disappearance of the lymphoid system in Bcl-2 homozygous mutant chimeric mice. Science 1993; 261:1584-1588.

105. Boise LH, Gonzalez-Garcia M, Postema CE et al. bcl-x, a bcl-2-related gene that functions as a dominant regulator of apoptotic cell death. Cell 1993; 74:597-608.

106. Oltvai ZN, Milliman CL, Korsmeyer SJ. Bcl-2 heterodimerizes in vivo with a conserved homolog, bax, that accelerates programed cell death. Cell 1993; 74:609-619.

107. Nikolic-Zugic J, Moore MW, Bevan MJ. Characterization of the subset of immature thymocytes which can undergo rapid in vitro differentiation. Eur J Immunol 1989; 19:649-653.

108. Nikolic-Zugic J, Moore MW. T-cell receptor expression on immature thymocytes with in vivo and in vitro precursor potential. Eur J Immunol 1989; 19:1957-1960.

109. Lane DP. A death in the life of p53. Nature 1993; 362:786-787.

110. Lowe SW, Schmitt EM, Smith SW et al. p53 is required for radiation-induced

apoptosis in mouse thymocytes. Nature 1993; 362:847-849.

111. Clarke AR, Purdie CA, Harrison DJ et al. Thymocyte apoptosis induced by p53-dependent and independent pathways. Nature 1993; 362:849-852.

112. Adachi M, Watanabe-Fukunaga R, Nagata S. Aberrant transcription caused by the insertion of an early transposable element in an intron of the Fas antigen gene of lpr mice. Proc Natl Acad Sci USA 1993; 90:1756.

113. Chu JL, Drappa J, Parnassa A et al. The defect in Fas mRNA expression in MRL/lpr mice is associated with insertion of the retrotransposon, Etn. J Exp Med 1993; 178:723-730.

114. Watanabe-Fukunaga R, Brannan CI, Copeland NG et al. Lymphoproliferation disorder in mice explained by defects in Fas

antigen that mediates apoptosis. Nature 1992; 356:314.

115. Zhou T, Bluethmann H, Eldrige J et al. Origin of CD4⁻CD8⁻B220⁺ T cells in MRL-lpr/lpr mice. J Immunol 1993; 150:3651.

116. Russell JH, Rush B, Weaver C et al. Mature T cells of autoimmune lpr/lpr mice have a defect in antigen-stimulated suicide. Proc Natl Acad Sci USA 1993; 90:4409.

117. Chan SH, Cosgrove D, Waltzinger C et al. Another view of the selective model of thymocyte selection. Cell 1993; 73:225.

118. Davis CB, Killeen N, Crooks MEC et al. Evidence for a stochastic mechanism in the differentiation of mature subsets of T lymphocytes. Cell 1993; 73:237.

119. Meerwijk JPMvan, Germain RN. Development of mature CD8⁺4⁻thymocytes: Selection rather than instruction?. Science 1993; 261:911-915.

INDEX

Items in italics denote figures (f) or tables (t).